Gunzburg et al. (Eds.) **Arthroplasty of the Spine**

Springer
Berlin
Heidelberg
New York
Hong Kong
London
Milan
Paris
Tokyo

R. Gunzburg · H. M. Mayer · M. Szpalski · M. Aebi
(Editors)

Arthroplasty of the Spine

With 159 Figures and 29 Tables

Springer

Dr. Robert Gunzburg
Eeuwfeestkliniek
Harmoniestraat 68
2018 Antwerp
Belgium

Dr. Heinz Michael Mayer
Orthopädische Klinik
München-Harlaching
Wirbelsäulenzentrum
Harlachinger Str. 51
81243 München
Germany

Prof. Dr. Marek Szpalski
Centre Hospitalier Molière
Longchamps
Rue Marconi 142
1180 Brussels
Belgium

Prof. Dr. Max Aebi
Maurice E. Müller Institute
for Evaluative Research
and Documentation
in Orthopaedic Surgery
Murtenstr. 35
3008 Bern
Switzerland

ISBN 3-540-20295-1 Springer-Verlag Berlin Heidelberg New York

Also published as Volume 11, Supplement 2, October 2002
of the European Spine Journal
ISSN 0940-6719

Library of Congress Cataloging-in-Publication Data

Arthroplasty of the spine / R. Gunzburg ... [et al.] (eds.).
p. ; cm. – (European spine journal, ISSN 0940-6719 ; v. 11, suppl. 2)
Includes bibliographical references and index.
ISBN 3-540-20295-1 (alk. paper)
1. Spine–Surgery. 2. Arthroplasty. I. Gunzburg, Robert. II. Series
[DNLM: 1. Intervertebral Disk–surgery. 2. Arthroplasty, Replacement–methods.
3. Prostheses and Implants. WE 740 A7866 2002]
RD768.A785 2002 617.4'71–dc22 2003066402

Springer-Verlag is a part of Springer Science+Business Media

springeronline.com

Printed in Germany

Cover design: e STUDIO CALAMAR, Pau/Girona
Typesetting, printing and bookbinding: ROTABENE, Rothenburg o. d. T.

Printed on acid-free paper 24/3150/PF 5 4 3 2 1 0

Contents

Robert Gunzburg
H. Michael Mayer
Marek Szpalski
Max Aebi

Arthroplasty of the spine: the long quest for mobility

R. Gunzburg
Eeuwfeestkliniek, Antwerp, Belgium

H.M. Mayer
Orthopädische Klinik
München-Harlaching,
Munich Spine Center, Munich, Germany

M. Szpalski
Centre Hospitalier Molière Longchamp,
Brussels, Belgium

M. Aebi
Division of Orthopaedic Surgery,
McGill University,
Royal Victoria Hospital,
Montreal, Quebec, Canada

Joint replacement is a logical step in the treatment of severe joint pathologies with irreversible lesions resisting conservative therapy. While hip arthrodesis brought relief to many patients, total replacement opened a new era in orthopedics and revolutionized the quality of life for coxarthrosis sufferers. These pioneering efforts were soon followed by similar techniques being proposed for other peripheric joints, sometimes with only qualified success. Knee replacement is now routine surgery, whereas shoulder arthroplasty is less common, while ankle, elbow and wrist arthroplasties have given disappointing results because of their more complex structural and functional properties.

At the spinal level, arthrodesis became, very early, the gold standard of treatment for severe intervertebral disc pathologies. The next logical step was to envision functional replacement, and this step was taken as early as 1956, when the first intervertebral implant was described. However, it took many more years and a great variety of proposed implant designs before clinical applications could be attempted.

The problems in designing a successful intervertebral implant are linked to the three-column structure of the spine, which involves three separate joints at each level. Furthermore, the intervertebral disc is not a true joint, and serves a double function of mobility and damping, with load repartition properties. To add to the complexity, the center of rotation constantly moves along the three axes. Reproducing this complex structure and function is a challenge well beyond the design of the hip implant, which is mainly a simple ball joint structure. Whereas hip implants represent mainly multiple variations around a common theme, the principles governing the different spinal arthroplasty designs are multiple and totally distinct. The same can be said about the materials used in those designs. This challenge has stimulated the productive imagination of both surgeons and engineers. The ratio between the number of patents and publications and the number of designs that reached the animal implantation level, not to mention clinical use, is enormous. This wide heterogeneity of designs reflects well the complexity of the task involved in the creation of an artificial implant mimicking the nature and function of the disc.

The few designs that are in commercial production and current human use have to withstand the test of time and of evidence-based medicine. There are few prospective studies on this topic, and no true randomized control trial demonstrating the superiority of spine arthroplasty over fusion has been published to this day. We should also be guided by the experience in other areas of joint replacement, showing that a great number of problems and complications only become apparent through a process of true long-term follow-up.

Clinical experience with different implants, principles of design and surgical techniques are presented in this volume. Although not a true joint arthroplasty, ligamentoplasty, nevertheless, uses implants to maintain mobility and is also discussed here.

The different approaches presented in this volume reflect current thought on the subject. New ideas will probably arise and, in the more distant future, the solutions will probably lie more in possibilities of disc repair by cell biology than in replacement by mechanical hardware.

In the meantime, we hope that the techniques described here will prove their efficacy in methodologically sound studies, and that spinal surgery will join the rest of orthopedic care in the quest for motion.

Marek Szpalski
Robert Gunzburg
Michael Mayer

Spine arthroplasty: a historical review

M. Szpalski (✉)
Department of Orthopedics,
Centre Hospitalier Molière Longchamp,
142 rue Marconi, 1190 Brussels, Belgium
e-mail: marek.szpalski@win.be

R. Gunzburg
Euwfeestkliniek, Antwerp, Belgium

M. Mayer
Orthopädische Klinik-München-Harlaching,
Munich Spine Center, Germany

Abstract Degenerative disc disease is one of the most frequently encountered spinal disorders. The intervertebral disc is a complex anatomic and functional structure, which makes the development of an efficient and reliable artificial disc a complex challenge. Not only is the disc function arduous to reproduce, but there are important consequences associated with the conception and the choice of materials that will have to bear the loads. Biochemical problems have complicated things even more. Two different principles have been applied in the realisation of a discal replacement: a metallic and/or polyethylene prosthesis allowing mainly mobility or a prosthesis enabling the reproduction of viscoelastic properties. Of course some devices attempt to combine both principles. In this paper we will try to present, in chronological order, an overview of the designs published in the literature as well as in the patents granted in this field. The very fact that such a long list of implants, based on highly varied principles, has been proposed, and that only very few have reached the level of animal models, let alone human implantation, clearly demonstrates how challenging the task of designing an intervertebral disc replacement is. Proper randomized controlled trials are now on the way, and should help in assessing the efficacy and real place of spine arthroplasty in the treatment of spinal disorders. Only then will spinal surgery join the list of successful joint replacements.

Keywords Spine · Arthroplasty · Artificial disc · Intervertebral disc · Degeneration

Introduction

Degenerative disc disease is one of the most frequently encountered spinal disorders. Disc arthrosis, segmental instability and spondylolisthesis are the principal indications for spinal fusion. However, there is a lack of precision concerning the definition of certain "pathologies" [175], and the relation between degenerative lesions, actual low back pain and the need for fusion is, at best, open to debate [138].

The pain generated by a degenerative joint is linked to its mobility, and the suppression of the latter should induce pain relief at the cost of impaired function. Hence, fusion became the standard treatment in many severe joint disorders (e.g. knee, hip) until the advent of reliable arthroplasty techniques. Arthroplasty allows for pain relief while keeping or restoring function. It was therefore seen as appealing to apply this principle to the spine by replacing a degenerated disc instead of fusing a segment.

Conception of disc arthroplasty

The structure, function and aetiopathogenesis of peripheral joints such as the hip or the knee are fundamentally different from those of the functional spinal unit. The function of a peripheral joint is to allow a wide range of mainly rotatory movements by means of cartilaginous interfaces. The hip biomechanics is relatively simple, and allowed quite early the development of highly efficient and reliable prostheses. The biomechanics of the knee are more complex, and adequate (although still less reliable) implants followed years later.

The intervertebral disc is not a simple cartilaginous interface joint. It is a mixed structure consisting of a peripheral collagenous band (annulus fibrosus) uniting the adjacent vertebral endplates. This band is composed of 15–20 concentric layers of alternating oblique fibres. In the centre lies a core (nucleus pulposus) made of a mucopolysacharide gel and proteoglycans. It is extremely hydrophilic, thus generating a tension on the peripheral annulus like air in a tyre, even in the absence of external loading. This preloading enhances the resistance to external forces and provides a very efficient repartition of compression forces [70]. The highly complex structure of the disc allows small movements along and around the three main axes. As a result, the centre of rotation is constantly modified along two axes simultaneously. These movements are both allowed and constrained by the discal structure itself. Contrary to the case with peripheral joints, whose stability is essentially achieved by ligamentous structures, the disc provides, on its own, a major part of its stability. For instance, the alternating arrangements of collagen fibres in the annulus creates a very efficient system to control and restrict rotation.

Peripheral joint degeneration consists essentially of destruction of the cartilaginous surfaces followed, in time, by subchondral bone destruction and deformation of surfaces. The movement on destroyed cartilaginous surfaces generates pain. Replacement of those surfaces restores function and abolishes pain. In the disc, however, degenerative lesions are much more complex and consist of a decrease in the hydrophilic properties of the nucleus as well as the appearance of annulus tears. Furthermore, the disc is not the sole mobile structure of the functional unit: secondary osteo-arthrosic modifications of the facet joints influence disc degeneration, and vice versa [103].

To complicate matters, the origin of pain in the functional unit is ill understood, and appears to be more complex than in peripheral joints.

All these structural, functional and pathogenic factors make the development of an efficient and reliable artificial disc a complex challenge. Not only is the disc function arduous to reproduce but there are important consequences associated with the conception and choice of materials that will have to bear the loads. The strains are very different from those supported by peripheral implants. In a correctly implanted hip prosthesis, long-term problems arise from surface wear, and recent advances have been achieved in the field of friction coefficients improvement. Implant fracture is mostly due to poor placement or construction faults.

The complex strains supported by an intervertebral disc make it a different challenge. It is estimated that the spine undergoes approximately 100 million flexion cycles during a lifetime [189], not taking into account the slight motion occurring when breathing, estimated to be 6 million a year [105]. Thirty million cycles appears to be the optimal life length of an implant, and 10 million should be the minimum [106]. This represents a very severe demand both for the metallic and elastomer components.

Biochemical problems have complicated things even more. Whereas silicones appeared to be promising composites in the making of viscoelastic implants, they form molecular links with lipids, making them rigid and brittle in the long term [150].

Two different principles have been applied in the realisation of a discal replacement: a metallic and/or polyethylene prosthesis allowing mainly mobility or a prosthesis enabling the reproduction of viscoelastic properties.

Specific challenges are related to the insertion technique: whereas it is relatively easy to cut or ream an acetabulum, a femur or a tibia in order to adapt the surface to the implant, it is much more complex to prepare two vertebrae, where it advisable not to damage the endplates in order to avoid subsidence of the prosthesis. Yet, as osteointegration is facilitated by contact with subchondral bone, the implant has to have a perfect fit.

Finally, there are major problems at the level of implant/bone fixation, which is much more complex than the cementing or press fitting techniques used in peripheral joints. An additional challenge is presented by the significant osteopoenia often found in severe low back pain sufferers [83]. It is desirable to cover the entire surface of the disc to create a better load repartition structure, as this will minimize surface stress. However, it makes the implant bulkier, which makes the surgical technique more arduous.

All these problems largely explain why disc replacement surgery was slow to develop. There is also a difference in the consequence of loss of function. Whereas a hip or knee joint fusion is highly debilitating, the absence of motion of one or even several intevertebral units is of little consequence for the global mobility of the spine, and therefore for the quality of life.

Principles behind disc replacement concepts

Among the different design proposals for intervertebral disc replacement, two key principles can be differentiated:

- Some prostheses mainly aim to reproduce the viscoelastic properties of the disc. These are usually manufactured from various silicones or polymers, although some rely on springs and/or piston systems. Some are injected in monomer form and polymerised in-situ.
- Other prostheses mainly aim at the reproduction of the motion characteristics of the disc. These are usually mechanical devices made from metal and sometimes polyethylene couples. These designs are inspired by the basic principles of peripheral joints prosthesis.

Of course some devices attempt to combine both principles. We will try to present, in chronological order, an overview of the designs published in the literature as well as in the patents granted in this field. At times the choice may seem arbitrary, and some designs touch on different principles. In some cases the patent documents appear a little unclear as to what the real nature of the described device is. Different variations on the basic principle are also often described. While we feel that this is a fairly complete overview of devices designed in this field, there are probably other existing implants that we did not come upon. We will first present implants for which, to our knowledge, no clinical use has been published, and then those, much scarcer, for which clinical data have been reported. In the first category are also implants for which clinical trials are ongoing, but where no results have yet been presented.

Implants patented or published but never clinically used

Devices aimed mainly at restoring the viscoelastic function

In the late 1950s, Nachemson injected self-hardening liquid silicone rubber into cadaver discs and did some basic biomechanical testing to demonstrate a relative restoration of some disc properties. Later, he tried out silicon testicular prostheses, but found that the implants rapidly disintegrated after 20 to 30 thousand cycles of walking load [135, 136, 137].

1955, [181]: van Steenbrugghe patented a series of joint replacement implants spanning nearly all the major joints. Among those drawings is one related to the disc. This prosthesis consists of two cushions which, according to the inventor, can be made in a wide variety of materials.

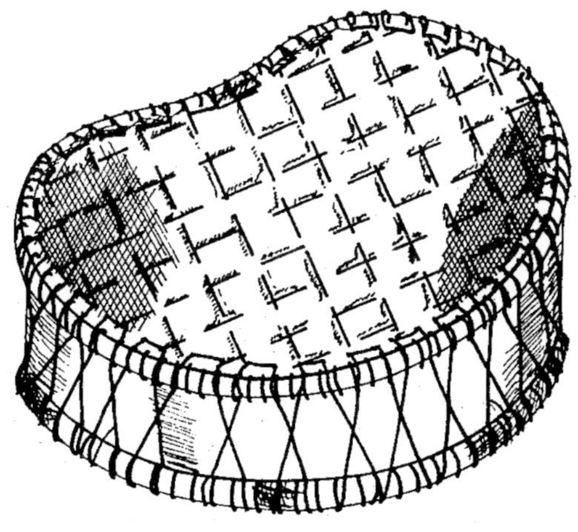

Fig. 1 Original Stubstdat design

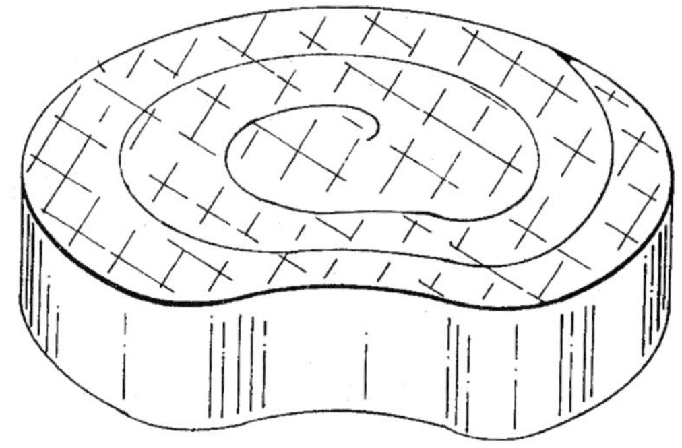

Fig. 2 Variant of the Stubstadt design, showing first helicoidal design

1973, [173]: Stubstad et al. [132] developed several designs approximating the shape and structure of a disc and made of reinforced elastic polymer (Fig. 1). A primate study was undertaken [179], but there does not appear to have been human use. In the same patent application, the authors also propose a coiled implant which, after introduction, wraps into a disc-shaped prosthesis. The same team also describes a spiral implant with elastic memory properties. The width of the coil varies so that it forms an oval shape (Fig. 2). This is the first of the multiple coiled or spiraled implants.

- 1974, [160]: Schneider and Oyen published an experimental work on silicon disc replacement.
- 1974, [92, 93]: Hoffman-Daimler patented an implant consisting of metal endplates with a complex plastic spacer.
- 1975, Froning [57]: discoid bladder-like implant filled with liquid after insertion. It is fixed to the vertebrae with a spike (Fig. 3).
- 1978, Roy-Camille et al. [156]: pre-made silicon disc.
- 1980, Kuntz [109]: simple wedge-shaped implant made of "biologically acceptable material" and inserted by "friction fit". It may be made of metal, hard plastic or elastomers. It enables motion in a sagittal plane.
- 1981, Edeland [42]: folded diaphragm-like device introduced in the disc where it unfolds. Looks like a wheel with four spokes. He also describes a disc containing a hydroscopic agent, which is used to expand the disc after introduction.

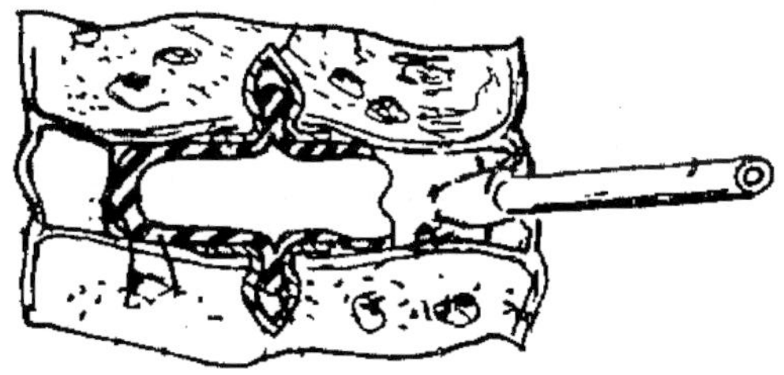

Fig. 3 Bladder-like Froning prosthesis

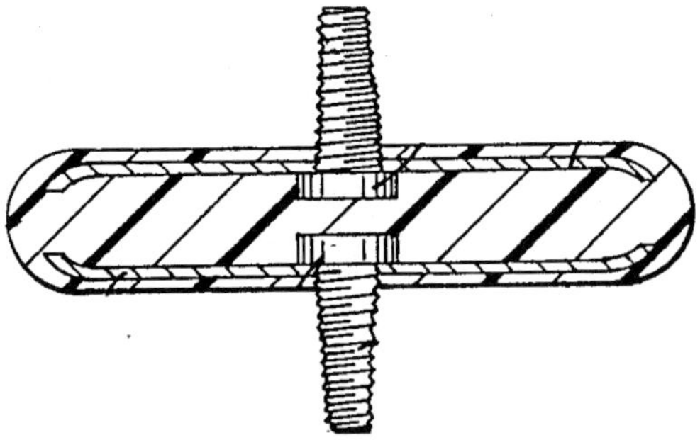

Fig. 4 Downey prosthesis

- 1982, Khvisuyk [102]: silicon cushion between two metallic plates fixed to the adjacent vertebrae with pins.
- 1987, Downey [39]: "flying saucer" shaped cushion made of silicon or polyethylene with an inner core in a more fluid material. Two large central screws attach to the endplates. The screws have opposite-direction threading, so that by rotating the device it threads simultaneously in both adjacent endplates. The placement of such a device would certainly be arduous (Fig. 4).
- 1987, Monson [133]: rubber or silicon implant made of two hollow moulded parts joined and glued together and containing a cavity in which saline solution is injected after implanting, in order to create resiliency and restore height. Suction cup like structures are placed on the upper and lower surfaces of the implant to ensure fixation.
- 1989, Ojima et al. [141]: hydroxyapatite-covered plates with a synthetic polymeric body. Inverted frustum cones are used to anchor the device to the vertebral bodies.
- 1989, Main et al. [118]: a device to replace disc and vertebral body. It consists of two thick rigid housings fixed by anchoring pins and an expandable connecting structure (Fig. 5).
- 1990, Harms et al. [86]: disc consisting of a biocompatible support layer (i.e. silicon rubber) covered on both sides with fibre-reinforced plastic plates. The endplates are made of triazin resin coated with hydroxyapatite-tricalcium phosphate mixture.
- 1990, Frey et al. [54, 55, 56]: compressible elastic hollow body between two anchoring plates. The hollow cavity is compartmented and filled with fluid, which is allowed to circulate.
- 1990, Clemow et al. [34]: disc-shaped spacer made of elastomeric material of varying hardness.
- 1990, Schoppe [162]: fluid inflatable device.
- 1990, Downey [40]: vertebral body replacement including an elastic disc screwed in the endplates.
- 1990, Lee et al. [112, 113, 144]: functional biocompatible intervertebral disc spacer. Laminated horizontal or axial polymer sheets in which changes in the physical parameters modify the flexibility of the disc. This has been one of the most studied devices over time. Many materials were experimented with, mostly silicon composites (C-Flex) or polyurethane (Biothane). In later modifications, porous coatings and hydroxyapatite particles were added to help bone ingrowth. Implantation in rabbits gave encouraging results [16] Hydroxyapatite models were experimented with in a canine model and the results were published in 1994. Poor bonding and high migration frequency was found [183]. Extensive development was conducted in later years with different design variations and materials (e.g. carbon fibres, Dacron), but no clinical use has ever been reported. Insufficient tear and fatigue strength of most rubbers used appeared to be the main stumbling block. The biocompatibility of materials was also not optimal; for example C-Flex has been reported to contain mineral oil, which could leach out [184] and potential carcinogenicity of certain polyurethane composites is talked about.

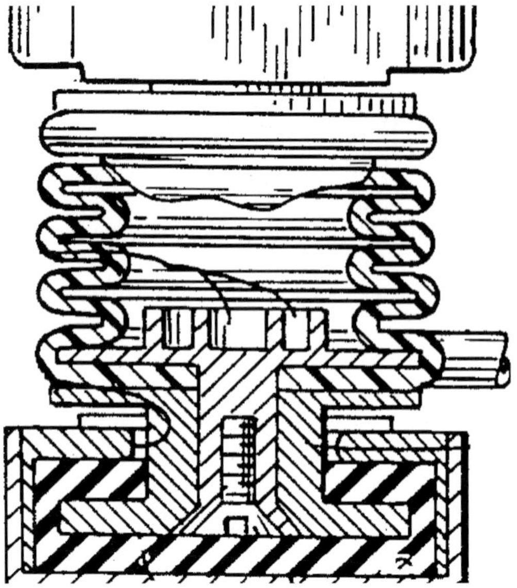

Fig. 5 Main prosthesis

- 1991, Pisharodi [147]: expandable device designed to fill the disc space. It is made of a hollow bag containing springs and small external spikes at both ends of each spring. The prosthesis is folded into a small rectangular package in order to be inserted. Once in place, it opens and expands by filling with liquid or gas (Fig. 6).
- 1991, Bao and Higham [5]: hydrogel beads covered by a semi-permeable membrane to fill the disc, permitting fluids to flow in and out of the implant. The hydrogel beads have a water content of at least 30% and can be made from many different composites. The membrane is made of Dacron or Nylon in a woven form. The surface of the implants can be either smooth or have grooves to increase stability in the intervertebral space, and can be slightly convex. Devices for minimally invasive insertion of beads have also been described [2].

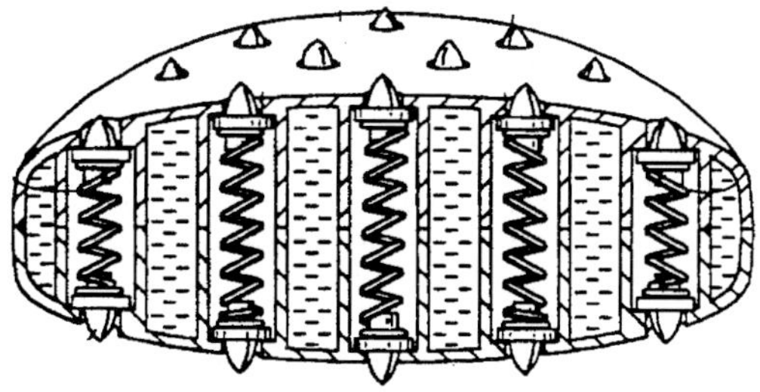

Fig. 6 Pisharodi expandable prosthesis

- 1991, Baumgartner [10]: flexible elastic body coiled in the intervertebral space with a valve capable of receiving a filling medium. The device is filled after being introduced and coiled in the disc space (Fig. 7). Further modifications on the same principles were patented later [95, 96]. The procedure has been baptized "spiral nucleoplasty". It seems to be in clinical experimentation by Husson, but nothing has been published to date.
- 1991, Kaden et al. [99]: a circular or elliptical corrugated tube filled with a viscoelastic material. The ends of the tube are sealed by rigid cover plates. Those plates have holes to allow screwing to the vertebral bodies.
- 1992, Baumgartner [9, 11]: a small elastomeric cylinder core with metallic endplates which have ascending and descending portions that act as stops for compression, translation and bending. The elastomeric core is placed after fixation of the endplates and can be removed.
- 1994, Baumgartner [12]: elastic beads introduced in the disc space, preserving the annulus. They may be introduced directly into the nucleus space or be enclosed within a membrane (Fig. 8).
- 1993, Fuchs et al. [59]: disc-shaped cushion made from elastic material with a bulging periphery (tyre like) sandwiched between two metallic plates screwed into the adjacent vertebrae.

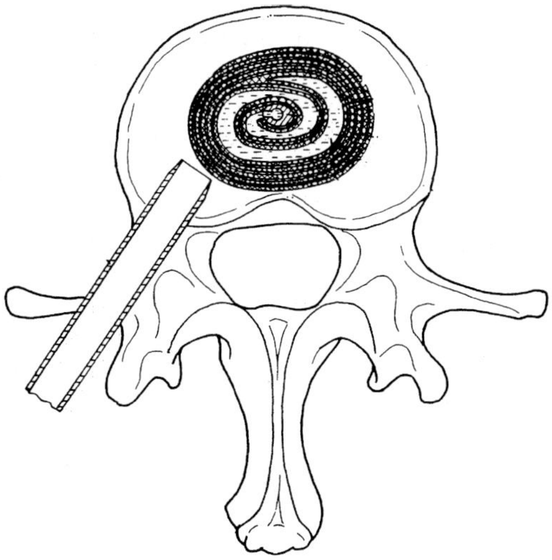

Fig. 7 The first of the Baumgartner and Husson helicoidal discs (spiral nucleoplasty)

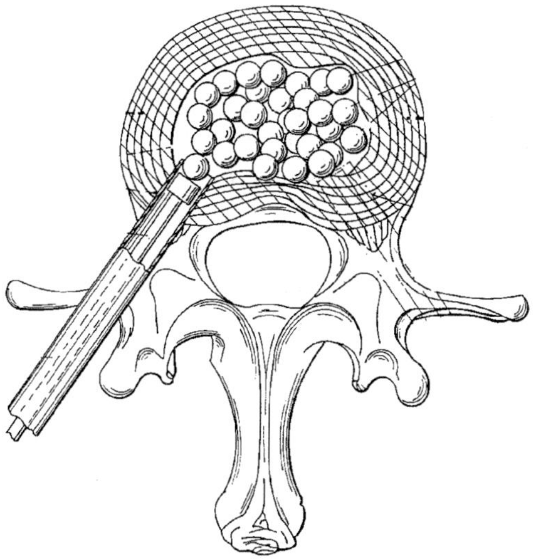

Fig. 8 Baumgartner elastic beads design

- 1994, Oka et al. [142]: composite body comprising layers of polyvinyl alcohol hydrogel and ceramic or metallous porous body allowing bone ingrowth.
- 1994, Grundei [78]: rounded silicon sleeve fitting to a metallic body enabling "partial replacement" of the disc.
- 1994, Popp et al. [148]: disc-shaped device made from a "biocompatible" material. This device has a U or W lateral shape and functions as a spring.
- 1995, Beer and Beer [13]: disc-shaped screwed plates joined by springs protected by an elastomeric covering. The plates have a compressible polymeric core (Fig. 9).
- 1995, Simon et al. [167]: spiraled device rolled around a central core. It has self-adhesive sides and a lengthwise reinforcing radio-opaque structure.
- 1996, Dumas et al. [41]: pair of plates with a helicoidal spring with exponentially increasing stiffness as the space between plates narrows.
- 1996, Bao et al. [6, 7, 8]: hydrogel prosthetic rods absorbing body fluids to fill the interbody nuclear cavity. The hydrogel contains approximately 70% of its uncompressed absorption capacity under physiological

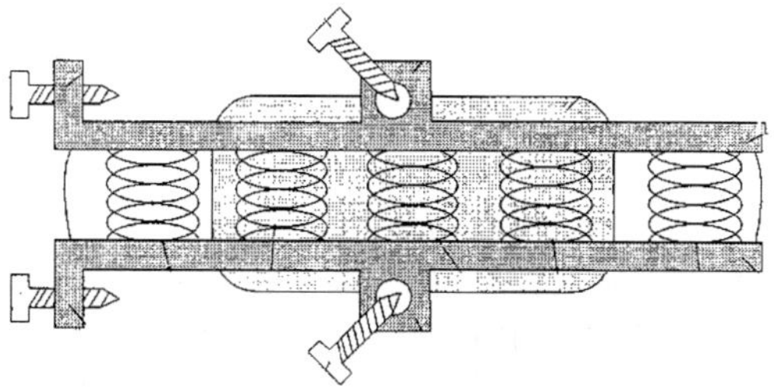

Fig. 9 Beer and Beer spring based implant

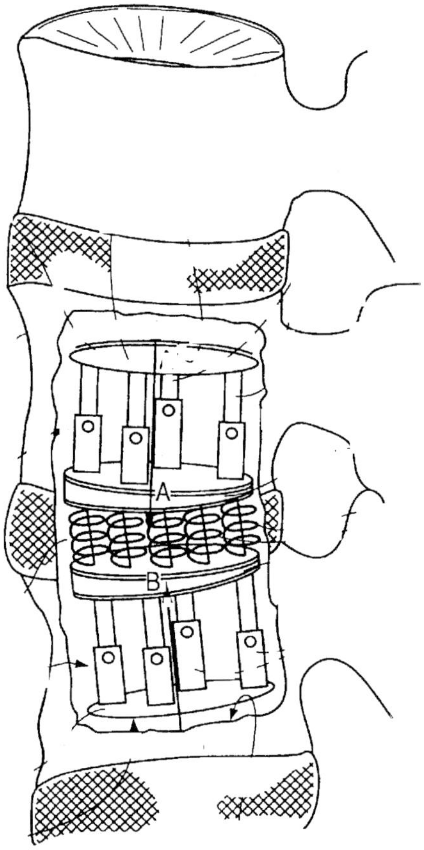

Fig. 10 Buttermann complex spring and pistons prosthesis

load. They reported that this hydrogel nucleus can absorb and release water when submitted to cyclic loading. Another hydrogel prosthetic nucleus shaped implant is also described [90, 91]. It appears that unpublished primate implantations have been realized and showed no adverse reactions, whether local or systemic. A preliminary human study is planned.

- 1996, Buttermann [27]: complex system with preloaded springs allowing preservation of the annulus fibrosus (sic). Looking at the patent drawing, one wonders about the insertion of the implant (Fig. 10).
- 1996, Grammont and Gauchet [75]: deformable capsules with rigid plates and connected by a deformable envelope.
- 1996, Pigg and Cassidy [146]: resiliently deformable material such as a hydrophilic polymer reinforced with physically discreet structures in order to form an in-situ composite.
- 1997, Monteiro et al. [134]: hollow flexible and inflatable capsule filled with radio-opaque "swelling" fluid.
- 1997, Ratron [149]: two plates joined by elastic partitions, implanted in pairs.
- 1997, Dios Seoane [38]: a flexible structure made of osteointegrating material.
- 1997, Bisserie [15]: mirror-like left/right half disc prosthesis consisting of rigid upper and lower spiked plates with elastic cushions in between.
- 1997, Bainville et al. [3]: two metal half envelopes confining a compression cushion with a controlled differential compression. It also utilises an anti-expulsion system to limit the expansion of the elastic cushion.
- 1997, Bouvet [17]: two rigid plates fixed to the bone separated by leaf spring in the shape of a cross and made of elastic material. This device is described as a hip and intervertebral prosthesis.
- 1997, Krapiva [108]: cylindrical flexible hollow nucleus prosthesis, which is folded for insertion and expands in situ. It is then filled with a gel.
- 1999, Graf [71, 72, 73]: three designs. One design consists of an elastic conical core with two grooved rigid covers, the conical shape being meant to help preserve lordosis [71]. The second design appears to be based on the same plates/core principles, but the core is limited to the anterior two-thirds of the disc, and this design allows a greater degree of motion [72]. In a third design, Graf describes a composite device consisting of a posterior damping system fixed with pedicular screws combined with an intervertebral implant (Fig. 11). The latter could be based on different principles: a posterior pivot axis with an anterior damping spring, a rigid ball between concave plates, a ball with hydrophilic gel surrounded by a membrane or an elastic cushion [73].
- 1999, Harrington [87]: pivot ball and socket with shock-absorbing devices between plates screwed into the endplates (Fig. 12).
- 1999, Wardlaw [185]: nucleus-shaped transudative material cover filled with hydrogel material.

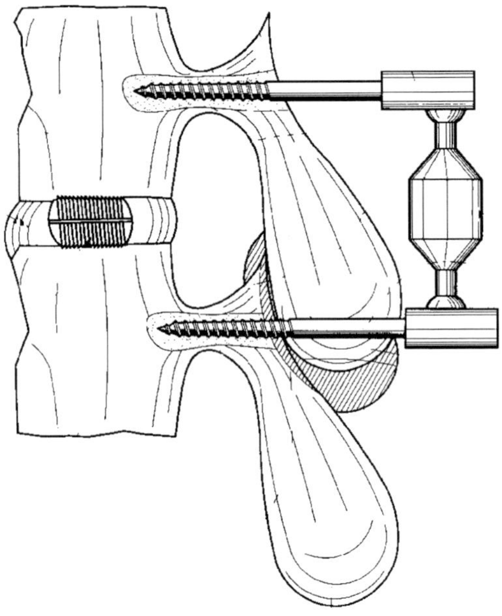

Fig. 11 Graf combined antero-posterior implants

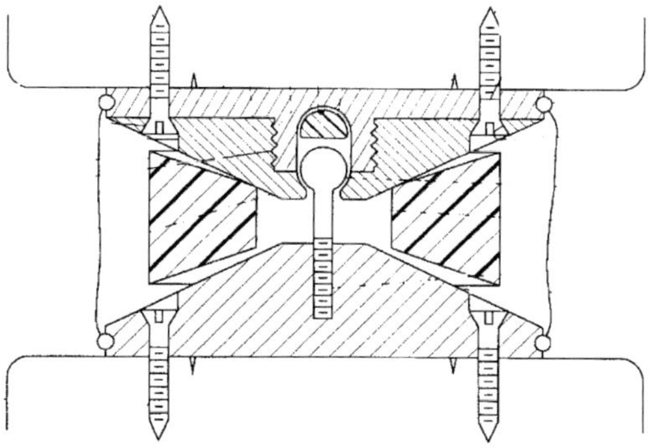

Fig. 12 Harrington ball and socket prosthesis

- 1999, Savchenko et al. [159]: porous titanium plates with an intermediate fluoroplastic nucleus.
- 2000, Cochet [35]: two titanium plates linked by a core and connecting piece with through cells arranged in honeycomb shape.
- 2000, Bryan and Kunzler [22, 23]: resilient intervertebral body maintained by two articulating anterior plates (Fig. 13).

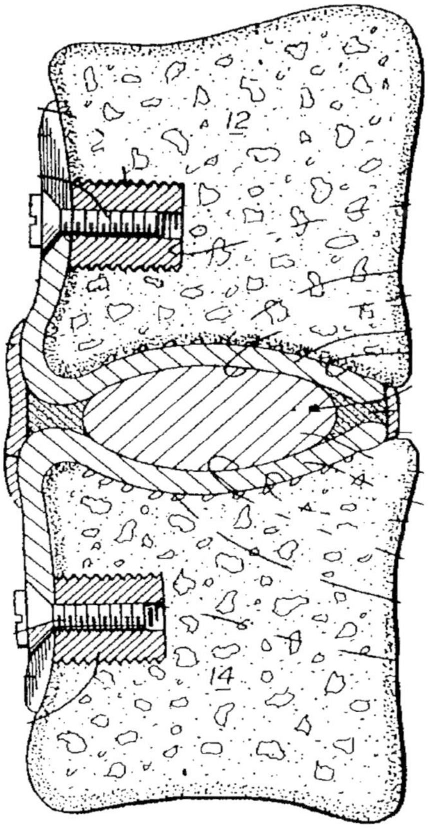

Fig. 13 Bryan and Kunzler prosthesis with disc replacement by "resilient body"

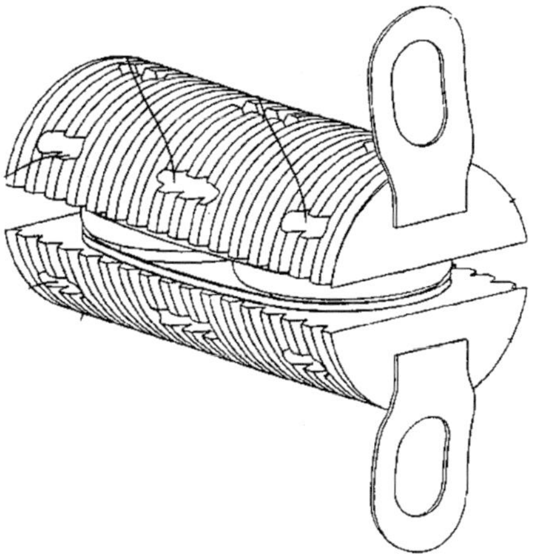

Fig. 14 Bryan and Kunzler cylindric implant

- 2000, Bryan and Kunzler [24]: two threaded hollow half-cylinders screwed to the bodies and containing multiple discoid resilient bodies (Fig. 14).
- 2000, Bryan [20]: "Peanut spectacle" shaped device made of two half "peanut" shells containing resilient bodies.
- 2000, Bryan and Carver [21]: an implant that looks like a combination of the two previous designs: half cylinders filled with peanut shaped resilient bodies.
- 2000, Gauchet and Le Couëdic [64]: disc made of two metal blades screwed to the vertebral bodies surrounding a compressible cushion (Fig. 15).
- 2000, Gauchet [62]: elastic material cylinder surrounding a liquid-filled nucleus between two plates screwed to the bodies.
- 2000, Gauchet et al. [65]: construct of two round plates and an intermediate deformable body in the shape of a four-leaf clover.
- 2000, Lawson [110]: semi-ovoid design. The lower surface is slightly convex and comprises a short peg for cemented fixation in the upper endplate of the inferior vertebra. The superior surface is more convex and ar-

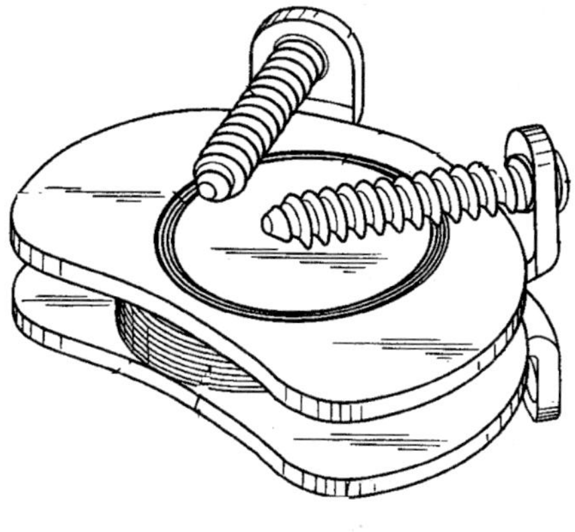

Fig. 15 Prosthesis of Gauchet and Le Couedic

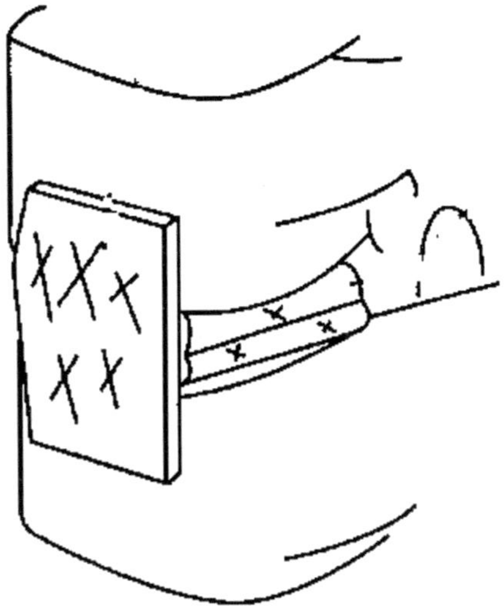

Fig. 16 Jackowski and McLeod elastomeric prosthesis

ticulates with the upper vertebra. The device is placed through an annular flap after curetting nucleus material. The annulus is preserved.

- 2000, Middleton [128]: complex multi-slit disc-shaped device.
- 2000, Jackowski and McLeod [98]: elastomeric material compressed by textile encapsulation and laid in the intervertebral space (Fig. 16).
- 2000, Gauchet [63]: compressible bladder filled with liquid and a compressible material between two plates.
- 2000, Zdeblick and McKay [194]: two rectangular shells with grooved biconvex surfaces for contact with the endplates. A spacer made from an elastic material is sandwiched between the shells.
- 2001, Viart and Marin [182]: two spiked convex plates with a viscoelastic biconcave "tyre like" core.
- 2001, Gau [61]: one or several spheres made from "biocompatible" material moving in a conic cage-like enclosure.
- 2001, Studer and Schärer [174]: another variation of a spiraled device. The spiral is made of "plastic material" containing small hydrogel cylinders. It is meant to be implanted following discectomy.
- 2001, Marcolongo and Lowman [119]: prosthetic nucleus made from blends of polyvinylalcohol and polyvinyl pyrollidone.
- 2001, Minda and Schmidt [131]: fillable soft container or balloon to be filled with fluid or air.
- 2001, Weber and Da Silva [188]: prosthesis including an annulus and a nucleus which can be adapted to the anatomical configuration by stereotactic forming after imaging studies (MRI, CT). The nucleus includes an empty cavity for the introduction of fluid or gel. An optional fibre-optic carriage could transmit laser or electromagnetic rays to stimulate tissue ingrowth from adjacent vertebrae into porosities on the upper and lower surfaces.

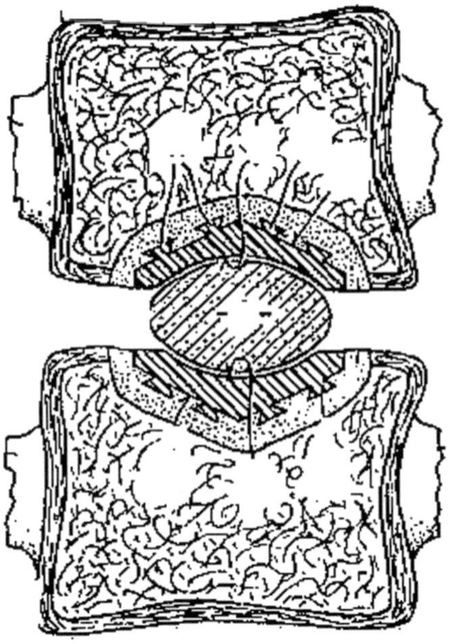

Fig. 17 Weber lumbar prosthesis

- 2001, Banks et al. [4]: implants of different shapes made from synthetic polyamide, polyester, polyethylene, collagen or other plastics. They may have bone fixation anchor and annulus closing features.
- 2002, Kotani et al. [107]: a disc made from a three-dimensional fabric woven from polyethylene fibers and coated with bioactive ceramic on the surfaces. The authors describe biomechanical studies and sheep implantation. They report that the best motion results are achieved when a temporary rigid fixation is used over 6 months.

Devices aimed mainly at restoring the motion function

- 1978, Weber [186]: two polyethylene box-like structures anchored in the adjacent vertebrae, each having a shell-shaped cavity in which a ceramic ovoid core is introduced to enable motion (Fig. 17).
- 1987, Hedman et al. [48, 88]: this is the Kostuik team implant. Made of two titanium springs between cobalt-chromium-molybdenum hinged alloy plates screwed to the bodies. This implant allows good sagittal motion (15°–20°) with very restricted lateral motion (3°–6°). It is designed in six sizes. Fatigue tests to 100 million cycles showed that springs tended to break [89]. Implantation in sheep did not show fibrous ingrowth in the mechanisms [104]. It was never implanted in humans.
- 1989, Keller [101]: two concave spiked stop plates with a biconvex metallic core (Fig. 18).
- 1992, Bullivant [25]: two plates and a core with an inferior convex surface sliding in a concave shape of the inferior plate. A superior flat surface slides against the upper flat plate. It appears to be inspired by the Charité concept.

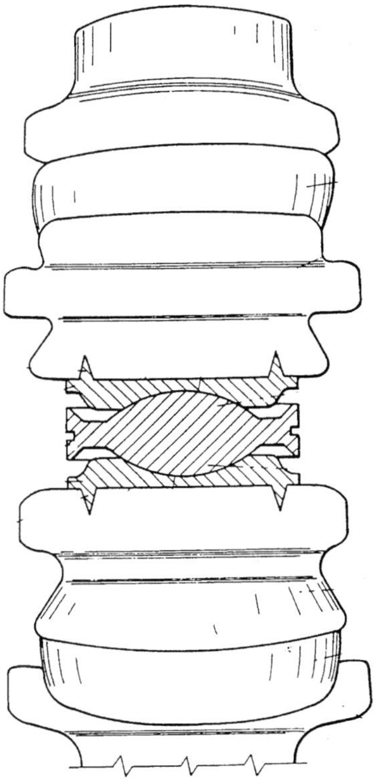

Fig. 18 Keller prosthesis

- 1992, Graham [74]: ball and socket joint fixed to cylinders and flexible spacers inserted in the vertebral body and locked by hemicylindrical plates and screws. The ball and socket provides motion and the spacers compressive function (Fig. 19).
- 1992, Salib and Pettine [158]: eccentric ball and socket joint screwed to the vertebral bodies. It is designed to have six degrees of freedom but no compressive properties (Fig. 20).

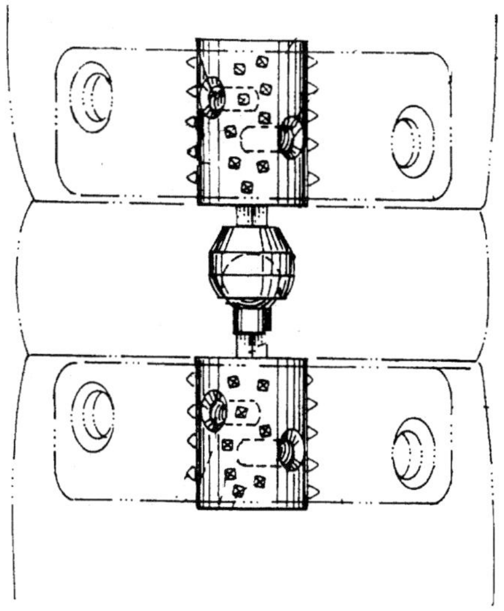

Fig. 19 Graham ball and socket joint

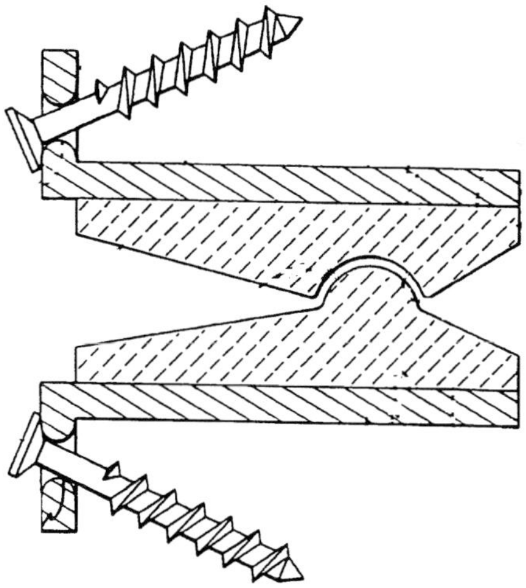

Fig. 20 Salib and Pettine ball and socket design

- 1994, Mazda [124]: two spiked plates between which is placed a centred ball joint with an elastic surrounding cushion.
- 1996, Teule [178]: low-friction prosthesis with a lens-shaped spacer.
- 1997, Yuan et al. [193]: articulated convex/concave implant enabling motion in all planes and fixed through spikes in the endplates.
- 1997, Shinn and Tate [166]: two plates anchored with pins in the endplates and screwed into the anterior wall of adjacent vertebrae. A partial socket is attached to the lower plate and a partial ball is attached to the upper plate to articulate with and be retained by the socket. A peripheric membrane can be added.
- 1998, Xavier et al. [191]: vertebral body replacement allowing motion. Two spiked plates are screwed to the bodies with an articulated ball surrounded by an elastic annulus. They attempt to restrain rotational motion by X-pattern wires between the two plates (Fig. 21).

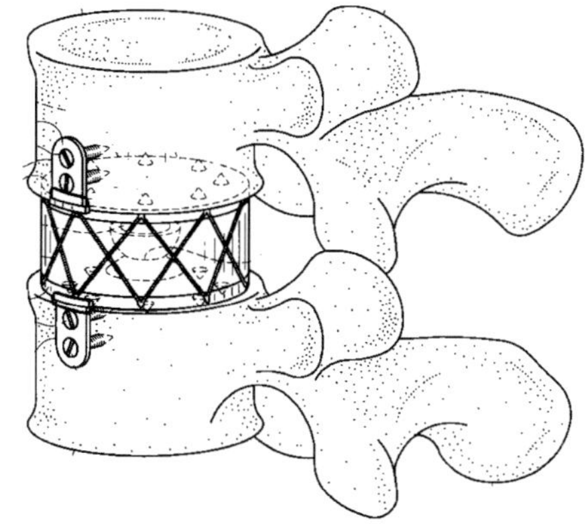

Fig. 21 Xavier wire stabilized prosthesis

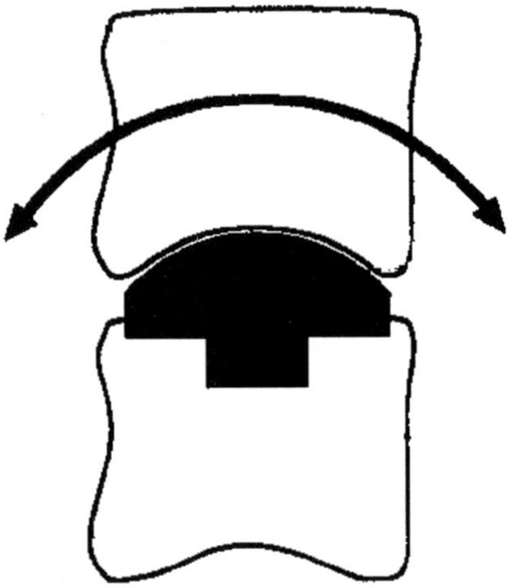

Fig. 22 Sabitzer prosthesis

- 1999, Sabitzer and Fuss [157]: this device has a flat inferior side with a rod for fixation in the inferior vertebra. The upper side is convex and articulates with the lower endplate of the superior vertebra (Fig. 22).
- 1999, Rogozinski [155]: self-centering system with a biconvex core sliding in two concave plates.
- 2000, Shelokov [164]: prosthesis resembling a knee implant with two condyles. An upper double-convex element slides on an inferior double-concave one.
- 2000, Griffith and Erickson [76]: spiked plates with one curved bearing and one plane bearing surface and an intermediate core adapted to those surfaces. It allows for rotation and, optionally, for certain amount of translation.
- 2000, Gordon et al. [69]: two plates, one with a male concave element placed in a female flat element fixed on the other plate. A hemispheric bearing is sandwiched between the two elements. The plates are screwed to the anterior walls of the adjacent vertebrae.
- 2001, Cauthen [31]: two hemi-cylindrical elements with a longitudinal slit on the inferior element in which a rounded ridge on the upper element articulates, enabling sagittal motion (Fig. 23).
- 2001, Betisor et al. [14]: articulated frame with rods and axes and a toothed contact surface.

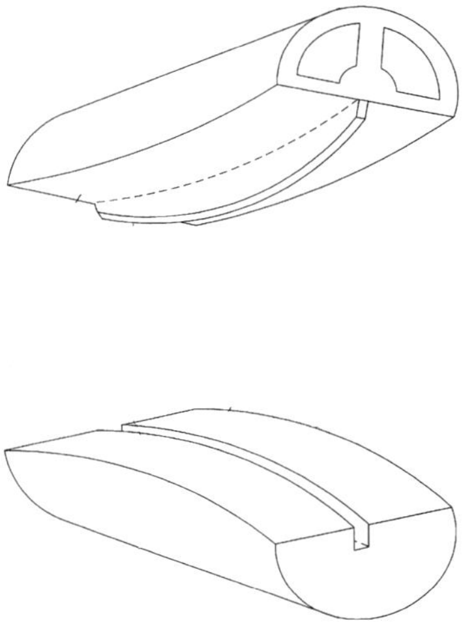

Fig. 23 Cauthen cylindrical slit and rib implant

Cervical disc prosthesis

- 1979, Weber [187]: this implant is similar to his lumbar implant. Two concave structures are anchored in the vertebral bodies with cemented grooved spikes, between which lies a central ovoid core. In the cervical model, the holding plates have a guiding system linking them to avoid expulsion of the core during movements. Each superior and inferior component is fixed with a single cemented spike, which is eccentric in the frontal plane (Fig. 24).
- 1980, Patil [145]: interlocking spiked plates, resembling box cover, linked with springs (Fig. 25).

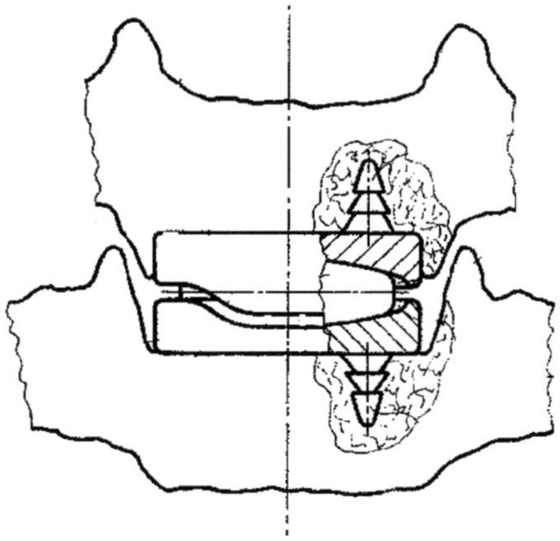

Fig. 24 Weber cervical implant with eccentric cementing

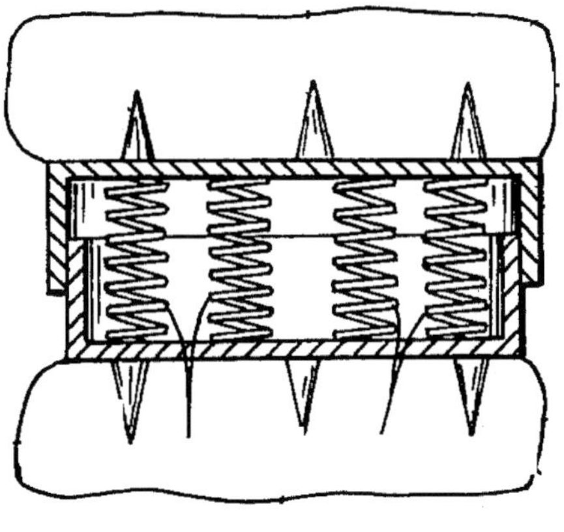

Fig. 25 Patil cervical interlocking plates and springs

- 1995, Lesoin et al. [116]: two plates screwed in the bodies with a large concave/convex articulation.
- 1996, Kehr et al. [100]: sliding prosthesis made of an inferior plate screwed on the side of the vertebra on which is mounted a convex element. The latter can articulate either with the inferior endplate of the upper vertebra or with a concave element fixed to that upper vertebra (Fig. 26).

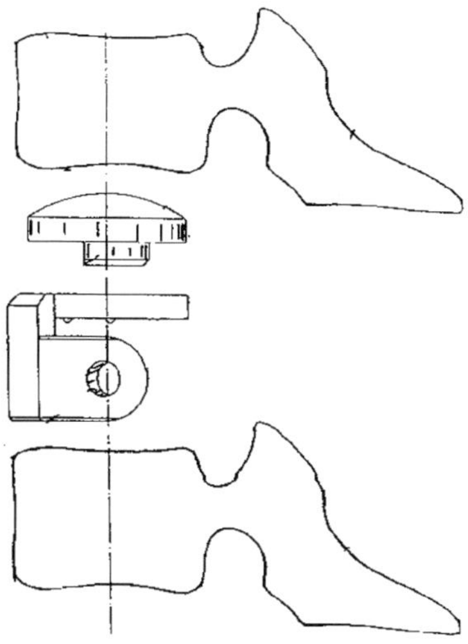

Fig. 26 Kehr cervical implant

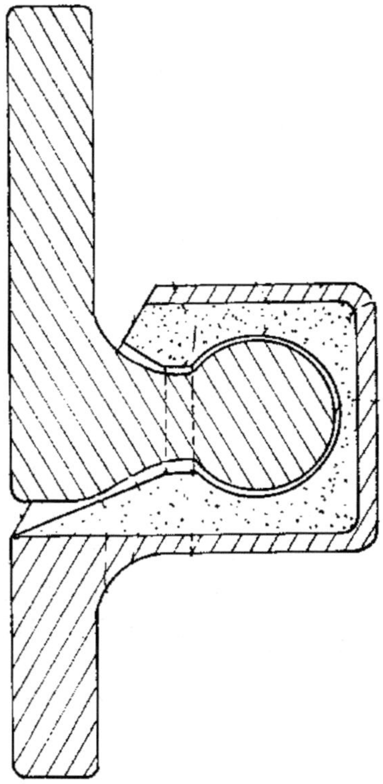

Fig. 27 Ibo "inversed hip" ball and socket implant

- 1998, Ibo and Pierotto [97]: a ball and socket joint screwed in the bodies. It looks like a small total hip replacement (Fig. 27).
- 2000, Cauthen [30]: two threaded half-cylinders with a ball and socket joint in the centre (Fig. 28).
- 2001, Buhler and Ramadan [25]: two spiked plates with ceramic articulation.
- 2001, Medizadeh [127]: two threaded half-cylinders linked by small springs. It looks like a longitudinally split cylindrical cage in which springs have been inserted.

Other designs

- 1996, Navas [139]: two ball joints with a dampening element screwed into adjacent vertebral bodies and linked together to try to reproduce disc behaviour.

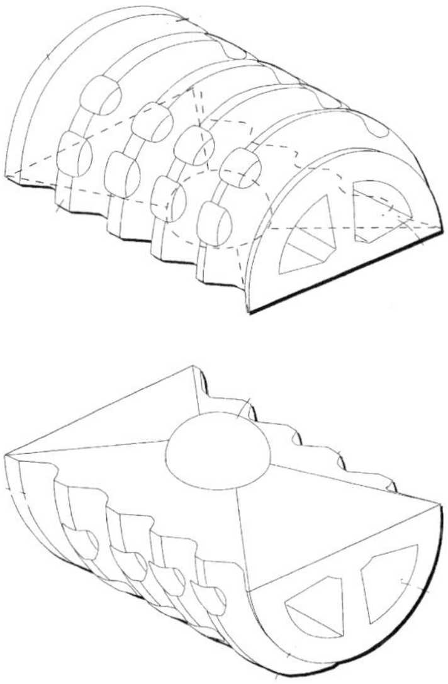

Fig. 28 Cauthen cylindrical ball and socket designs

Fig. 29 Fitz articular facet covers implant

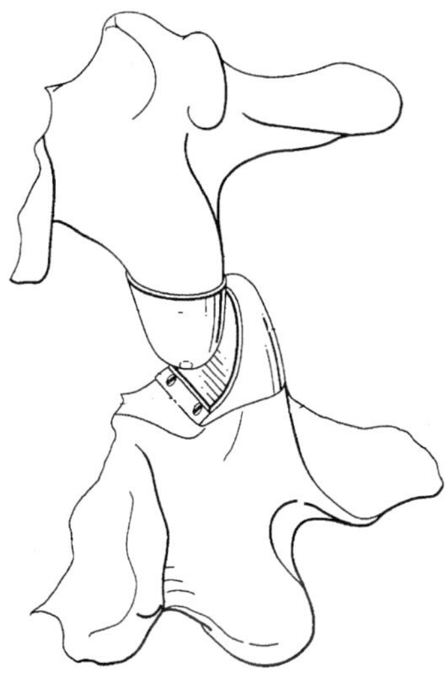

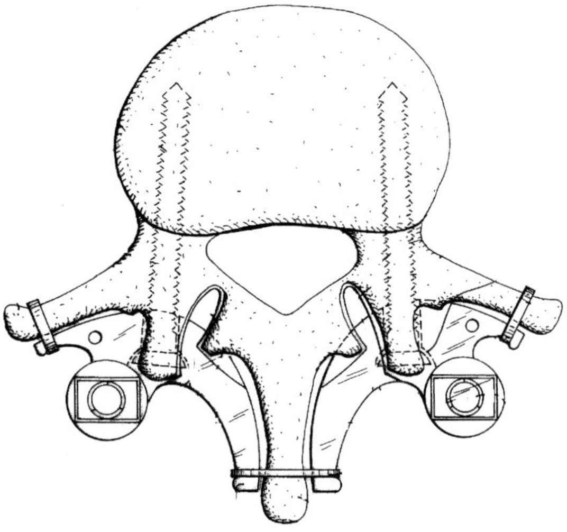

Fig. 30 Martin complex facet replacement

- 1990, Stone [171, 172]: prosthetic disc acting as a scaffold for regrowth of disc tissue made of a dry porous volume matrix of biocompatible and bioresorbable fibres. This matrix establishes a scaffold for ingrowth of intervertebral fibrochondrocytes.
- 1996, Fitz [51]: facet prosthesis with two metal elements capping the superior and inferior facets (Fig. 29).
- 2000, Martin [122]: complex facet joint prosthesis with the joint construct attached to pedicular screws and to the lateral and spinous processes (Fig. 30).
- A number of Chinese patents relating to disc prostheses exist, although we have no precise description [81, 84, 117, 165].

In situ polymerizing devices

A number of attempts to inject substances that polymerize in situ in the intervertebral space in order to restore viscoelastic function have been proposed.

Garcia [60] and Shepperd [18] have described such a procedure. Recently, Felt et al. [47] described a minimally invasive technique to deliver a curable biomaterial such as a two-part polyurethane system. The delivery balloon used also allows for expansion during polymer injection, thus restoring disc height. Preliminary clinical testing is to begin.

Arrowsmith and Milner [1, 129, 130] propose materials that would cross-link upon contact with water or moisture, such as isocyanate prepolymers or silane functionalised polymers or precursors.

However, all in situ curing formulations contain monomer, prepolymers and catalysts, which are generally cytotoxic and/or carcinogenic. Furthermore, they are exothermic. Permanent anchoring may also be a problem.

Some attempts have been made at trying to reform a degenerate disc. Chin Chin Gan et al. [32] describe a disc-shaped porous hybrid device made of disc cells and a bioactive biodegradable material like bioactive glass or synthetic materials coated with bioactive substances.

Experimental animal reinsertions of allograft nucleus pulposus have also been described [140, 143].

Clinical use

Artificial discs that have been used clinically

In spite of the very large amount of different disc replacement designs, only a few have reached the level of clinical implantation, even in primate animal models.

The first human implantation of artificial disc was performed by Fernström in the late 1950s [49]. He was using a metal ball – in fact an SKF ball bearing – and tried to reproduce the “ball joint” mechanism of the disc. Along the same line of thought, Harmon utilises Vitalium spheres, which were commercialised for a short period of time. The Harmon spheres could also have been used as instrumen-

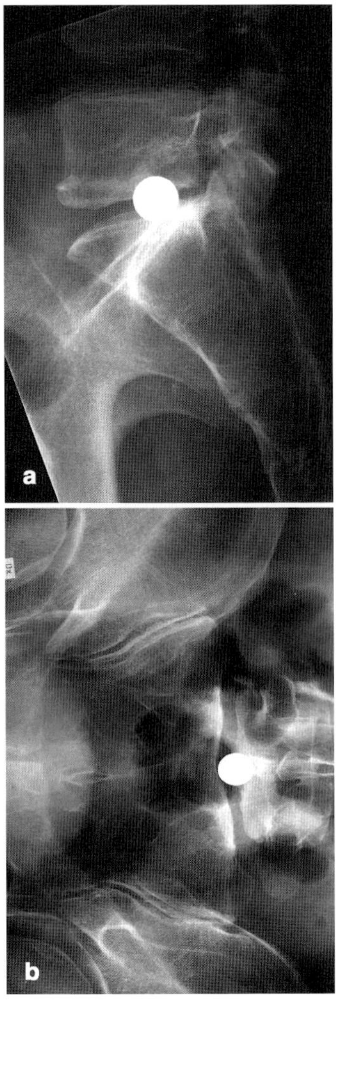

Fig. 31 **A** Lateral and **B** antero-posterior view of an implanted Fernström ball. Note the sinking of the device in the upper endplate (courtesy T. Hansson)

tation for fusion [85]. The Fernström balls seem to have been used in about 250 patients. They created a segmental hypermobility and had a marked tendency to subside into the vertebral endplates and bodies (Fig. 31). McKenzie presented good preliminary results [125] and good long-term results, but the latter in a methodologically dubious paper published in a non indexed and non peer reviewed journal [126]. Fernström himself admitted poor results; the implant was withdrawn and no long-term studies are available [50].

Reitz and Joubert, from South Africa, implanted a metal prosthesis in the cervical spine in the treatment of intractable headache and cervico-brachialgia. No long-term follow-up is available [154].

Fassio designed and patented an elastic, which has a "flying saucer shape" [45]. The central sphere is in silastic and the lateral plateau in uncompressible synthetic resin (Fig. 32). After laboratory testing and primate implantation, they implanted it in three patients in 1977 (Fig. 33) [46]. They stopped because of the destructive posterior approach and subsidence of the implant in the endplates, which created an intraspongious hernia. After 4 years follow-up, there was a marked disc narrowing and absence of motion.

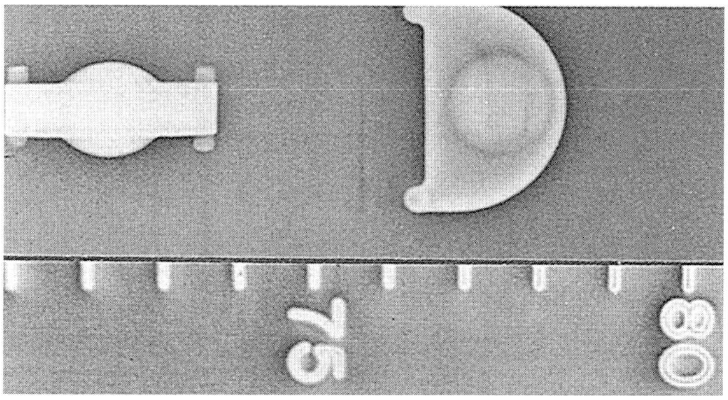

Fig. 32 Fassio silicon implant (courtesy B. Fassio)

It appears that Hou and co-workers used a silicon prosthesis in about 30 patients. Results were not published [94].

Steffee designed a lumbar implant [168, 169, 170], the Acroflex, consisting of a hexen-based polyolefin rubber cushion attached to two titanium endplates. Six patients were implanted and followed up for 3 years, with very average results [43]. Possible carcinogenic properties of a chemical used in the rubber vulcanisation process caused the withdrawal of the implant.

A new design using HP-100 silicon elastomer was proposed by Steffee, Fraser, and co-workers [53, 163] (Fig. 34). Those new implants were third-generation AcroFlex artificial discs. The initial implant, referred to as the Pilot 1 device, had flat endplates and a crescent-shaped protruberance for bony fixation and was used in 11 patients; the subsequent version, with contoured endplates and fins, was called the Pilot 2 device (used in 29 patients). Apart from the metal endplate surfaces, the devices were identical. However, after those first 40 implantations (Fig. 35), it was decided to stop, because of the failure of the device in vivo to live up to the performance demonstrated in laboratory testing, with the development in a number of cases of minor defects in the polyolefin, which were displayed on fine-cut computed tomography scans (accurate to 0.25 mm) after 1 or 2 years [52].

The SB Charité prosthesis was designed in former East Germany in the early 1980s by Schellnac and Büttner-Jans, and was first implanted by Zippel in 1984. Problems of migration and metal fatigue fractures led to the aban-

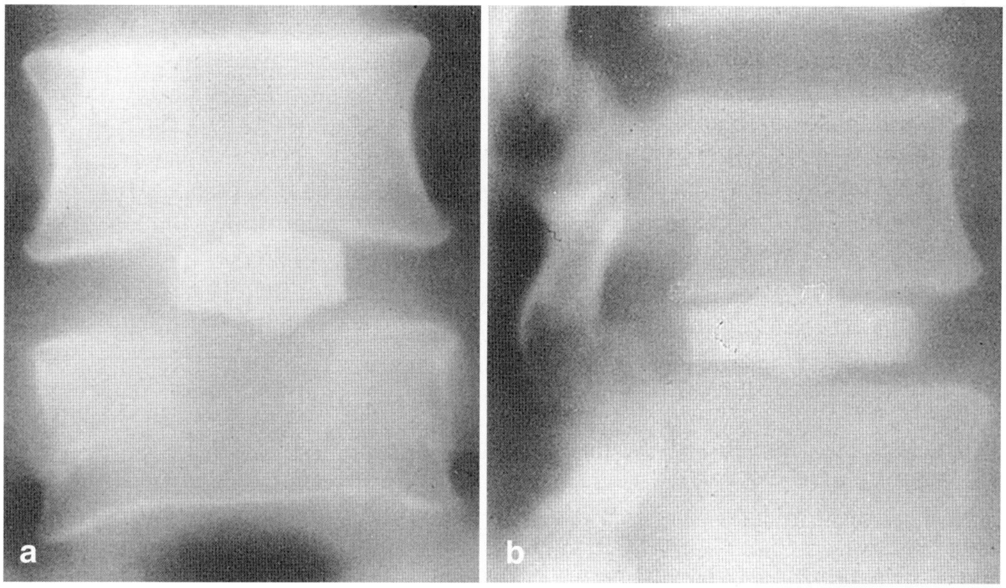

Fig. 33 **A** Antero-posterior and **B** lateral radiograph of the Fassio implant (courtesy B. Fassio)

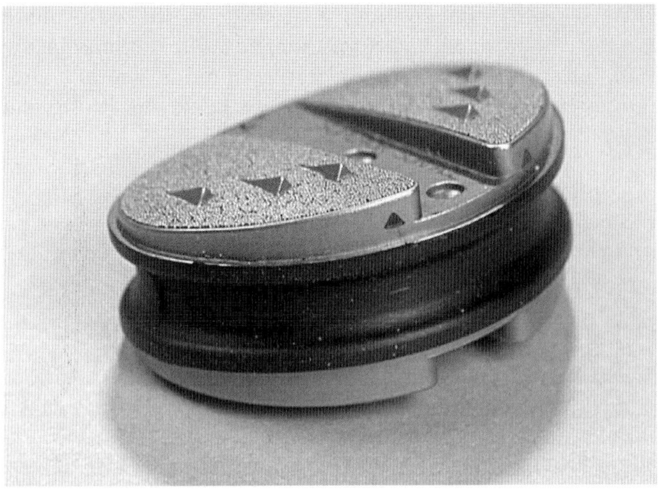

Fig. 34 The Fraser/Steffee second Acroflex implant (courtesy R.D. Fraser)

donment of versions I and II [28, 29]. The Charité III, introduced in 1987, consists of a biconvex ultra-high-molecular-weight polyethylene nucleus with a radio-opaque metallic ring. It interfaces with two endplates of cobalt-chromium-molybdenum alloy coated with titanium and hydroxyapatite and primarily fixed through ventral and dorsal teeth. It has been widely implanted [33, 77, 115, 195], and clinical results are presented elsewhere in this volume.

Ray and Corbin developed a nucleus replacement [151, 152] consisting of dual-threaded cylinders made of semi-permeable, flexible and high-tensile polymeric fibres containing a hydroscopic semi-fluid. Probably due to technical problems in manufacturing a perfectly sealed semi-fluid, this concept was abandoned. Ray et al. then developed the PDN (Prosthetic Disc Nucleus), also a nucleus replacement. It consists of a hydrogel core enclosed in an elastic woven polyethylene jacket, resembling a pillow. Different designs have been patented and used. The annulus fibrosus is conserved during implantation. The hydrogel has hydrophilic properties: it absorbs fluids and expands, and therefore tries to mimic the behaviour of the nucleus pulposus. The design has led to several modifications after a number of device migrations [153]. Preliminary clinical reports have been published [161] and longer-term clinical results are presented elsewhere in this issue.

The Pro-Disc is an articulating disc with polyethylene core. The metal endplates are plasma sprayed with titanium and have two vertical fins for fixation in the endplates. Various clinical trials are currently under way [120, 121], and results are published elsewhere in this issue.

Mathews, Le Huec and al. [123] conceived the Maverick prosthesis, a metal/metal (chrome cobalt) interface implant with a posterior rotation axis. It allows normal motion in sagittal and frontal planes. A multicentric clinical trial is ongoing (Fig. 36).

The Bryan Total Cervical Disc is designed as a low-friction, wear-resistant elastic nucleus. This nucleus is set between and articulates with two titanium plates covered with a porous coating and screwed to the vertebral bodies. A flexible membrane surrounds the construct. It allows range of motion in all planes. The device has been used by several authors, and a paper has been submitted for publication [68]. Another report about this device can be found elsewhere in this issue.

In 1998, Gill and co-workers patented the Bristol cervical disc [66] (Fig. 37). This is a ball and socket type de-

Fig. 35 Lateral radiographic view of implanted second Acroflex prosthesis (courtesy R.D. Fraser)

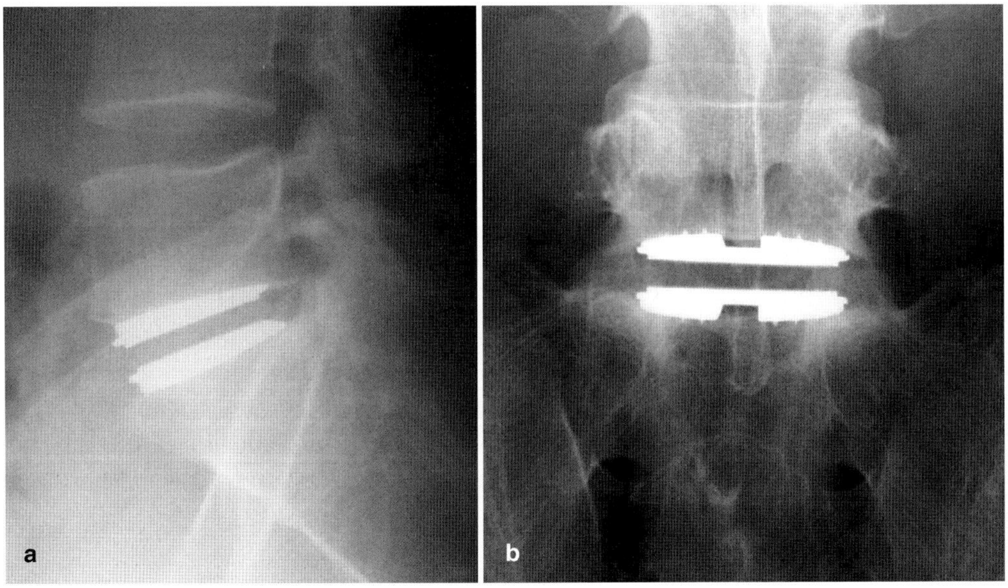

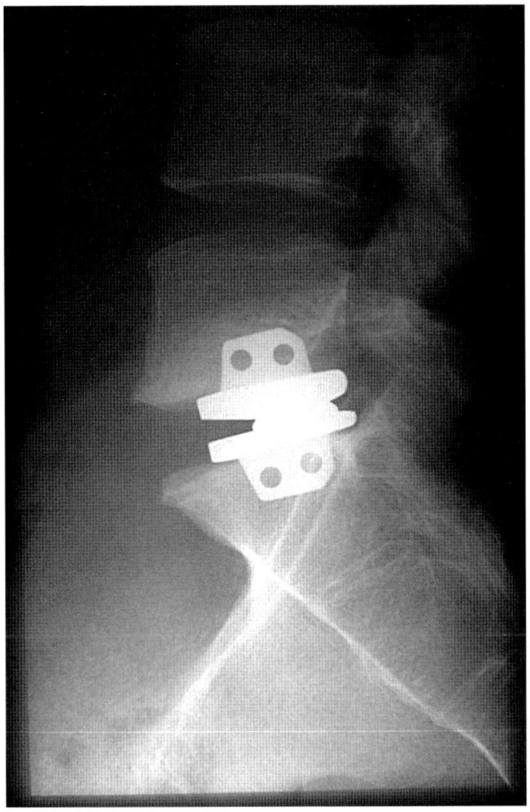

Fig. 36 Antero-posterior radiographic view of the Maverick prosthesis (courtesy J.C. Le Huec)

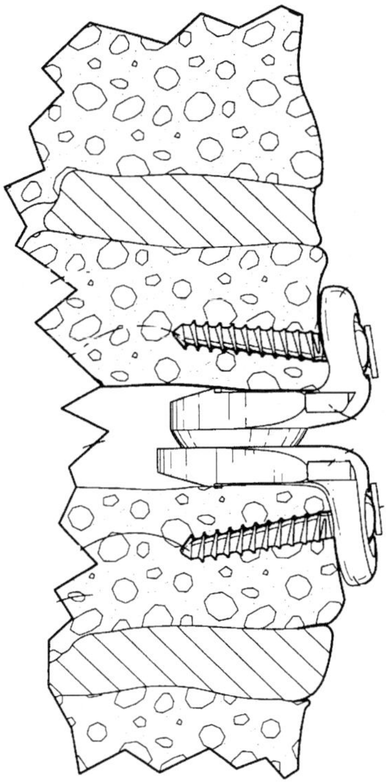

Fig. 37 The Bristol/Gill cervical implant

vice made of stainless steel, which is screwed to the anterior sides of the adjacent vertebral bodies. Cummins reported on 20 patients implanted with the device, and found good results. The device is being clinically evaluated [36].

In 1992, Gjunter [67], from Russia, patented a device with a coiled design. But whereas previous such implants spiraled around a transversal axis, this one spirals around an antero-posterior sagittal axis, to form a resilient flexible cylinder made of a rolled sheet of superelastic porous TiNi alloy [79]. It can be ready coiled or rolled on itself to enable a variation in the diameter. At least one patient has undergone a cervical implantation at the C6/C7 level in Novosibirsk. Results are not known.

Discussion

Proponents of disc prosthesis advance several reasons in favour of spine arthroplasty:

- Preservation of function
- Immediate pain relief
- Frequency of failed fusions
- Possible absence of degeneration at adjacent levels
- Absence of drawbacks linked to autologous bone harvesting

Preservation of function is appealing. However, whereas loss of mobility of a hip or knee is extremely incapacitating, the loss of motion in one, or even several, spinal units is of little functional consequence.

The disc is not, by a long way, the only spinal structure at the origin of nociception [192]. Pain can originate at any of the components of the three-joint complex [103]. In the case of fusion, all structures capable of nociception are fixed, which is not so in arthroplasty. We know that clinical outcome is not necessarily linked to a successful fusion, and that non-union does not preclude a good result [44, 58]. In the literature published to date, the success rate of arthroplasties is comparable to that of fusions. Furthermore, psycho-social factors [82, 190] are known to play a major role in the outcome of any spinal surgery, and the nature of arthroplasty should have a major influence on this aspect. This shows the complex nature of back pain and its relation to surgery. One may wonder whether the poor outcomes are not related to poor indications rather than to the techniques themselves [176].

Some studies have shown a higher degeneration frequency at levels adjacent to a fusion [19, 111]. However, other publications have shown that if imaging does indeed show degeneration, the relation with clinical complaints is very weak [114], and the importance of low back pain is not higher than that in matching-age non-operated patients [37].

Graft harvesting does indeed carry its load of complications and irritations. However, the development in biomaterials and molecular biology will make it possible to use reliable bone substitutes [80, 177].

The very fact that such a long list of implants, based on highly varied principles, has been proposed, and that only very few have reached the level of animal models, let alone human implantation, clearly demonstrates how challenging the task of designing an intervertebral disc replacement is. In the current days of evidence based medicine, adequate prospective clinical trials are imperative. Very recently, leading Dutch orthopaedic surgeons representing the Dutch Orthopaedic Society and the Dutch Spine Society published a warning about uncontrolled clinical implantation in Europe of disc prostheses. They stress the fact that those devices are labelled experimental in the US. In the absence of proper clinical evidence, they consider it should also be seen as experimental in Europe. They denounce the commercial hype through the media, which tends to present these techniques as miracle cures [180].

Proper randomized controlled trials are on the way, and should help in assessing the efficacy and real place of spine arthroplasty in the treatment of spinal disorders. Only then will spinal surgery join the list of successful joint replacements.

Acknowledgements We wish to thank R.D. Fraser, J.C. Le Huec, B. Fassio, T. Hansson ... and the World Wide Web (www.uspto.gov, www.european-patent-office.org, www.depatisnet.de) ... for providing us with precious information and illustrations.

References

1. Arrowsmith P, Milner R (1995) Intervertebral disc implant, World Patent 9531946, 30–11–1995
2. Bagga CS, Higham PA, Yuan HA, Bao QB (1998) Method and apparatus for injecting an elastic spinal implant, United States Patent 5800549, 01–09–1998
3. Bainville D, Laval FR, Roy-Camille R, Saillant G, Lavaste F (1997) Intervertebral disk prosthesis, United States Patent 5674294, 07–10–1997
4. Banks T, Vidal CL, Lambrecht GH, Moore RK, Redmond RJ (2001) Devices and methods of vertebral disc augmentation, World Patent 0112107, 22–02–2001
5. Bao Q-B, Higham PA (1993) Hydrogel bead intervertebral disc nucleus, United States Patent 5192326, 09–03–1993
6. Bao Q-B, Higham PA (1999) Hydrogel intervertebral disc nucleus, United States Patent 5976186, 02–11–1999
7. Bao Q-B, Higham PA (2001) Hydrogel intervertebral disc nucleus implantation method, United States Patent 6280475 B1, 28–08–2001
8. Bao QB, McCullen GM, Higham PA, Dumbleton JH, Hyuan HA (1996) The artificial disc: theory, design and materials. Biomaterials 12:1157–1167
9. Baumgartner W (1992) Intervertebral spinal disc, European Patent EP 0566810 A1, 04–04–1992
10. Baumgartner W (1992) Intervertebral prosthesis, United States Patent 5171280, 15–12–1992
11. Baumgartner W (1994) Artificial intervertebral disk member, United States Patent 5370697, 06–12–1994
12. Baumgartner W (1994) Intervertebral prosthesis and method of implanting such a prosthesis, European Patent 0621020, 26–10–1994
13. Beer JM, Beer JC (1995) Synthetic intervertebral disc, United States Patent 5458642, 17–10–1995
14. Betisor A, Corlateanu M, Hurmuzache E, Hurmuzache V, Glavan I, Moroz P, et al (2001) Device for intervertebral decompression and prosthesis, Moldova Patent MD1736F, 30–09–2001
15. Bisserie M (1997) Intervertebral disk prosthesis, United States Patent 5702450, 30–12–1997
16. Boone PS, Zimmerman MC, Guttling E, Lee CK, Parsons JR, Langrana N (1989) Bone attachment to hydroxyapatite coated polymers. J Biomed Mater Res 23:183–199
17. Bouvet JC (1997) Prothèse destinée à restaurer une articulation entre deux os et application, notamment comme prothèse de hanche et intervertébrale, French Patent 2761878, 11–04–1997
18. Brock M, Mayer HM, Weigel K (1989) The artificial disc. Springer, New York Hedielberg Berlin
19. Brodsky AE (1976) Post laminectomy and post fusion stenosis of the lumbar spine. Clin Orthop 115:130–139
20. Bryan V (2000) Peanut spectacle multi discoid thoraco-lumbar disc prosthesis, World Patent 0013619, 16–03–2000
21. Bryan V, Carver K (2000) Cylindrical hemi-lunar parallel array threaded disc prosthesis, World Patent 0013620, 16–03–2000
22. Bryan V, Kunzler A (1999) Human spinal disc prosthesis, United States Patent 5865846, 02–02–1999
23. Bryan V, Kunzler A (2000) Human spinal disc prosthesis, United States Patent 6156067, 05–12–2000
24. Bryan V, Kunzler A (2000) Threaded cylindrical multidiscoid single or multiple array disc prosthesis, World Patent 0004851, 03–02–2000
25. Buhler M, Ramadan A (2001) French Patent 2805733, 07–09–2001
26. Bullivant M (1993) Improvements in or relating to spinal vertebrae implants, World Patent 93/10725, 10–06–1993
27. Buttermann GR (1998) Intervertebral prosthetic device, United States Patent 5827328, 27–10–1998
28. Büttner-Jans K (1999) Artificial disc and instability: biomechanical principles In: Szpalski M, Gunzburg R, Pope MH (eds) Lumbar segmental instability. Lippincott Williams & Wilkins, Philadelphia
29. Büttner-Janz K, Schellnack K, Zippel H (1989) Biomechanics of the SB Charité lumbar intervertebral disc endoprosthesis. Int Orthop 13:173–176
30. Cauthen JC (2000) Articulating spinal implant, United States Patent 6019792, 01–02–2000
31. Cauthen JC (2001) Articulating spinal implant, United States Patent 6179874 B1, 30–01–2001
32. Chin Chin Gan J, Ducheyne P, Vresilovic E, Shapiro I (2001) Compositions and methods for intervertebral disc reformation, United States Patent 6240926 B1, 05–06–2001
33. Cinotti G, David T, Postachinni F (1996) Results of disc prosthesis after a minimum follow-up period of 2 years. Spine 21:995–1000
34. Clemow AJ, Langrana NA, Lee CK, Parsons JR, Chen EH (1990) Biocompatible elastomeric intervertebral disc, European Patent 0356112, 28–02–1990

35. Cochet R (2000) Intervertebral disc prosthesis has connecting pieces with through cells between plates and core, French Patent 2784291, 14–04–2000
36. Cummins BH, Robertson JT, Gill SG (1998) Surgical experience with an implanted artificial cervical joint. J Neurosurg 88:943–948
37. Dennis D, Watkins R, Landaker S, Dillin W, Springer D (1989) Comparison of disc space heights after anterior lumbar interbody fusion. Spine 14:876–878
38. Dios Seoane J (1997) Intervertebral disc prosthesis, Spanish Patent 2107377, 16–11–1997
39. Downey EL (1989) Replacement disc, United States Patent 4874389, 17–10–1989
40. Downey EL (1990) Vertebra prosthesis, United States Patent 5147404, 24–10–1990
41. Dumas B, Chanchole S, Lahille M (1996) Spinal intervertebral disc replacement prosthesis, French Patent 2734148, 22–11–1996
42. Edeland HG (1981) Suggestions for a total elasto-dynamic intervertebral disc prosthesis. Biomater Med Devices Artif Organs 9:65–72
43. Enker P, Steffee A, McMillin C, Keppler L, Biscup R, Miller S (1993) Artificial disc replacement. Preliminary report with a 3 year minimum follow-up. Spine 18:1061–1080
44. Evans JH, Gilmore KH, O'Brien JP (1981) How does fusion relieve low back pain? Annual Meeting of the International Society for the Study of the Lumbar Spine, Paris
45. Fassio B (1978) French Patent 2372622, 30–06–1978
46. Fassio B, Ginestie JF (1978) Prothèse discale en silicone. Etude experimentale et premières observations cliniques. Nouv Press Med 21:207
47. Felt JC, Bourgeault CA, Baker MW (1999) Articulating joint repair, United States Patent 5888220, 30–03–1999
48. Fernie GR, Hedman TP, Maki BE (1988) Artificial spinal disc, European Patent 0282161, 14–09–1988
49. Fernström U (1966) Arthroplasty with intercorporal endoprosthesis in herniated disc and in painful disc. Acta Orthop Scand Suppl 10:287–289
50. Fernström U (1972) Der bandscheibenersatz mit erhaltung der beweglichkeit. In: Herdman H (ed) Zukunftaufgaben für die erforschung und behandelung von Wirbelsaülenleiden. Die wirbelsaüle in forschung und praxis. Hippokrates, Stuttgart
51. Fitz WR (1996) Artificial facet joint, United States Patent 5571191, 05–11–1996
52. Fraser RD (2002) Personal communication
53. Fraser RD, Ross ER, Lowery GL, Steffee AD (2000) Spinal disc, United States Patent 6139579, 31–10–2000
54. Frey O, Koch R (1990) Intervertebral prosthesis, United States Patent 4917704, 17–04–1990
55. Frey O, Koch R (1990) Metallic intervertebral prosthesis, United States Patent 4955908, 11–09–1990
56. Frey O, Koch R, Planck HMF (1993) Joint endoprosthesis, United States Patent 4932969, 12–06–1990
57. Froning EC (1975) Intervertebral disc prosthesis. United States Patent 3,875,595, April 8, 1975
58. Frymoyer JW, Hanley EN, Howe J, Kuhlman D, Matteri RW (1978) A comparison of radiographic findings in fusion and non fusion patients ten or more years following lumbar disc surgery. Spine 3:1–6
59. Fuchs J, Luderschmidt W, Mehler K, Weib C (1993) Bandscheibenendoprothese, German Patent 4213771 C1, 30–09–1993
60. Garcia A (1990) Replacement of the nucleus of the intervertebral disc by a polyurethane polymerised in situ, French Patent 2639823, 08–06–1990
61. Gau M (2001) Intervertebral nucleus prosthesis and surgical procedure for implanting the same, World Patent 0108612, 02–08–2001
62. Gauchet F (2000) Prothèse de disque interverterbral à frottements réduits, French Patent 2787014, 16–06–2000
63. Gauchet F (2000) Prothèse de disque interverterbral à enceinte de liquide, French Patent 2787018, 16–06–2000
64. Gauchet F, Le Couëdic R (2000) Intervertebral disc prosthesis with improved mechanical behaviour, World Patent 00/35385, 22–06–2000
65. Gauchet F, Saint Martin PH, Kelly W (2000) Intervertebral disc prosthesis with contact blocks, World Patent 0035387, 22–06–2000
66. Gill SS, Walker C, van Hoeck J, Gause L (2000) Artificial intervertebral joint permitting translational and rotational motion, United States Patent 6113637, 05–09–2000
67. Gjunter VE (2002) Artificial disc, World Patent 0230336, 18–04–2002
68. Goffin J. Initial results with the Bryan cervical disc prosthesis. J Neurosurg (Submitted)
69. Gordon DP, Maya WE, Roberts RD, Thomas JC (2000) Multiaxis intervertebral prosthesis, United States Patent 6146121, 14–11–2000
70. Gosh P (1988) The biology of the intervertebral disc. CRC Press, Boca Raton
71. Graf H (1999) Partial posterior intervertebral disc prosthesis, French Patent 2772594, 25–06–1999
72. Graf H (1999) Partial posterior intervertebral disc prosthesis, French Patent 2775891, 17–09–1999
73. Graf H (1999) Dispositif de stabilisation intervertebral. French Patent 2801782, 01–12–1999
74. Graham D (1993) Artificial disk, United States Patent 5246458, 21–09–1993
75. Grammont P, Gauchet F (1996) Lumbar vertebral disc prosthesis, French Patent 2723841, 01–03–1996
76. Griffith SL, Erickson RA (2000) Intervertebral disc prosthesis and method, World Patent 0053127, 14–09–2000
77. Griffith SL, Shelokov AP, Büttner-Janz K, LeMaire JP, Zeegers WS (1994) A multicentre retrospective study of the clinical results of the Link SB Charité intervertebral prosthesis. The initial European experience. Spine 15:1842–1849
78. Grundei H (1994) Partial spinal disc replacement, German Patent 4323595, 07–07–1994
79. Gunther V (1998) Medical materials and implants with shape memory effect. Tomsk University, Tomsk, pp 460–463
80. Gunzburg R, Szpalski M (2002) Use of a novel b-tricalcium phosphate-based bone void filler as a graft extender in spinal fusion surgeries. Orthopaedics 25:S591–S595
81. Han D (1999) Artificial vertebral disc, Chinese Patent 2315923U, 28–04–1999
82. Hanley EN, Levy JA (1989) Surgical treatment of isthmic lumbosacral spondylolisthesis: analysis of variables influencing results. Spine 14: 48–50
83. Hansson T, Sandström J, Roos B, et al (1985) The bone mineral content of the lumbar spine in patients with chronic low back pain. Spine 12: 158–160
84. Hao S, Liu S, Huang D (1999) Artificial lumbar intervertebral disc, Chinese Patent 2333369U, 18–08–1999
85. Harmon PH (1963) Anterior excision and vertebral body fusion operation for intervertebral disc syndromes of the lower lumbar spine. Clin Orthop 26:107–111
86. Harms J, Oberle J, Esper FR, Gohl W (1990) Künstliche bandschiebe, German Patent 3911610, 18–10–1990
87. Harrington M (1999) Artificial disc, United States Patent 5893889, 13–04–1999
88. Hedman TP, Kostuik JP, Fernie GR, Maki BE (1988) Artificial spinal disc, United States Patent 4759769, 26–07–1988

89. Hellier WG, Hedman TP, Kostuik JP (1992) Wear studies for development of an intervertebral disc prosthesis. Spine 17:S86–S96
90. Higham PA, Bao Q-B (1993) Hydrogel bead intervertebral disc nucleus, United States Patent 5192326, 09–03–1993
91. Higham PA, Bao Q-B (1996) Hydrogel intervertebral disc nucleus with diminished lateral bulging, United States Patent 5534028, 09–07–1996
92. Hoffman-Daimler S (1974) Intervertebral disk replacement. Z Orthop Ihre Grenzgeb 112:792–795
93. Hoffmann-Daimler S (1974) Bandscheibenprothese, German Patent 2263842, 04–07–1974
94. Hou TS, Tu KY, Yu YK, et al (1991) Lumbar intervertebral disc prosthesis. An experimental study. Chin Med J (Engl) 104:381–386
95. Husson JL, Schärer N, Le Nihouannen JC, et al (1997) Nucléoplastie per-discetomie: concept et étude experimentale. Rachis 9:145-152
96. Husson JL, Baumgartner W, Freudiger S (1999) Intervertebral prosthesis, United States Patent 5919235, 06–07–1999
97. Ibo I, Pierotto E (1998) Prosthesis of the cervical intervertebralis disk, United States Patent 5755796, 26–05–1998
98. Jackowski A, Mcleod ARM (2000) Surgical implant, United States Patent 6093205, 25–07–2000
99. Kaden B, Fritz T, Gross U, Kranz C, Fuhrmann G, Schmitz HJ (1991) Intervertebral disk endoprosthesis, United States Patent 5002576, 26–03–1991
100. Kehr P, Feron J-M, Graftiaux A, Nazarian S, Ricart O (1996) Sliding intervertebral prosthesis, especially cervical intervertebral prosthesis, European Patent 0699426, 06–03–1996
101. Keller A (1991) Surgical instrument set, United States Patent 4997432, 05–03–1991
102. Khvisyuk NI, Prodan AI, Lygun LN (1982) Intervertebral disc prosthesis, USSR Patent 895433, 07–01–1982
103. Kirkaldy-Willis WH (1983) Managing low back pain. Churchill Livingstone, New York
104. Kostuik JP (1997) Intervertebral disc replacement. Experimental study. Clin Orthop 37:27–41
105. Kostiuk JP (1997) Intervertebral disc replacement. In: Bridgwell KH, De Wald RL (eds) The textbook of spinal surgery. Lippincott-Raven, Philadelphia, pp 2257–2266
106. Kostuik JP, Hedman T, Hellier W, Fernie G (1991) Design of an intervertebral disc prosthesis. Spine 16: S256-S260
107. Kotani Y, Abumi K, Shikinami Y, et al (2002) Artificial intervertebral disc replacement using bioactive three dimensional fabric: design, development and preliminary animal study. Spine 27:929–936
108. Krapiva PL (1997) Disc replacement method and apparatus, United Sates Patent 5645597, 08–07–1997
109. Kuntz JD (1982) Intervertebral disc prosthesis, United States Patent 4349921, 21–09–1982
110. Lawson KJ (2001) Prosthetic nucleus replacement for surgical reconstruction of intervertebral disc and treatment method, United States Patent 6146422, 14–11–2001
111. Lee CK (1988) Accelerated degeneration of the segment adjacent to a lumbar fusion. Spine 14:1324–1331
112. Lee CK, Langrana NA, Alexander H, Clemow AJ, Chain EH, Parsons JR (1990) Functional and biocompatible intervertebral disc space, United States Patent 4,911,718, March 27, 1990
113. Lee CK, Langrana LA, Parsons JR, Zimmerman MC (1991) Development of a prosthetic intervertebral disc. Spine 16:S253–S255
114. Lehman TR, Spratt KF, Tozzi JE, et al (1987) Long term follow-up of lower lumbar fusion patients. Spine 12:97–104
115. Lemaire JP, Skalli W, Lavaste F, et al (1997) Intervertebral disc prosthesis. Results and prospects for the year 2000. Clin Orthop 337:64–76
116. Lesoin F, Villette L, Marnay Th, Caenen J, Michel O (1995) Vertebral cervical prosthesis, French Patent 2718635, 20–10–1995
117. Lu J (1998) Artificial intervertebral disc, Chinese Patent 2288707, 26–08–1998
118. Main JA, Wells ME, Keller TS (1990) Vertebral prosthesis, United States Patent 4932975, 12–06–1990
119. Marcolongo MS, Lowman AM (2001) Associating hydrogels for nucleus pulposus replacement in intervertebral discs, World Patent 0132100, 10–05–2001
120. Marnay T (1991) L'arthroplastie intervertebrale lombaire. Med Orthop 25:48–55
121. Marnay T (1994) Prosthesis for intervertebral discs and instruments for implanting it, United States Patent 5314477, 24–05–1994
122. Martin J-R (2000) Vertebral joint facets prostheses, United States Patent 6132464, 17–10–2000
123. Mathews H, Le Huec JC, Bertagnoli R, Friesem T, Eisermann L (2002) Design rationale and early multicenter evaluation of Maverick total disk arthroplasty. International Meeting on Advanced Spine Technologies, 2002, Montreux
124. Mazda K (1994) Prothèse discale intervertébrale, French Patent, 2694882, 25–02–1994
125. McKenzie AH (1972) Steel ball arthroplasty of lumbar intervertebral discs: a preliminary report. J Bone Joint Surg Br 54:S766
126. McKenzie AH (1995) Fernström intervertebral disc arthroplasty: a long term evaluation. Orthopedics International Edition 3B:313–324
127. Mehdizadeh HM (2001) Disc replacement prosthesis, United States Patent 6231609, 15–05–2001
128. Middleton LM (2000) Artificial intervertebral disc, United States Patent 6136031, 24–10–2000
129. Millan EJ, Arrowsmith P, Milner R (1997) Intervertebral disc implant, British Patent 2303555, 26–02–1997
130. Millan EJ, Arrowsmith P, Milner R (2001) Intervertebral disc implant, United States Patent 6187048, 13–02–2001
131. Minda R, Schmidt H (2001) Befüllbare künstliche bandscheibe, European Patent 1157675, 28–11–2001
132. Mitscherlich H, Körber W (1975) Prothese zum Ersatz einer beschädigten oder degenerierten Bandscheibe und Verfahren zu ihrer Herstellung, German Patent 2203242, 09–10–1975
133. Monson GL (1989) Synthetic intervertebral disc prosthesis, United States Patent 4863477, 05–09–1989
134. Monteiro A, Morgenstern Lopez R (1997) Prosthesis for intervertebral disc nuclei and process for using same, Spanish Patent 2094077, 01–01–1997
135. Nachemson A (1962) Some mechanical properties of the lumbar intervertebral disc. Bull Hosp Joint Dis 23: 130–132
136. Nachemson A (1976) The lumbar spine – an orthopedic challenge. Spine 1:59–71
137. Nachemson A (1992) Challenge of the artificial disc. In: Weinstein JW (ed) Clinical efficacy and outcome in the diagnosis and treatment of low back pain. Raven, New York, pp 271–278
138. Nachemson A (1996) Instrumented fusion of the lumbar spine for degenerative disorders: a critical look. In: Szpalski M, Gunzburg R, Spengler D, Nachemson A (eds) Instrumented fusion of the degenerative lumbar spine. Lippincott Raven, Philadelphia
139. Navas F (1996) Extra-discal inter-vertebral prosthesis for controlling the variations of the inter-vertebral distance by means of a double damper, United States Patent 5480401, 02–01–1996

140. Nishimura K, Mochida J (1998) Percutaneous reinsertion of the nucleus pulposus. An experimental study. Spine 14:1531–1538
141. Ojima S, Haruko I, Yasuhiko H, Matsuzaki H (1989) Artificial intervertebral disc, European Patent 0317972, 31–05–1989
142. Oka M, Gen S, Ikada Y, Okimatsu H (1995) Artificial intervertebral disc, United States Patent 5458643, 17–10–1995
143. Olson JE, Hanley EN, Rudert JM, Baratz ME (1991) Vertebral column allografts for the treatment of segmental spine defects. An experimental investigation in dogs. Spine 16: 1081–1088
144. Parsons JR, Lee CK, Langrana NA, Clemow AJ, Chen H (1992) Functional and biocompatible intervertebral disc spacer containing elastomeric material of varying hardness, United States Patent 5171281, 15–12–1992
145. Patil AA (1982) Artificial intervertebral disc. United States Patent 4,309,777, April 8, 1982
146. Pigg W, Cassidy JJ (1996) Prosthetic devices, World Patent 9601598, 25–01–1996
147. Pisharodi M (1992) Artificial spinal prosthesis, United States Patent 5123926, 23–06–1992
148. Popp E, Sajda W, Bohnenberger J, Bolte E, Möller F (1994) Wirbelkörperimplantat, German Patent 4315757 C1, 10–11–1994
149. Ratron YA (1997) Elastic disc prosthesis, United States 5676702, 14–10–1997
150. Ray CD (1974) Medical engineering. Mosby Year Book Medical Publishers, Chicago
151. Ray CD, Assell RL (2000) Tapered prosthetic spinal disc nucleus, United States Patent 6132465, 17–10–2000
152. Ray CD, Corbin TP (1990) Prosthetic disc containing therapeutic material, European Patent 0353936, 07–02–1990
153. Ray CD, Sachs BL, Norton BK, Mikkelsen SM, Clausen N (2002) Prosthetic disc nucleus implants. An update. In: Gunzburg R, Szpalski M (eds) Intervertebral disc herniation. Lippincott Williams & Wilkins, Philadelphia
154. Reitz H, Joubert MJ (1964) Intractable headache and cervicobrachialgia treated by a complete replacement of cervical intervertebral discs with a metal prosthesis. S Afr Med J 38:881–889
155. Rogozinski C (2000) Intervertebral prosthetic disc, United States Patent 5888226, 30–03–1999
156. Roy-Camille R, Saillant G, Lavaste F (1978) Etude experimentale d'un remplacement discal lombaire. Rev Chir Orthop 64 [Suppl]:106–107
157. Sabitzer RJ, Fuss FK (1997) Wirbelsaülen-Prothese, Austrian Patent 405237B, 28-08–1997
158. Salib RM, Pettine KA (1993) Intervertebral disk arthroplasty, United States Patent 5258031, 02–11–1993
159. Savchenko PA, Fomichev NG, Gjunter VEH, Jasenchuk JUF, Khodorenko VN, Shemetov VP, Koroshchenko SA (1999) Prosthesis of intervertebral disc, Russian Patent 2140229, 27–10–1999
160. Schneider PG, Oyen R (1974) Surgical replacement of the intervetebral disc. First communication: replacement of intervertebral discs with silicon rubber. Z Orthop Ihre Grenzgeb 112:1076–1086
161. Schönmayr R, Busch C, Lotz C, Lotz-Metz G (1999) Prosthetic disc nucleus implants – the Wiesbaden feasibility study: 2 years follow-up in ten patients. Riv Neuroradiol 12 [Suppl]: 163–170
162. Schoppe F (1990) Chirurgisches Instrument zur Implantation einer Bandscheibenkernprothese, German Patent 3922203 C1, 25–10–1990
163. Serhan H, Kuras J, Mcmillin C, Persenaire M (1999) Spinal disc prosthesis, World Patent 99/20209, 29–04–1999
164. Shelokov AP (2000) Articulating spinal disc prosthesis, United States Patent 6039763, 21–03–2000
165. Shen Q (2001) Human intervertebral disc prosthesis, Chinese Patent 2445722U, 09–05–2001
166. Shinn GL, Tate JD (1997) Artificial intervertebral disc prosthesis, United States Patent 5683465, 04–11–1997
167. Simon G, Caton P, Rossin R, Lazannec JY, Breslave P (1995) Prothèse intervertébrale, French Patent 2712486, 24–05–1995
168. Steffee AD (1991) Artificial disc, United States Patent 5071437, 10–12–1991
169. Steffee AD (1990) Artificial spinal disc, European Patent 0392076, 17–10–1990
170. Steffee AD (1992) The Steffee artificial disc. In: Weinstein JN (ed) Clinical efficacy and outcome in the diagnosis and treatment of low back pain. Raven Press, New York
171. Stone KR (1991) Prosthetic intervertebral disc, World Patent 9116867, 14–11–1991
172. Stone KR (1992) Prosthetic intervertebral disc, United States Patent 5108438, 28–04–1992
173. Stubstad JA, Urbaniak JR, Kahn P (1975) Prosthesis for spinal repair, United States Patent 3867728, 25–02–1975
174. Studer A, Schärer N (2001) Bandscheibenerstz für den kern einer bandscheibe, European Patent 1157676, 28–11–2001
175. Szpalski M (1996) The mysteries of segmental instability. Bull Hosp Joint Dis 55:147–148
176. Szpalski M, Gunzburg G (1998) The role of surgery in the management of low back pain. Baillière's Clin Rheumatol 12:141–159
177. Szpalski M, Gunzburg R (2002) Applications of calcium phosphate-based cancellous bone void fillers in trauma surgery. Orthopaedics 25:S601–S609
178. Teule JG (1996) Intervertebral disc prosthesis for reduced stress and natural movement, French Patent 2730159, 09–08–1996
179. Urbaniak JR, Bright DS, Hopkins JE (1973) Replacement of intervertebral discs in chimpanzees by silicon-dacron implants: a preliminary report. J Biomed Mater Res 7:165–186
180. Van Roermund PM, Plasmans CMT, Donk R, Oner FC, de Kleuver M, van Ooij A, Verbout AJ (2002) Orthopedic miracle device (in Dutch). Med Contact 57:670
181. Van Steenbrugghe MH (1956) Perfectionnements aux prothèses articulaires, French Patent 1.122.634, 28 May 1956
182. Viart G, Marin F (2001) Intervertebral disc prosthesis comprises two plates anchored to vertebrae, central core and viscoelastic ring. French Patent 2805985, 14–09–2001
183. Vuono-Hawkins M, Zimmerman MC, Parsons JR, Langrana NA, Lee CK (1993) Environmental effect on a thermoplastic elastomer (TPE) for use in a composite intervertebral disc spacer. In: Jamison RD, Gilbertson LN (eds) Composite materials for implant applications in the human body. ASTM Philadelphia, pp 17–26
184. Vuono-Hawkins M, Zimmerman MC, Lee CK, Carter FM, Parsons JR, Langrana NA (1994) Mechanical evaluation of a canine intervertebral disc spacer: in situ and in vivo studies. J Orthop Res 12:119–127
185. Wardlaw D (1999) Intervertebral disc nucleus prosthesis, World Patent 9902108, 21–01–1999
186. Weber BG (1978) Zwischenwirbel Prothese, Swiss Patent 624573, 01–02–1978
187. Weber BG (1979) Zwischenwirbel Totaprothese, Swiss Patent 640131, 03–10–1979

188. Weber PJ, Da Silva LB (2001) Prosthetic Spinal disc, World Patent 0190786, 01–01–2001
189. White AA, Panjabi MM (1978) The basic kinematics of the human spine. Spine 3:12–20
190. Wiltse LL, Rochio PD (1975) Preoperative psychological tests as predictors of success of chemonucleolysis in the treatment of low back syndrome J Bone Joint Surg Am 57:478–483
191. Xavier R, Xavier S, Xavier S (2000) Vertebral body prosthesis, United States Patent 6063121,16–08–2000
192. Yamashita T, Cavanugh JM, et al (1990) Mechanosensitive afferent units in the lumbar facet joint. J Bone Joint Surg Am 72:865–870
193. Yuan HA, Chih-I L, Davidson JA, Small LC, Carls TA (1997) Low wear artificial spinal disc. United States Patent, 5,676,701, 14–10–1997
194. Zdeblick TA, McKay WF (2000) Artificial disc implant, World Patent 0074606, 14–12–2000
195. Zeegers WS, Bohnen LM, Laaper M, Verhaegen MJ (1999) Artificial disc replacement with the modular type SB Charite III: 2 year results in 50 prospectively studied patients. Eur Spine J 8:210–217

H. Michael Mayer
Andreas Korge

Non-fusion technology in degenerative lumbar spinal disorders: facts, questions, challenges

Abstract Although surgical fusion of the painful degenerating functional spinal unit (FSU) of the lumbar spine has always been a matter of debate, it has become a gold-standard procedure for all cases that lack an alternative treatment. However, a detailed and honest review of the clinical data reveals a considerable number of undesired side effects, complications and poor outcomes. The continuous search for alternative surgical treatment modalities has led to the development of numerous ideas for surgical reconstruction of the anterior and/or posterior column. The term "spine arthroplasty" summarises all procedures that have the goal of restoring function. This article describes the principles of the most current surgical techniques and implants, it points out potential challenges and poses a number of questions that need evidence-based answers before the incorporation of these innovations into surgical routine can be justified.

Keywords Spinal fusion · Spine arthroplasty · Artificial disc · Lumbar spine

H.M. Mayer (✉) · A. Korge
Spine Center,
Orthopedic Clinic Munich-Harlaching,
Harlachinger Strasse 51,
81547 Munich, Germany
e-mail: MMayer@schoen-kliniken.de,
Tel.: +49-89-62112011,
Fax: +49-89-62112012

Introduction

Surgical treatment of the painful degenerating spine has been continuously debated throughout the last 50 years. Although there is little evidence from the scientific literature that surgery can positively influence the course of degenerative spinal disorders, the number of surgical procedures is increasing continuously [5, 7, 39]. On the other hand, the same observations can be made about non-surgical therapeutic options, whose justification mainly stems from empirical results, and where an evidence base is also lacking. Whereas the acceptance of conservative measures is higher, especially in countries with medical and social security networks that allow long therapy periods with only minor negative socio-economic consequences, it is hard to convince patients to take "the long way" if there seems to be a surgical "short way" to get rid of the pain. The pressure "from the street" to resolve patients' pain or improve their symptoms as quickly as possible has triggered the use of a variety of so-called "semi-invasive" procedures such as peridural injections, catheters, intradiscal electrothermal therapy (IDET) and laser therapy to achieve these goals [17, 22, 32, 33].

However, a considerable number of patients with painful degenerative disc disease end up as candidates for spinal fusion, either primarily or after various unsuccessful semi- and/or minimally invasive procedures. This article will discuss the role of spinal fusion in the light of upcoming potential alternative treatments.

Spinal fusion in degenerative lumbar disc disorders

There is no doubt about the place of spinal fusion in deformities or unstable conditions of the lumbar motion segment. However, spinal fusion in degenerative disc disease without signs of instability or disturbed curvature, though performed quite frequently, is not generally accepted [13, 14, 19, 24]. In most cases, the indication is based on unsuccessful conservative therapy, and the lack of reasonable therapeutic alternatives. This lack of alternatives often leads surgeons to accept potential risks, side-effects and complications to help patients get rid of their symptoms [10, 20, 36]. However, the results seem to not always justify these decisions.

Own data

Between April 1998 and January 2000, a total of 134 patients (84 female; 50 male, age range: 20.4–87.2 years, mean age: 56.2 years) were treated with fusion for degenerative disorders of the lumbar spine. The diagnoses are listed in Table 1. Spinal fusion was performed in all patients; in 91 cases it was combined with segmental decompression. Posterior-anterior 360° fusion was performed in 94.8%, posterior lumbar interbody fusion (PLIF) in 3% and posterolateral fusion in 2.2%. In all patients, fusion was performed using autologous bone graft from the iliac crest, which was augmented by a titanium cage in only 4.5% of the patients. All operations were performed by an experienced team of surgeons, each of them having performed a minimum of 300 spinal fusions. After a minimum follow-up time of 24 months, the overall fusion rate was 97.0%. The clinical results were analysed according to the economic/functional rating (EFR) score published by Prolo et al. in 1986 [28]. They are shown in Fig. 1 and Fig. 2, and are comparable with the results published in the literature [13, 19, 23]. A meticulous analysis of negative side-effects and complications was performed retrospectively. There were a total of 74 complications or adverse side-effects in 44 of the 134 operated patients (33%) (Table 2). While there were ten general complications, the majority related to the surgery (Table 3). Detailed analysis of these surgery-related complications showed an implant failure rate of 4.5%, 3% non-union and a rate of superficial wound-healing disturbances of 4.5% (Table 4). There was no deep wound infection. Revision surgery had to be performed in ten patients (7.5%). Approach-related complications occurred in 7.5% of the posterior and 5.2% of the anterior approaches (Table 5, Table 6). These compli-

Table 1 Diagnosis for spinal fusion (n=134)

Diagnosis[a]	n
Degenerative disc disease	82
Degenerative spondylolisthesis	29
Failed back (following discectomy)	23
Total	134

[a] Spinal stenosis was an additional diagnosis in 91 of the patients

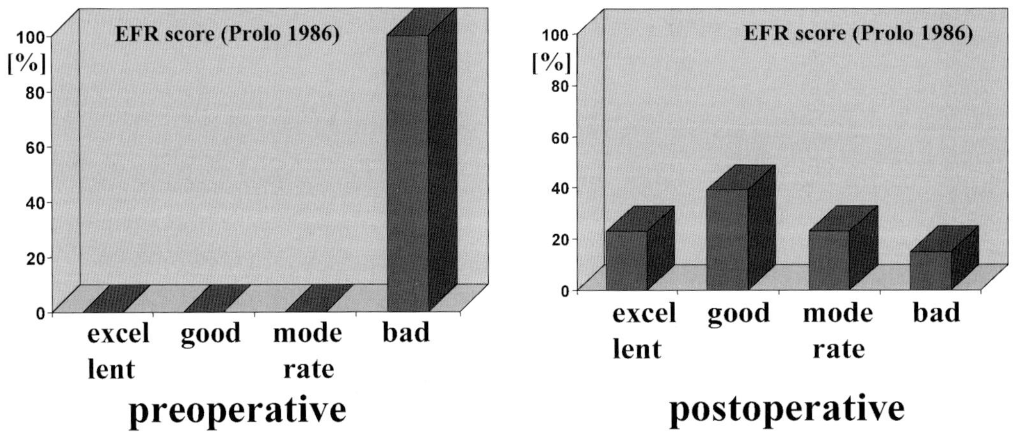

Fig. 1 Results of spinal fusion at the lumbosacral junction

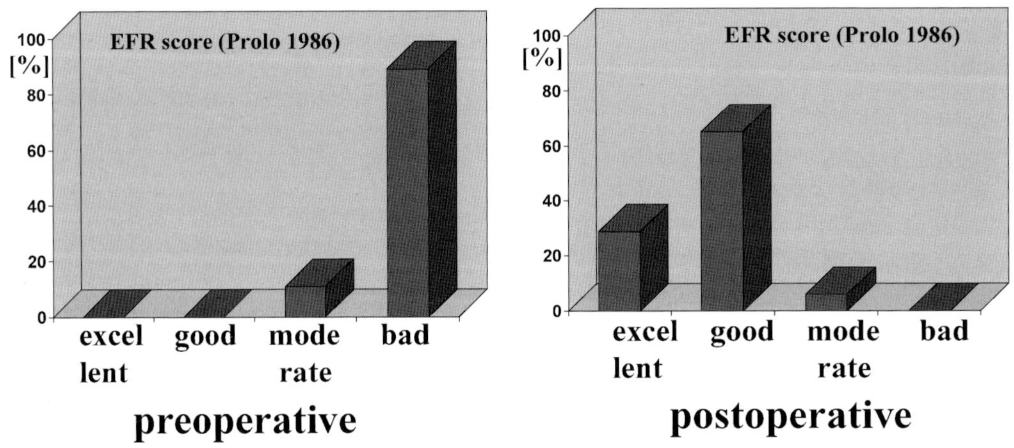

Fig. 2 Results of spinal fusion at levels L2/3, L3/4, L4/5

Table 2 Complications following lumbar spinal fusion (n=134)

No. (%) of patients without complications	99 (67%)
No. (%) of patients with complications	44 (33%)
No. of complications	74
General: n (%)	10 (7.5%)
Surgery-related: n (%)	64 (47.6%)
Independent from approach: n (%)	10 (7.5%)
Approach/Fusion-related: n (%)	48 (35.9%)

Table 3 General complications following lumbar spinal fusion (n=134) (*GIT* gastro-intestinal tract, *DVT* deep vein thrombosis, *UT* urinary tract)

Total	10 (7.5%)
Cardiac (arrhythmia, infarction)	4
Pulmonary (pneumonia)	1
GIT (GI bleeding)	2
Vascular (DVT)	1
Urinary (UT infection)	1
Neural arm plexus	1

Table 4 Surgery-related complications (independent from approach) following lumbar spinal fusion (n=134)

Total	10 (7.5%)
Non-union	4 (3.0%)
Wound healing disturbance	6 (4.5%)

Table 5 Posterior approach-related complications following lumbar spinal fusion (n=134)

Total	10 (7.5%)
Sensory deficit	4
Motor deficit	5
CSF fistula (1/91 decompressions)	1

Table 6 Anterior approach-related complications following lumbar spinal fusion (n=134)

Total	7 (5.2%)
Irritation n. genitofemoralis	6
Sexual dysfunction	1

Table 7 Fusion technique-related complications (n=134)

Total	37 (27.6%)
Implant failure	6
Loosening	4
Screw breakage	2
Pain at iliac crest at discharge	11
Meralgia paraesthesia	8
Numbness iliac crest	7
Fracture spina il. ant. sup.	5

cation rates are well below those published in the literature [10, 36]. The vast majority of complications were specific to the fusion-technique, being associated with the harvesting of the autologous bone graft from the iliac crest (Table 7).

The following conclusions can be drawn from these data. The surgical goal (spinal fusion) was achieved in 97% of the patients with the fusion technique described (pedicle screw fixation and interbody fusion with iliac crest bone) (excellent radiological result). The clinical results according to the EFR-score were acceptable, and compare well to the results published in the literature (acceptable clinical result). However, whereas the rate of general complications was acceptable as well, the price for the clinical and radiological result seems to be high in the light of the complications produced by the surgical procedure(s). Looking at other surgical specialties, it is rare to find procedures in which an "acceptable" clinical result can be justified in the presence of such a high rate of complications and adverse side-effects in the first 2 years postoperatively. We have not analysed late effects of segmental fusion, such as accelerated degeneration of the adjacent level. However, the problem is obvious: it is neither the surgical approach nor the general complications that produce the complication and co-morbidity level, it is the fusion procedure itself that obliges us to search for alternative procedures.

Reconstruction versus fusion

The historical aspects of reconstructive procedures have been described extensively in the article by Szaplski et al. in this issue [38]. A variety of experimental and clinical applications will be presented in the following papers, which all have one thing in common: they represent partial solutions for the multi-factorial problem of degeneration of the functional spinal unit (FSU) and they can only be considered as part of a step-by-step treatment philosophy, which has as its goal avoiding any use of spinal fusion at all for this condition.

Nucleus pulposus reconstruction (biological concept)

Principle: The experience with autologous chondrocyte transplantation (ACT) in peripheral joints has recently been applied to the lumbar spine (autologous disc chondrocyte transplantation; ADCT) (Meisel, personal communication, and [2, 11, 27]). Nucleus pulposus tissue is harvested during lumbar disc operations, the cells are cultured and re-implanted through a minimal-invasive percutaneous route several weeks following discectomy, with the goal of a biological reconstruction of the nucleus pulposus.

Facts and Questions: Although animal experiments suggest a potential regeneration of the nucleus pulposus as compared to the non-transplanted control groups, results of an ongoing clinical pilot study are not yet available. Though a fascinating idea, ADCT poses many questions such as: Does the nucleus re-grow? and if it does: How does it re-grow? Which qualities does the new nucleus have? Does it even make sense to re-grow the nucleus in a lumbar disc with a weakened or destroyed posterior annulus? Does ADCT influence the reintegration of the annulus fibrosis? All these questions need to be answered in the ongoing clinical and experimental studies. The idea of revitalising the nucleus pulposus at an earlier stage of the degenerative process with cell culture techniques or with genetic engineering techniques should draw our scientific attention. Looking even more into the future, the pre-implantation diagnosis will make corrective actions possible at a very early stage of life.

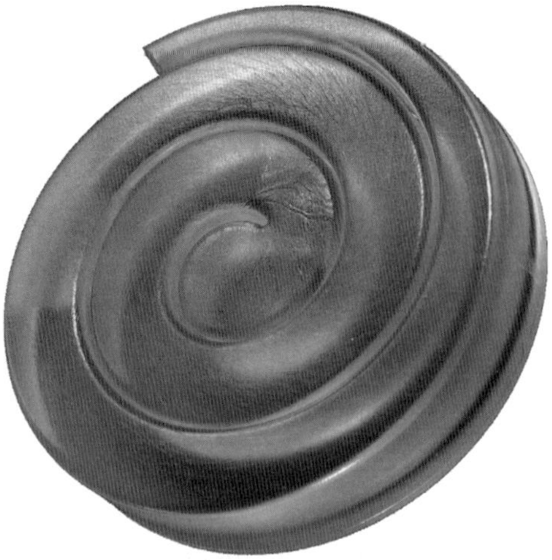

Fig. 4 Spiral implant for nucleoplasty (Sulzer Medica)

Nucleus pulposus replacement

Principle: Replacement of the degenerated or excised nucleus pulposus has been performed in experimental and clinical studies using different materials such as hydrogel cushions (Prosthetic Disc Nucleus, PDN RayMedica Inc., Fig. 3; Aquarelle, Stryker Spine); or polyurethane spirals (Sulzer Medica Inc.; Fig. 4) [1, 16, 29]. Empirical data are now accumulating very rapidly from the first clinical applications. Only two nucleus implants are currently used, with different indication criteria: the Nucleoplasty Spiral (Sulzer Medica) is indicated after simple microdiscectomy for lumbar disc herniation. It serves as a spaceholder and is supposed to prevent early disc height loss following discectomy [16, 18]. The indication for implantation of the Prosthetic Disc Nucleus (PDN) is different. It is used in patients with discogenic low-back pain without previous operations. It can be implanted through a traditional PLIF approach [31]. However, due to the higher risk of extrusions into the spinal canal, the minimally invasive anterior retroperitoneal route is preferred by the protagonists of this implant [1].

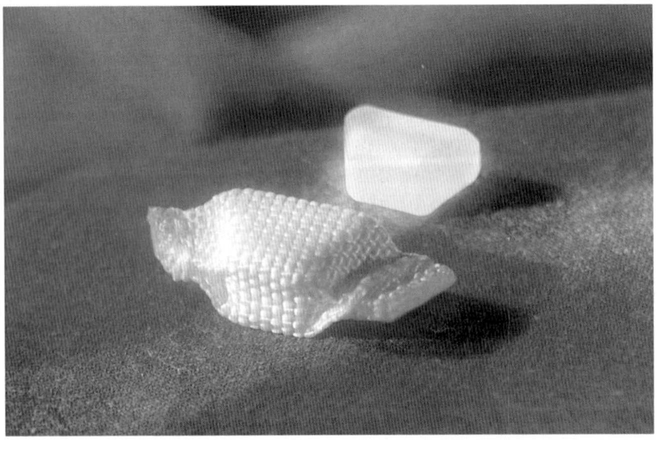

Fig. 3 PDN prosthetic disc nucleus (RayMedica Inc.)

Facts and Questions: The PDN and Aquarelle are "hydro-active" implants, which are able to behave in a manner similar to the natural nucleus pulposus by increasing their water content when unloaded and decreasing it under load [9]. Although there have been extrusions of the PDN device after implantation through a posterior surgical approach, the initial results of the anterior implantation technique seem to be acceptable [1, 30, 31, 34]. There are still only few data on the long-term effects and behaviour of the implants in the intervertebral disc space. Implantation through a posterior route seems to be associated with a high extrusion rate.

In discogenic low-back pain, the pain is generated by nociceptors in the tears of the outer annulus fibrosus or in the cartilaginous endplates (often associated with Modic type I changes) [26]. This means that, at the time the patient becomes symptomatic, the nucleus is no longer the primary morphologic problem. This leads to fundamental questions: Does it make sense to replace the nucleus pulposus if its "container" (annulus fibrosus; cartilaginous endplates) is insufficient? Can replacement of the nucleus pulposus by a hydro-active implant restore disc height and thus (temporarily) protect the annulus from further degeneration? How will the cartilaginous endplates of the lumbar vertebrae tolerate the new load distribution initiated by artificial nucleus? No standards have been elaborated with regard to the degree of annulus degeneration or disc height loss up to which a nucleus replacement can still be accepted.

Total disc replacement (TDR)

Principle: The easiest reconstructive philosophy is total disc replacement. The implant model currently in use resembles the principles of total joint replacement of the hip or knee joint. This also means that, from a biomechanical point of view, preservation of motion is considered to be superior to load distribution and damping effect. Both implants that are on the world market today are characterized by a three-component modular design, which includes two metallic endplates and a nucleus pulposus made out of polyethylene (PE). In the Prodisc II implant (ProDisc II, Spine Solutions Inc.), the PE inlay is fixed in the lower endplate by a snap-lock mechanism. In the SB III Charité Disc (SB III Charité, Link Inc.), the nucleus moves freely between the endplates (Fig. 5, Fig. 6) [6, 21, 25]. With both implants, distraction of the intervertebral space is one of the main surgical goals. Disc height and foraminal height as well as segmental lordosis can be restored even in "collapsed" segments, and segmental motion is preserved. The latest disc generation (ProDisc) can be implanted through a minimal invasive anterior approach [24, 25].

Facts and Questions: TDR is he most advanced reconstructive concept of the anterior column of the lumbar spine. More than 3000 implantations have been performed with the two systems described above [6, 15, 21, 25]. The clinical results seem to be promising, although there has been no prospective randomised study comparing this procedure with the "gold standard" of lumbar fusion. The advantage of the latest implant generation (ProDics II) is that it can be implanted through less invasive anterior approaches [25], and that peri- and post-operative morbidity seem to be dramatically reduced as compared to lumbar fusion procedures. Many questions remain to be answered, and provide the motivation for further scientific work: Which morphological factors influence the indication and outcome? Special attention has to be focussed on the posterior column, especially on the degenerative status of the facet joints. How do the implants behave in the long term? How do the adjacent segments behave and react after disc replacement? Can total disc replacement relieve the load on the facet joints, and can a slightly degenerated facet joint recover? How does the implant design and the surgical approach influence post-operative mobility, clinical result and long-term behaviour ? How does the position of the implant in the intervertebral space (centred, anterior or posterior deviation) influence the range of motion, implant behaviour and clinical result? etc.

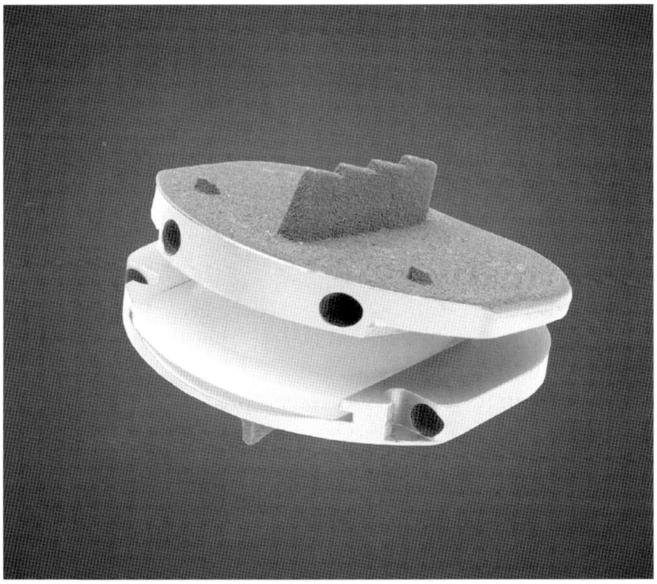

Fig. 5 ProDisc modular total disc (Spine Solutions Inc.)

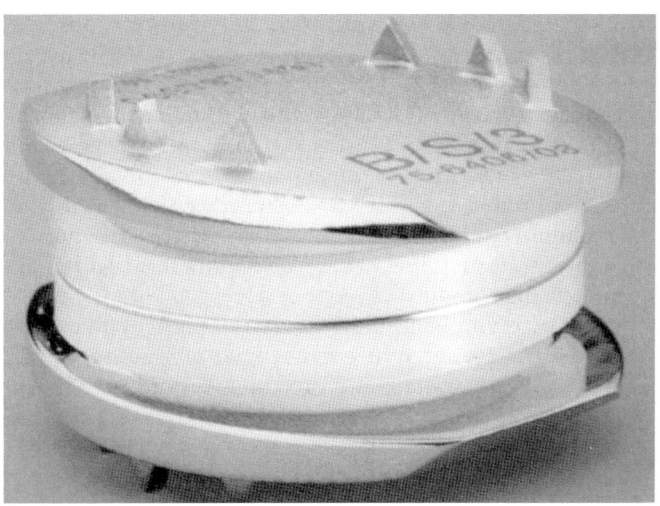

Fig. 6 Link SB III Charité total disc prosthesis (Link Inc.)

Reconstruction of the posterior column

Principles: Compared to disc replacement techniques, attempts to reconstruct the posterior elements (ligaments, facet joints) have been rare. The most advanced technology is the so-called "dynamic neutralization" concept, with the Dynesys Implant (Dynesys, Sulzer Medica Inc.) [8, 37], which is a combination of a pedicle screw system with dynamic posterior stabilisation. The combination of slight distraction and posterior tension-banding allows segmental mobility, but obviously restricts it towards the physiological "neutral zone". It thus represents an improvement over the initial "Graf" ligamentoplasty concept [12].

The distraction effect to ameliorate mild forms of spinal stenosis is the main rationale behind other concepts such as the Wallis system [35] or the posterior shock absorber [3]. These H-shaped implants are placed between the spinous processes with a minimal invasive approach. They do not provide rotational stability and are merely segmental distractors, which provide a positive stop in extension and keep the segment in a slightly kyphotic position. The latter effect accounts for the expected relief of symptoms in spinal stenosis cases.

Facts and Questions: These implant systems are promoted for different indications. The Dynesys concept is mainly indicated for dynamic stabilisation in cases where lumbar fusion procedures might be associated with a high surgical risk and/or bad results. It is, however, again a partial solution for a multi-factorial problem. Its efficacy strongly depends on the behaviour and integrity of the anterior column.

Interspinous space-holders are distractive devices proposed for the treatment of slight forms of spinal stenosis. There are no controlled studies available nor have any reliable clinical results been published to date. Looking at the pathology of degenerative lumbar spinal stenosis (hypertrophic facet osteoarthritis, yellow ligament hypertrophy, annular protrusion, kyphotic deformity), doubts can be raised as to whether these concepts can lead to acceptable clinical outcomes. However, they represent current developments that need to be discussed and evaluated using scientific criteria.

Conclusions

This survey describes the main developments in the field of lumbar spinal arthroplasty. It is probably not complete (since a considerable number of new devices are currently being developed), nor does it allow any final conclusions to be drawn. However, we are facing a change of paradigms in the surgical treatment of degenerative disorders of the lumbar spine. The progress in implant development, the acceptance of, and clinical routine in, less invasive surgical approaches, as well as the results of lumbar spinal fusion procedures have triggered a willingness for scientific discussion and clinical acceptance of ideas that are, in fact, not so new [29, 38]. We are at the beginning of another period of fundamental progress in the field of spine surgery, which can be compared to the "Charnley era" in the development of the total hip joint replacement more than 50 years ago [4]. We are looking at a variety of new concepts, some of which will disappear, but some of which will stay and will definitely be accepted as basic new therapeutic concepts. The more we learn about these new techniques, the more we realise how little we know. It is our responsibility to our patients and our scientific duty to critically elaborate the solutions to all these open questions.

References

1. Bertagnoli R, Schönmayr R, Vazquez R J (2002) Surgical and clinical results with the PDN prosthetic disc-nucleus device. Eur Spine J DOI 10.1007/s00586-002-0424-8
2. Brittberg M, Tallheden T, Sjögren-Jannson E, Lindahl A, Peterson L (2001) Autologous chondrocytes used for articular cartilage repair. Clin Orthop 391 [Suppl]:337–348
3. Caserta S et al (2002) Elastic stabilisation alone or combined with rigid fusion in spinal surgery. Eur Spine J DOI 10.1007/s00586-002-0426-6
4. Charnley J (1974) Total hip replacement. JAMA 230:1025–1028
5. Danish Institute for Health Technology Assessment (1999) Low-back-pain – frequency, management and prevention from an HTA perspective. Danish Institute for Health Technology Assessment series, vol 1(1)
6. David T (1993) Lumbar disc prosthesis – surgical technique, indications and clinical results in 22 patients with a minimum of 12 months follow-up. Eur Spine J 1:254–259
7. Deyo RA (1998) Low-back pain. Sci Am 279:28–33
8. Dubois G, de Germay B, Schaerer N, Fennema P (1999) Dynamic neutralization: a new concept for restabilization of the spine. In: Szpalski M, Gunzburg R, Pope MH (eds) Lumbar segmental instability. Lippincott Williams & Wilkins, Philadelphia, pp 233–240
9. Eysel P, Rompe JD, Schönmayr R, Zoellner J (1999) Biomechanical behaviour of a prosthetic lumbar nucleus. Acta Neurochir (Wien) 141:1083–1087
10. Faciszewski T, Winter RB, Lonstein JE, et al (1995) The surgical and medical perioperative complications of anterior spinal fusion surgery in the thoracic and lumbar spine in adults. A review of 1223 procedures. Spine 20: 1592–1599
11. Ganey TM, Meisel H-J (2002) A potential role for cell-based therapeutics in the treatment of intervertebral disc herniation. Eur Spine J DOI 10.1007/s00586-002-0494-7
12. Gardner A, Pande K (2002) Graf ligamentoplasty: a 7-year follow-up. Eur Spine J DOI 10.1007/s00586-002-0436-4
13. Greenough CG, Taylor LJ, Fraser RD (1994) Anterior lumbar fusion: results, assessment techniques and prognostic factors. Eur Spine J 3:225–230
14. Greenough CG, Peterson MD, Hadlow S, Fraser RD (1998) Instrumented posterolateral lumbar fusion. Spine 23: 479–486
15. Griffith SL, Shelokov AP, Büttner-Janz K, Lemaire JP, Zeegers S (1994) A multicenter retrospective study of the clinical results of the LINK ™ – SB Charité Intervertebral Prothesis. Spine 19:1842–1849
16. Husson, JL, Schärer N, Le Nihouannen JC, Freudiger S, Baumgartner W, Polard JL (1997) Nucleoplasty during discectomy: concept and experimental study. Rachis 9:145–152
17. Ito S, Yamada Y, Tsuboi S (1990) An observation of ruptured annulus fibrosis in lumbar discs. J Spinal Disord 4: 462–466
18. Korge A, Nydegger Th, Polard JL, Mayer HM, Husson JL (2002) A spiral implant as nucleus prosthesis in the lumbar spine. Eur Spine J DOI 10.1007/s00586-002-0444-4
19. Kozak JA, Heilman AE, O'Brien JP (1994) Anterior lumbar fusion options. Clin Orthop 300:45–51

20. Larsen JM, Rimoldi RL, Capen DA, et al (1996) Assessment of pseudoarthrosis in pedicle screw fusion: a prospective study comparing plain radiographs, CT scanning, and bone scintigraphy with operative findings. J Spinal Disord 9:117–120
21. Lemaire JP, Skalli W, Lavaste F, Templier A, Mendes F, Diop A, Sauty V, Laloux E (1997) Intervertebral disc prosthesis – results and prospects for the year 2000. Clin Orthop 337:64–76
22. Letcher F, Goldring S (1968) The effect of radiofrequency current and heat on peripheral nerve action potential in the cat. J Neurosurg 29:42–47
23. Mayer HM (1997) A new microsurgical technique for minimally invasive anterior lumbar interbody fusion. Spine 22:691–700
24. Mayer HM (1998) Microsurgical anterior approaches for anterior interbody fusion of the lumbar spine. In: McCulloch JA, Young PH (eds) Essentials of spinal microsurgery. Lippincott-Raven, Philadelphia, pp 633–649
25. Mayer HM, Wiechert K, Korge A, Qose I (2002) Minimally invasive total disc replacement – surgical technique and preliminary clinical results. Eur Spine J DOI 10.1007/s00586-002-0446-2
26. Modic MT, Steinberg PM, Ross JS, et al (1988) Degenerative disc disease: assessment of changes in vertebral body marrow with MR imaging. Radiology 166:193–199
27. Peterson L, Minas T, Brittberg M, Nilsson A, Sjögren-Jannson E, Lindahl A (2000) Two-to-9-year outcome after autologous chondrocyte transplantation of the knee. Clin Orthop 374:212–234
28. Prolo DJ, Oklund SA, Butcher M (1986) Toward uniformity in evaluating results of lumbar spine operations. A paradigm applied to posterior lumbar interbody fusions. Spine 11:601–606
29. Ray CD (1992) The artificial disc – introduction, history and socioeconomics. In: Weinstein JN (ed) Clinical efficacy and outcome in the diagnosis and treatment of low back pain. Raven, New York, pp 205–225
30. Ray CD (2002) The PDN prosthetic disc-nucleus device. Eur Spine J DOI 10.1007/s00586-002-0425-7
31. Ray CD, Schönmayr R, Kavangh SA, Assell R (1999) Prosthetic disc nucleus implants. Riv Neuroradiol 12 [Suppl]: 157–162
32. Saal JA, Saal JS (1998) Thermal characteristics of lumbar disc: evaluation of a novel approach to targeted intradiscal thermal therapy. Presented at the 13th Annual Meeting of the North American Spine Society. San Francisco, 28–31 October
33. Saal JS, Saal JA (2000) Management of chronic discogenic low back pain with a thermal intradiscal catheter. Spine 25:382–388
34. Schönmayr R, Busch C, Lotz C, Lotz-Metz G (1999) Prosthetic disc nucleus implants: the Wiesbaden feasibility study, 2 years follow-up in ten patients. Riv Neuroradiol 12 [Suppl 1]:163–170
35. Sénégas J (2002) Mechanical supplementation by non-rigid fixation in degenerative intervertebral lumbar segments (the Wallis system). Eur Spine J DOI 10.1007/s00586-002-0423-9
36. Spivak JM, Neuwirth MG, Giordano CP, et al (1994) The perioperative course of combined anterior and posterior spinal fusion. Spine 19:520–525
37. Stoll TM, Dubois G, Schwarzenbach O (2002) Dynamic neutralisation system for the spine – a non-fusion system. Eur Spine J DOI 10.1007/s00586-002-0438-2
38. Szpalski M, Gunzburg R, Mayer HM (2002) Spine arthroplasty: a historical review. Eur Spine J DOI 10.1007/s00586-002-0474-y
39. Viscogliosi AG, Viscogliosi MR, Viscogliosi JJ (2000) Artificial disc – market potential and technology update. Spine Industry Analysis Series, Viscogliosi Bros. LLC, New York

Vincent E. Bryan Jr

Cervical motion segment replacement

Abstract When symptoms bring to light a cervical spine degenerative disc process that requires surgical intervention, a symptom relieving procedure such as decompression, followed by functional restoration, arthroplasty, offers the benefit of prophylaxis of accelerated spondylosis at the operated level. In addition, by altering the biomechanical stress factors at adjacent levels, theoretically it should offer prophylactic benefit at these levels as well. The design requirements for a cervical disc prosthesis, the importance of precision instrumentation, and technique are described. Mechanical testing, animal testing, the study design for the EU clinical study, and the operative technique are discussed. The clinical 1- and 2-year data to date are presented.

Keywords Cervical vertebrae · Degenerative disc disease · Herniated disc · Intervertebral disc · Joint prosthesis implantation · Spinal fusion · Spondylosis

The clinical investigators involved in this study were: J Goffin, MD, PhD; A Casey, MD; P Kehr, MD; K Liebig, MD, PhD; B Lind, MD, PhD; C Logroscino; V Pointillart, MD, PhD; F Van Calenbergh, MD; and J van Loon, MD. The clinical data were gathered from the following sites: Universitaire Ziekenhuizen, Leuven, Belgium; the National Hospital for Neurology and Neurosurgery, London, UK; Centre de Traumatologie et d'Orthopedie, Illkirch, France; Orthopädische Abteilung des Waldkrankenhauses St. Marien, Erlangen, Germany; Sahlgrenska University Hospital, Gothenberg, Sweden; Piazza Madona Del Cenacolo, Rome, Italy; Unite de Pathologie Rachidienne, CHU Pellegrin, Bordeaux, France.

V.E. Bryan Jr (✉)
Spinal Dynamics Corporation,
9655 SE 36th St., Suite 110,
Mercer Island, WA 98040–3732, USA
e-mail: bryanv@spinedyn.com,
Tel.: +1-206-2752715/2197004,
Fax: +1-206-2752735

Introduction

Factors that qualify a degenerative disc process, including herniated nucleus pulposus (HNP), as a disease as opposed to a normal aging process include the age at which the degenerative disease process presents itself and the rate at which it progresses relative to the general population.

Once initiated, degenerative disc disease (DDD) is likely to progress at a more rapid rate than the normal degenerative disc aging process. Both the biomechanical and physiologic effects become increasingly more stressful on the component tissues of the functional spine unit (FSU). They may include: alteration in the axis of rotation, altered load sharing, loss of cushioning, hyper- or hypomobility of the FSU, and declining performance of the nutritional supply system.

Thus, the symptomatic presentation of DDD may lead to accelerated degeneration at the affected FSU and secondarily at the adjacent FSUs as well.

In time, the nature of the symptom(s), in combination with neurological impairment, may lead to surgical intervention. Surgical decompression of the neural structures usually results in symptomatic improvement in 6–12 weeks. In the cervical spine an anterior approach (including surgical fusion with grafts or devices) is commonly employed to foster lordosis, maintain intervertebral body spacing, and to address and/or potentially avoid axial pain and pseudarthrosis. Fusion, however, is often performed despite no radiographic evidence of mechanical instability. The need to assess surgical fusion outcome prolongs the outcome assessment period to 12–24 months.

Recently, longer-term outcome data (5–10 years) suggests that there are significant radiographic and clinical consequences associated with fusion. Hilibrand et al. [3] identified symptomatic adjacent-segment disease occurring at an average rate of 2.9% per year during the first 10 post-fusion years for patients in their study group, with two-thirds of those patients requiring reoperation. Goffin et al. [2] identified a 92% rate of adjacent-level radiological degeneration after fusion over a mean of 8.6 years. Brumley et al. [1] identified hypermobility at segments adjacent to a fused segment.

From a surgical perspective, the benefits of an anterior approach to the cervical spine are well appreciated, and for many surgeons it has become a satisfying and successful surgery. Posterior or anterior lateral partial discectomy approaches may be alternatives to an anterior approach as a means to avoid the biomechanical consequences of fusion. Nonetheless, even with decompression alone, the long-term degenerative disease process is left unattended in favor of symptomatic relief.

When deciding upon functional reconstruction, one is selecting a concept and treatment that addresses the symptomatic degenerative disc process as a disease rather than as a symptom that is simply part of the normal aging process. In doing so, one acknowledges the importance of addressing the long-term biomechanical and natural history issues in a prophylactic manner, at both the operated as well as the adjacent FSUs.

Hypothetically, the concept of a fully functional disc prosthesis, which re-establishes more nearly normal biomechanics to the FSU, if introduced early enough in the symptomatic DDD process, should return the biomechanical natural history of the FSU from that of a disease to that of the individual's normal aging process.

Materials and methods

Design requirements

Ideally, a fully functional disc prosthesis should provide a means to re-establish motion, elasticity, and more normal load sharing and rotational axes in a minimally constrained device with immediate, short- and long-term mechanical stability and durability.

Secondly, the device design should not contain features prone to frequent revisions (e.g. screws, etc.).

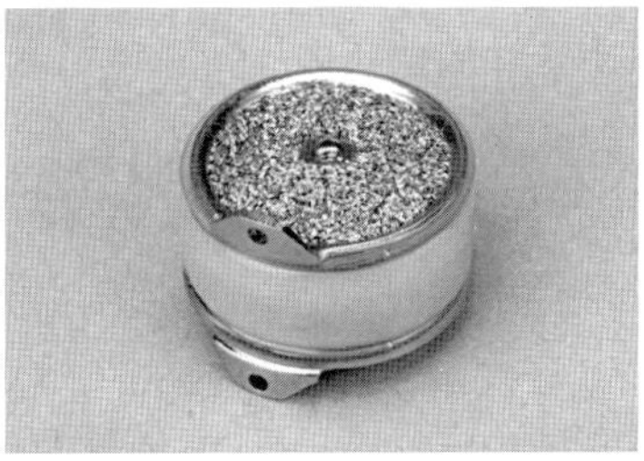

Fig. 1 Bryan Cervical Disc Prosthesis

Thirdly, the device should permit future interbody fusion options, should they become necessary.

Additionally, the prosthesis system must include precision instrumentation to ensure proper localization and preparation of the prosthesis interbody site.

Finally, the design requirements must recognize the critical role of the surgeon in applying appropriate indications to patient selection, employing prophylactic medications and closely adhering to prescribed surgical technique while, through knowledge, understanding, and skill, making adjustments for the variations in anatomic and degenerative conditions encountered from patient to patient.

The device

The Bryan Cervical Disc prosthesis (see Fig. 1) contains a proprietary, low-friction, wear-resistant, unique polyurethane nucleus. The nucleus is located between, and articulates with, shaped titanium plates (shells) that include convex porous ingrowth surfaces, to allow bony fixation to the adjacent vertebral endplates. The design provides for a normal range of motion (ROM) in flexion/extension, lateral bending, rotation and translation, as well as coupled motions. While prosthesis motion is unconstrained through the normal ROM, special geometric features provide soft limits to this range. Additionally, a unique flexible membrane surrounds the interior articulating shell surfaces, to separate the internal structures of the device from the external in vivo environment, and to contain a lubricant.

Testing

Extensive laboratory and animal testing was performed to adequately determine and demonstrate the safety of the functional cervical disc prior to initiating clinical trials. In vitro testing, including static and fatigue evaluations, was conducted on the components, subassemblies, and final devices to evaluate and establish the prosthesis' mechanical performance limits under "worst-case" conditions. The testing included evaluation of prosthesis stability, utilizing a mechanical cervical spine simulator to determine the long-term functionality and durability of the prosthetic system. This simulator subjected the device to dynamic load and motion profiles representative of normal in vivo conditions. Other bench and cadaver studies were conducted that included testing to ensure the functionality of the surgical instrumentation system.

Pre-clinical animal studies were conducted to study the in vivo performance of the prosthesis and the surgical instrumentation. The studies were conducted following the principles of laboratory animal care. An adult chimpanzee survivor model was selected as the most appropriate, because of its similarity to the human in cervical spinal anatomy, morphology, and biomechanics. Three independent studies evaluated device safety in a total of 12 animals, with up to 6 months follow-up. The results showed that the prosthesis was stable and provided motion at the operated level. Fluorochrome labeling demonstrated bone ingrowth into the prosthesis shells. Additionally, a goat study, utilizing 16 animals, was undertaken to evaluate the biologic response to any particulates in surrounding tissues, lymph nodes, liver, spleen, dura mater, and spinal cord. At 6 months, no inflammatory response was demonstrated in any of the tissues. When combined with extensive in vitro testing, the robust chimpanzee and goat study results collectively demonstrated device safety and supported the initiation of clinical trials during the first week of January 2000. The operative procedures represent the combined work of nine neuro- and orthopedic surgeons at seven centers in Europe.

Study design

Patients were concurrently enrolled in a multi-center evaluation of the prosthesis for the treatment of single-level DDD of the cervical spine. The prospective study was approved by the ethics committee and, as required, the regulatory agencies for each center. As such, the study was conducted in accordance with the Declaration of Helsinki. Patient inclusion criteria included disc herniation or spondylosis, with radiculopathy and/or myelopathy that had not responded to conservative treatment. Exclusion criteria included previous cervical spine surgery involving any other device, axial neck pain as the solitary symptom, significant cervical anatomical deformity or clinical instability, and active infection. Patients gave their informed consent before participating in the study.

Patient assessments are based on the evaluation schedule presented in Table 1. The primary endpoint is classification based on relief of preoperative symptoms, as assessed by the patient using the Cervical Spine Research Society (CSRS) and SF-36 patient questionnaires, and relief of objective neurological signs, as assessed by the physician in a neurological examination, associated with the treated level.

Data were entered into a database and, in accordance with a scoring algorithm, assessments were calculated to determine relief of neurological symptoms and signs. Results were scored according to a modified version of Odom's Criteria, and categorized as follows:

- *Excellent:* improvement in most (at least 80%) of the preoperative signs and symptoms, with little deterioration (not more than 10%)
- *Good:* improvement in some (at least 70%) of the preoperative signs and symptoms, with some deterioration (not more than 15%)
- *Fair:* improvement in half (at least 50%) of the preoperative signs and symptoms, with some deterioration (not more than 20%)
- *Poor:* improvement in few (less than 50%) of the preoperative signs and symptoms, or significant deterioration (more than 20%)

Radiographs were analyzed independently to determine ROM and assess device migration and/or subsidence.

Table 1 Patient assessments, carried out preoperatively, postoperatively, and at 6 weeks, 3 months, 6 months, 1 year, and 2 years

Motor strength on a five-point scale (right and left sides)
Deltoids
Biceps
Triceps
Wrist extensors
Wrist flexors
Finger flexors
Finger abductors
Gait on a four-point scale
Reflexes on a four-point scale (right and left sides)
Biceps
Triceps
Brachioradialis
Knees
Ankles
Sensory function on a four-point scale (right and left sides)
C4 dermatome
C5 dermatome
C6 dermatome
C7 dermatome
Neck pain severity on a six-point scale
Arm pain severity on a six-point scale
Ability to function with respect to activities of daily living on a four-point scale

Study enrollment

A total of 97 devices were implanted. In all cases, neural compression was verified using computed tomography (CT) or magnetic resonance imaging (MRI) and a neurological assessment. Complete clinical and radiographic data are available on 97 patients. As of late January 2002, 49 of the patients have been followed for 1 year and 10 patients have been followed for 2 years. Table 2 details the demographic variables of the patients.

The duration of preoperative symptoms ranged from 3 weeks to more than 2 years.

Operative technique

The prosthesis is implanted using a proprietary surgical procedure that is an extension of current anterior cervical discectomy and fusion (ACDF) procedures. Following initial discectomy, surgical instruments utilize a simple gravitational referencing system to establish a virtual axis in the intervertebral disc space that is used to position a milling fixture, which is then fastened to the anterior vertebral surfaces. This fixture controls the location and movement of the powered cutting instruments that prepare the vertebral end-

Table 2 Patient demographics (*n*=97)

Age range	26–79 years
Gender	41 men, 56 women
Clinical diagnosis[a]	Radiculopathy (*n*=90); myelopathy (*n*=13)
Primary etiology[a]	Herniation (*n*=75); spondylosis (*n*=33)
Duration of symptoms	6 wk. (*n*=6); 3 mo. (*n*=18); 6 mo. (*n*=24); 1 yr (*n*=15); 2 yr. (*n*=14); 2 yr. (*n*=20)
Levels implanted	C3–C4 (*n*=0); C4–C5 (*n*=11); C5–C6 (*n*=42); C6–C7 (*n*=44)
Size implanted	14 mm (*n*=22); 15 mm (*n*=21); 16 mm (*n*=25); 17 mm (*n*=20); 18 mm (*n*=9)

[a] Several patients presented with multiple diagnoses and/or etiology

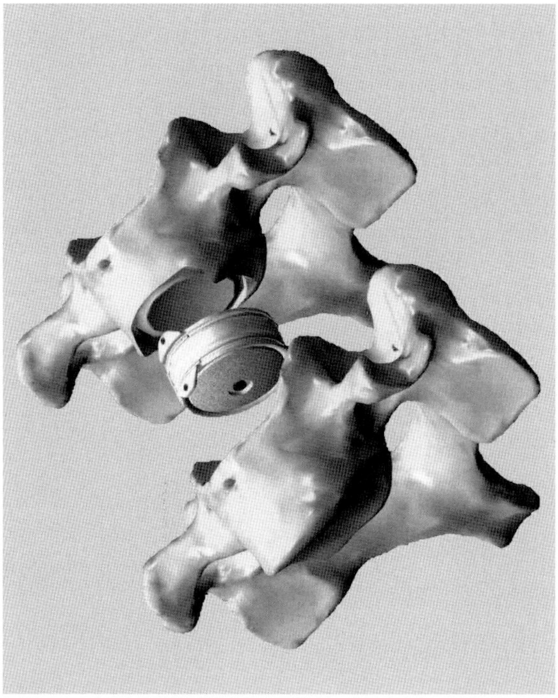

Fig. 2 Disc prosthesis and precisely milled concavity in the vertebral body

plates for placement of the prosthesis. The milled vertebral endplates exactly match the geometry of the shell's convex outer surface, capturing the rim of each shell inside a ridge of bone (see Fig. 2). This tight fit provides immediate antero-posterior and lateral stability.

Operative data were compiled on 97 procedures.

Results

Table 3 summarizes the clinical success results based on relief of preoperative symptoms (as assessed by the patient) and relief of neurological signs (as assessed by the surgeon) for the 1-year and 2-year follow-up periods.

Of the 46 patients rated for clinical success at 1-year follow-up, 40 (87%) were classified as a clinical success (excellent/good/fair). This result is better than the targeted success rate of 85% excellent/good/fair. Three patients with incomplete scores (one with an incomplete patient questionnaire, two with incomplete neurological forms) were disregarded in this scoring analysis.

At 2 years, the scores were excellent, good, or fair for eight out of nine, or 89%, of the patients. This result is better than the targeted success rate of 85%. One patient did not fully complete a patient questionnaire and was not evaluated for 2-year clinical success.

Complications

One patient experienced temporary dysphonia. One patient reported pain subsequent to the 3-month follow-up. This was due to failure to remove a lateral osteophyte, as well as to a 3-year history of preoperative dermatomal pain. A foraminotomy was performed in this case. The device, its position and its function remained good throughout, and it was considered to be unrelated to the symptom.

One patient reported pain in the right shoulder, right arm, and in the sternum region, approximately 6 months after surgery. An MRI examination ruled out any remaining neural compression. Another patient remarked on unresolved non-specific shoulder pain and left axial pain.

One surgical intervention at the target space occurred approximately 26 h post surgery. A standard drainage catheter had loosened and ceased draining. Subsequently, the patient experienced pain and shortness of breath. The re-operation revealed a hematoma, which was evacuated; no active bleeding was detected. The intervention was uneventful and the patient responded well.

There have been no device failures or device explants.

Radiographic results

Radiographic follow-up data were obtained for 43 (of 49) patients with 1 year's follow-up, and ten (of ten) patients with 2 years' follow-up. An independent radiologist assessed all radiographs.

Device position

After each follow-up visit, lateral radiographs were measured to ensure that device instability did not occur. Based on the accuracy of measuring plain radiographs, and as measured in fusion cage studies, 2 mm was considered the detection threshold. Subsidence has not been observed in any patients. Evidence of anterior/posterior device migration over 2 mm was detected in one patient; however, migration greater than 3 mm has not been observed. In this patient, the milled concavity had not been created, due to nearly mechanical failure in the cutting instrument.

Table 3 Clinical success results based on patient's assessment of relief of preoperative symptoms and surgeon's assessment of relief of neurological signs

Follow-up	Clinical success % (*n*)	Sample size	Excellent % (*n*)	Good % (*n*)	Fair % (*n*)	Poor % (*n*)
One year	87 (40)	46	70 (32)	4 (2)	13 (6)	13 (6)
Two years	89 (8)	9	78 (7)	–	11 (1)	11 (1)

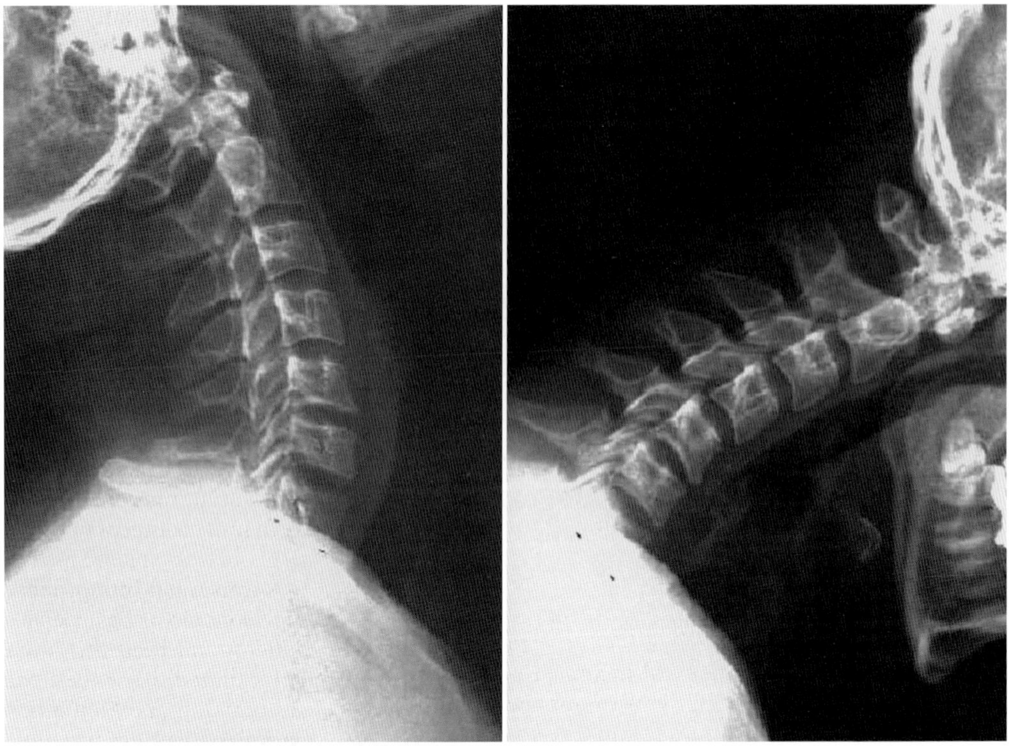

Fig. 3 Preoperative range of motion (ROM) in a 29-year-old man implanted with a 17-mm prosthesis at the C5-6 level

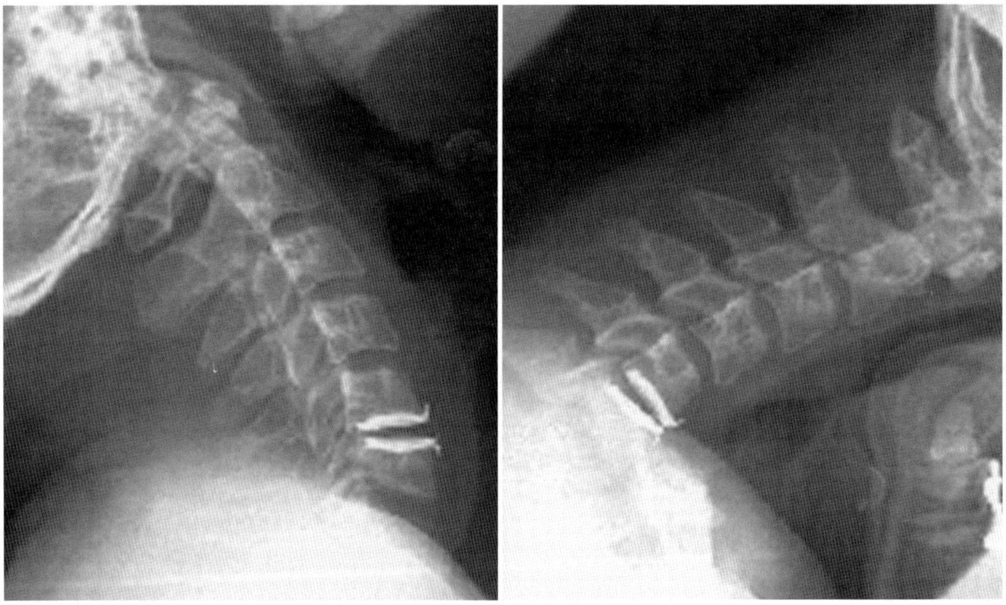

Fig. 4 Twelve-month postoperative ROM in the same man as Fig. 3

Range of motion results

Postoperative Cobb angles for flexion/extension of the FSU at the implant level demonstrated motion of the device in flexion/extension.

At 1 year, 38 out of 44 patients, or 86%, demonstrated flexion/extension ROM equal to or greater than 2°. In four patients ROM measured 1°; the radiograph for the remaining patient was not interpretable. The ROM for patients at 1 year averages just over 8°, with a standard deviation of 5°.

At 2 years, ten out of ten patients, or 100%, demonstrated flexion/extension ROM equal to or greater than 2°. The ROM for patients at 2 years averages just over 11°, with a standard deviation of 5°. Motion was observed in all patients, and there was no evidence of spondylotic bridging.

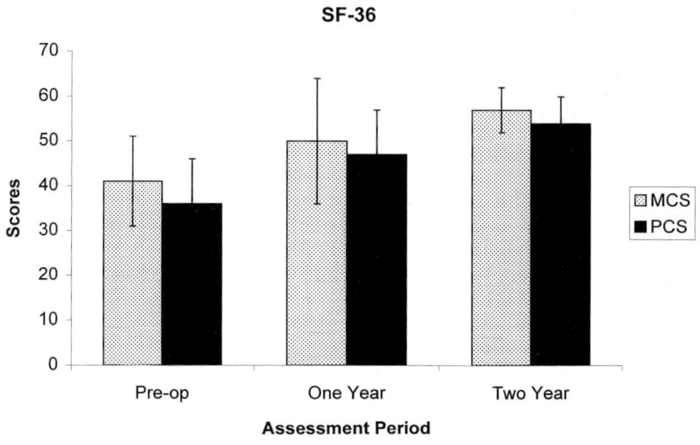

Fig. 5 SF-36 Quality of Life results for the patients reaching the 1-year and 2-year follow-up periods

Illustrative case

The patient illustrated in Fig. 3 and Fig. 4 – a 29-year-old man – was implanted with a 17-mm prosthesis at the C5-6 level. This patient's ROM increased by 4° (from 17° preoperatively to 21° at 12 months postoperatively).

Quality of life results

The SF-36 Health Survey results are presented in Fig. 5 for the patients reaching the 1-year and 2-year follow-up periods. Values for each period are presented in the SF-36 Physical Component Summary (PCS) and Mental Component Summary (MCS) scores, which utilize US population means to establish normalized scores. All PCS/MCS scores are norm based, with the general population mean equal to 50 and the standard deviation equal to 10. At 1-year post-implant, patients had PCS scores just under the US mean (47), but that represents a 31% improvement over the average preoperative PCS scores. At 2 years post-implant, patients with the Bryan prosthesis met or exceeded the US population mean for PCS and MCS scores.

Discussion

Though the 1- and 2 year data to date compare favorably with equivalent data for the ACDF procedure, this should come as no surprise, as the patient's symptomatic relief is obtained principally from the decompression, which is essentially the same in both ACDF and cervical spine arthroplasty procedures. What is noteworthy, however, is the fact that increased axial pain has not been noted in the prosthetic FSUs of DDD patients. This likely is related to facet unloading and movement of the axis of rotation to a location that is closer to normal, following insertion of an appropriately sized prosthesis.

Two of the poor outcomes noted in the 1-year results were in patients whose preoperative radicular symptom of pain had been present for 12–24 months. In two myelopathic patients whose outcome was fair, deficits persisted though no progression was observed (note: cases in which patients/investigators did not complete all 55 combined questions from the questionnaires and forms were automatically excluded from the outcome scoring).

Overall, motion of the FSU postoperatively was similar to that seen preoperatively. No subsidence, device migration or mechanical instability was noted when the device was implanted into properly prepared endplates. No bridging spondylosis has been seen to date, including the first ten patients followed for 2 years. Good movement, which did not diminish over time, has been demonstrated in all ten cases at 2 years. Patient satisfaction has been high, with no postoperative restrictions on activities of daily living (ADL). External orthoses were not required.Studies subsequent to the E.U. series showed the presence of some evidence of paravertebral ossification in about 30% of patients. This finding was profoundly reduced in frequency and degree in patients receiving NSAIDs postoperatively for 2 weeks.

Conclusion

Cervical spine arthroplasty can be expected to address the symptoms and signs of DDD within the outcome assessment period of 2 years at least as well as ACDF. The device instrumentation and technique offer the advantage of treating the disease aspects of the degenerative disc process by providing for continued motion and a more normal biomechanics. It would be desirable for cervical spine arthroplasty to favorably influence the rate of progress and age of onset of future symptoms. If this proves to be the case, it will in effect return the individual's degenerative disc disease process to that of their natural aging process. This will require at least 5–10 years to evaluate.

References

1. Brumley J, Komistek R, Jones A, Hajner M (2000) Handout at 2000 AAOS Conference, Orlando, Florida
2. Goffin J, Geusens E, Vantomme N, Quintens E, Waerzeggers Y, Depreitere B, Van Calenbergh F, van Loon J (2000) Long-term follow-up after interbody fusion of the cervical spine. Presentation at the 28th Annual Meeting of the Cervical Spine Research Society in Charleston, South Carolina
3. Hilibrand A, Carlson G, Palumbo M, Jones P, Bohlman H (1999) Radiculopathy and myelopathy at segments adjacent to the site of a previous anterior cervical arthrodesis. J Bone Joint Surg Am 81:519–528

Helmut D. Link

History, design and biomechanics of the LINK SB Charité artificial disc

H.D. Link (✉)
Waldemar Link GmbH & Co,
Barkhausenweg 10,
22339 Hamburg, Germany
e-mail: sekrhdl@linkhh.de,
Tel.: +49-40-539950,
Fax: +49-40-5383309

Abstract The SB Charité I artificial disc was developed in 1982 by Schellnack and Büttner-Janz and modified as the Mark II version in 1984. Both types were manufactured in the former German Democratic Republic (GDR). Today's design, the SB Charité III, was first produced by LINK in 1987. Five sizes of the artificial disc in various angulations are available today, with a double coating of titanium/calciumphosphate. Designed with a three-component set-up, the SB Charité mimics the physiological segmental motion. The possibility of translation in the SB Charité provides proper biomechanical function and protects the zygapophysial joints. Results of biomechanical testing showed a sufficient cold-flow resistance of the UHMWPE (**U**ltra **H**igh **M**olecular **W**eight **P**olyethylene) sliding core and confirmed the negligible abrasion rate. The LINK SB Charité disc is a safe and effective operative treatment for discogenic low back pain. Long-term results (10 years and more) have been published.

Keywords History · Materials · Bioactive coating · Translation · Zygapophysial joints

Introduction

In 1982 Schellnack and Büttner-Janz initiated the development of the functional artificial disc, the SB Charité I (Fig. 1A) at the Charité Hospital in Berlin [11]. The idea was based on the "low-friction" principle, which had proven to be successful in total joint replacement: an UHMWPE (**U**ltra **H**igh **M**olecular **W**eight **P**olyethylene) sliding core articulates between two highly polished metal endplates, imitating the movement of the nucleus within its annular containment.

In September 1984, following mechanical testing at the Institut für Leichtbau und ökonom, Verwendung von Werkstoffen, Dresden [10], the SB Charité I artificial disc was implanted for the first time at the Charité Hospital in Berlin. The endplates of this model were made of 1-mm-thick URX2CrNiMoN 18.12 steel and the sliding core was produced from Chirulen UHMWPE. For fixation in the bony vertebral endplates, the artificial disc incorporated first 11 and later 5 sharp anchoring teeth for cementless fixation.

In 1985, due to axial migrations, the artificial disc was modified to SB Charité II (Fig. 1B). It was based on the same functional principle as type I, but the metal endplates were enlarged with bilateral "wings", to improve the support of the implant on the bony endplates of the vertebral bodies. The endplates incorporated three ventral and two dorsal anchoring teeth. Mark II was manufactured of stainless steel and later of EMO titanium sheeting (only for biomechanical testing) [10]. Both the mark I and the mark II implants were manufactured in the former German Democratic Republic (GDR) only, and were never commercially available. The usage was confined to the Charité Hospital.

Fractures in Mark II endplates and insufficient instrumentation for implantation were the reasons that the authors contacted LINK for production of a state of the art implant version of the artificial disc, the design of which has basically remained unchanged since LINK started production in 1987.

The endplates of the LINK SB Charité III disc (Fig. 2) are of cast CoCrMo alloy (ISO 5832/IV; ASTM F75–82)

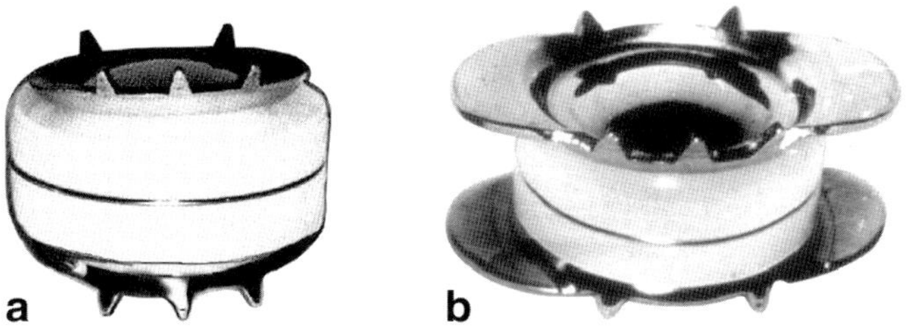

Fig. 1 **A** SB Charité I. **B** SB Charité II

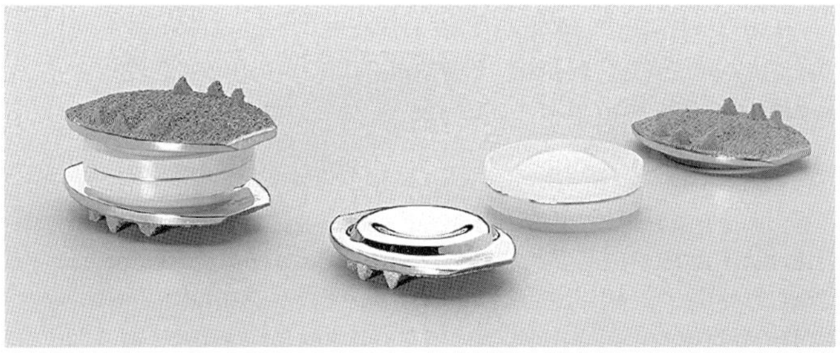

Fig. 2 SB Charité III

for optimal static mechanical properties, each with three anchoring teeth ventrally and dorsally. Originally three sizes of metal endplates in parallel and 5° angulation were produced [11]. In 1998 a size 4, and in 1999 an even larger size 5, was added to allow for an optimal choice of the largest endplate giving best possible support on the cranial and caudal vertebral body (Fig. 3).

To improve lordotic reconstruction, additional angulated endplates of 7.5° and 10° were introduced in 1999. Endplates of the same size but with different lordotic angulations may be combined with each other, allowing an even more precise reconstruction of the lumbar lordosis. UHMWPE sliding cores (ISO 5834/II; ASTM 648–83) of various heights are available for each endplate size to allow for physiological restoration of the intervertebral disc space (Fig. 3).

Since 1987, approximately 4000 SB Charité artificial discs have been implanted, and spine surgeons in Germany, France, the UK and the Netherlands have reported [12, 15, 16, 21] on results of 10 years or more follow-up.

The bioactive coating

To improve the anchoring of the endplates and to establish a mineralized connection between bone and implants, the endplates receive on their outside a "bioactive double coating" (Fig. 4). This concept has been successfully tested in an animal study [24, 25] and in non-cemented joint replacements such as pressfit hip cups, ankle joint prostheses and dental implants [23].

The coating consists of three layers. The first two layers are of commercially pure titanium (Ti) – the first layer provides a special strong bond between the cobalt-chrome endplate and the coating, and the second layer of plasma-sprayed Ti provides the desired pore size of 75–300 μm. The third coating consists of a layer of calcium phosphate

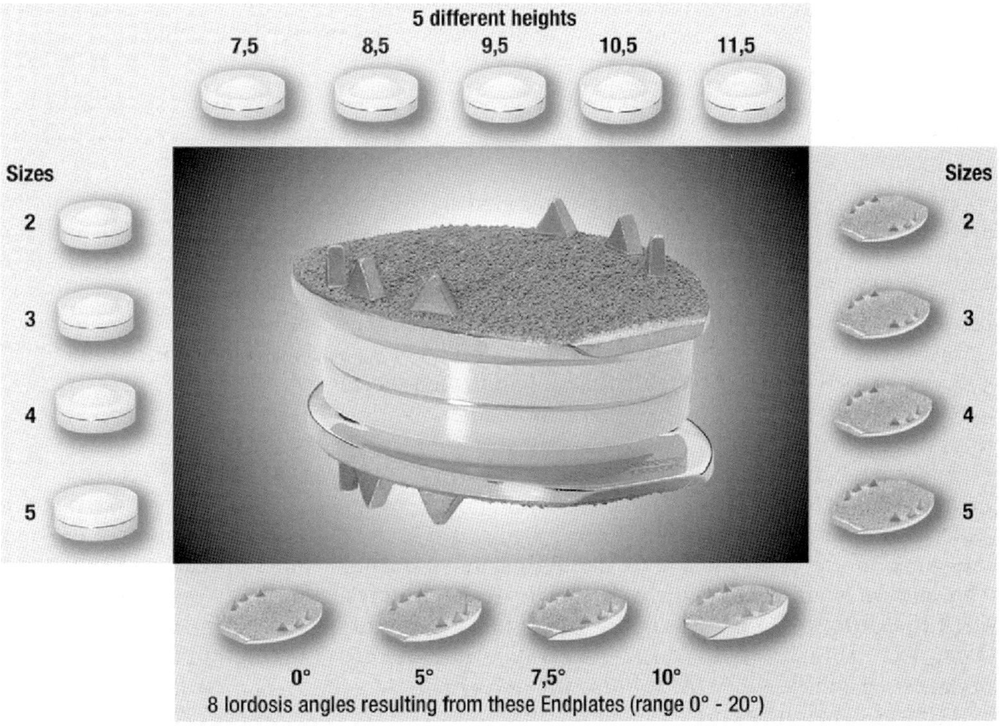

Fig. 3 Range of size, CoCr endplates and UHMWPE (**U**ltra **H**igh **M**olecular **W**eight **P**olyethylene) sliding cores

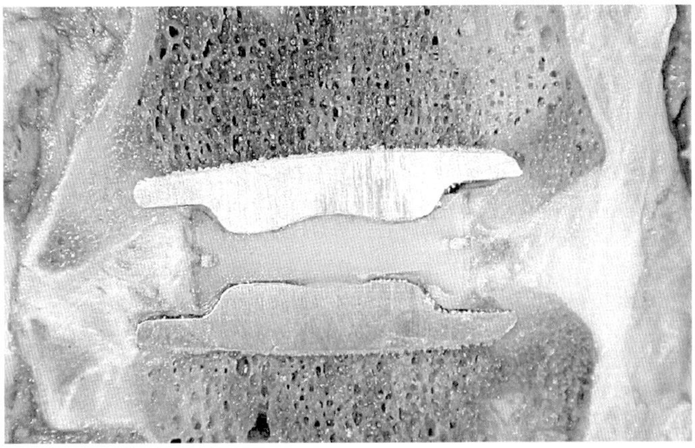

Fig. 4 The SB Charité "bioactive double coating" showed mean ingrowth of 47.9% in a baboon study (coronal diamond cut section, courtesy of Dr. McAfee, Baltimore)

(CaP). This is applied to the Ti surface in an electrochemical process that results in:

1. A thin layer of 10–25 μm
2. The retention of the open-cell structure of the Ti coating
3. A mechanically strong bond, which is necessary to cope with the stresses applied on the coating during implantation

The open-cell porous structure provides an optimal base for the ingrowth of bone cells. The attachment of osteoblasts on the structured surface is accelerated by the bioactive CaP coating (Fig. 5). This avoids at the same time the growth of connective tissues onto the implant.

Biomechanics

Sagittal rotation, lateral rotation, axial rotation and range of motion

Flexion and extension in the lumbar spine constitutes an arc-like motion combining sagittal rotation with sagittal translation [27]. The position of the instantaneous axis of rotation (IAR) point is not constant, and changes depending on the joint position.

This important aspect of spinal biomechanics is replicated in the functional motion of the SB Charité, due to its three-component set-up, which incorporates a floating sliding core, whose convex surfaces are encased in the concave cavities of the metal endplates (Fig. 6).

In vitro evaluations carried out by Ahrens [5, 24] of the mobility of the L4/L5 motion segment in fresh frozen cadavers with most ligamentous structures intact have revealed a similar mobility in those with and those without implanted SB Charité disc, in extension and flexion as well as right and left bending.

Only figures for the range of motion (ROM) in torsion (Table 1) for moments greater than 5 Nm were different. This seems to be related to the severed anterior ligament, the ventrally incised annulus fibrosis and the removed disc tissue. Clinical experience established that the soft-tissue structures adapt to that situation over a period of time.

Clinical evaluations have confirmed the values Ahrens found; David and Lemaire have both documented retained motion in their medium- and long-term follow-ups [14, 21].

Translation and the zygapophysial joints

Translation is a movement that causes all points in a body to move in parallel in the same direction and to the same extent as the force [7]. During flexion in an intervertebral segment two types of movement take place:

1. The center of nucleus moves dorsally
2. The cranial vertebral body translates ventrally

The major movements of an intervertebral segment in flexion and extension are sagittal rotation plus translation. The center of rotation changes and the path of the various centers of rotation is a centrode [8, 18] (Fig. 7).

In flexion and extension, the unconstrained sliding core of the SB Charité mimics this kind of movement (Fig. 8).

Fig. 5 CaP coating on porous implant surface

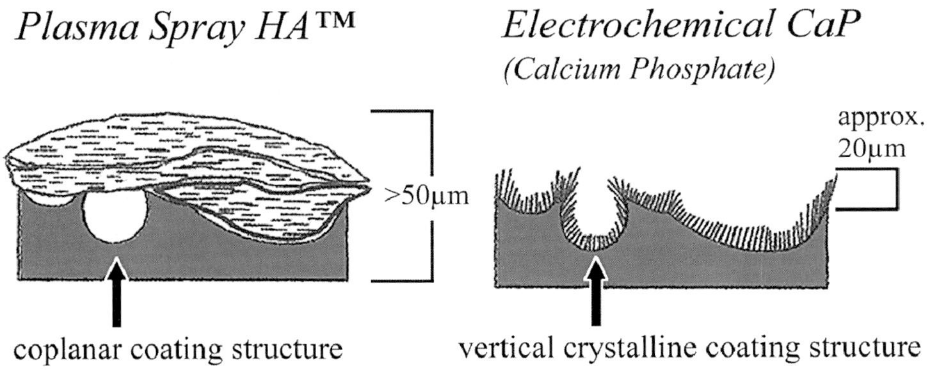

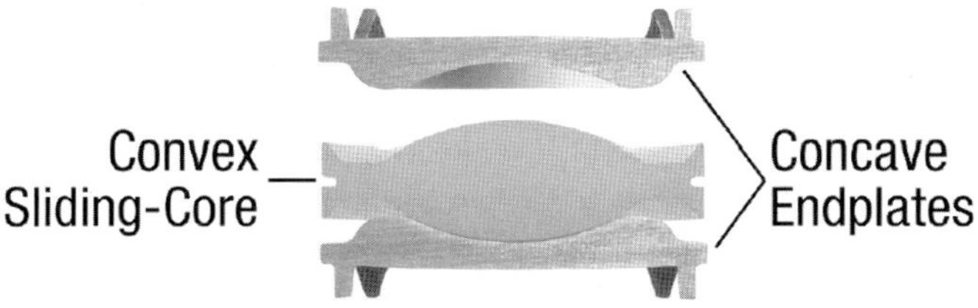

Fig. 6 Free-floating biconvex sliding core encased in concave endplates

Table 1 Mean range of motion in degrees (±SD) at level L4-L5, as published by Ahrens et al. [5]

	Maximum load (Nm)	Lumbar disc	Artificial disc
Extension	12	3.49 (0.82)	3.27 (0.83)
Flexion	12	7.72 (1.74)	9.78 (1.48)
Left flexion	8	2.78 (1.78)	2.37 (0.57)
Right flexion	8	5.24 (2.54)	7.41 (2.65)
Torsion	7	1.66 (0.74)	3.01 (0.73)

Fig. 7 Rotation and translation in the natural disc

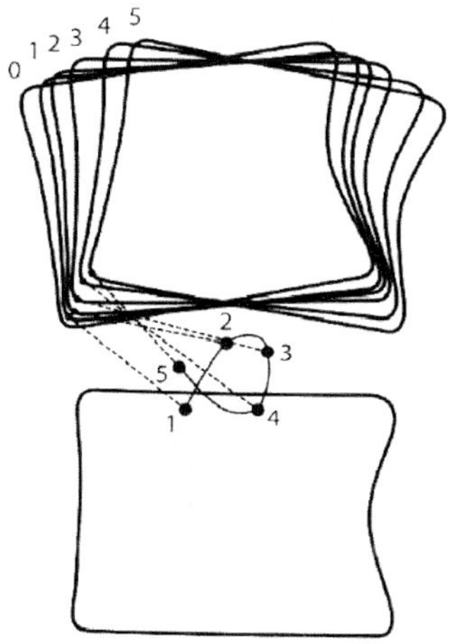

In lateral bending, coronal rotation is combined with translation. The mobile sliding core of the SB Charité mimics such movements as well.

In axial distraction or compression there is a possibility of axial translation. Such translation is possible in the sliding core of the modular SB Charité artificial disc, as it is attached to neither the superior nor the inferior endplate of the artificial disc.

If a vertebral body slides forward, the inferior articular processes are resisted by the superior articular processes of the inferior vertebral body. This resistance is transmitted to the vertebral body through the pedicles and the posterior elements and anterior vertebral column interact [9]. Such motion can be duplicated in the SB Charité without unphysiological stress, only due to the unconstrained three-component set-up. An artificial disc must allow the abovementioned motions simultaneously, otherwise zygapophysial joints and/or disc prostheses undergo un-

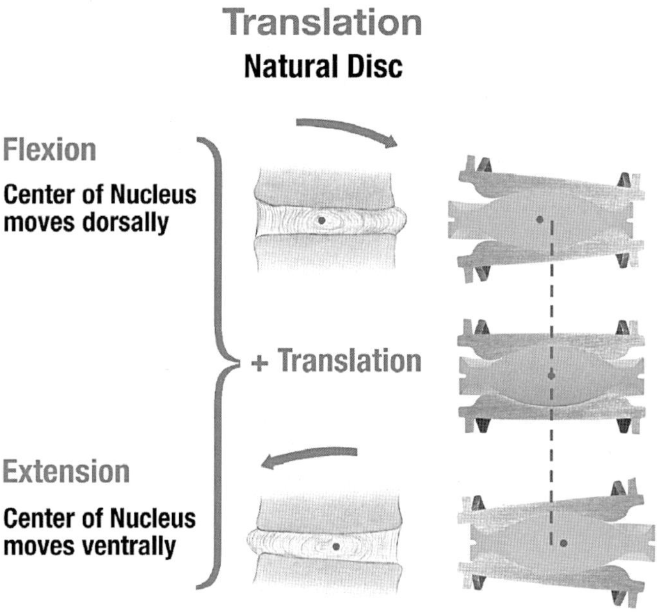

Fig. 8 SB Charité artificial disc showing rotation and translation

physiologic/mechanically unfavorable stresses. Flexion, for instance, combines [7, 9]:

1. Upward sliding movement of inferior articular processes
2. Tension of zygapophysial joint capsule
3. Tension of ligaments of intervertebral joint: (i) supraspinous and interspinous ligament, (ii) ligamentum flava
4. Contribution of longissimus thoracis pars lumborum muscle

Adams et al. calculated that the disc contributes 29% of resistance to flexion, while the capsule contributes 39% and the ligaments 32% [1]. Consequently, one can state that capsule and ligaments together dominate the action of movement. Thus the soft tissue structures under high stress must have a compensating counter element in the anterior vertebral column to avoid strain and noxious movement. In the natural disc it is the nucleomobility, in the SB Charité this compensating element is the unconstrained sliding core.

Joint replacement in diarthrodial joints has led this approach to mimicking physiologic movement. For instance, mobile bearing knee designs offer the advantage [19] of maximum conformal geometry, while protecting the interface between bone and implant from high stress, and by following the pattern of movement that the ligaments dictate, they offer advantages in cases of component malalignment.

And just like the contemporary mobile bearing knee designs (Fig. 9), the SB Charité artificial disc has a mobile sliding core which, in its degree of mobility, defines the required interaction between soft tissues, facet joints and

Fig. 9 Just like the contemporary "mobile bearing" knee designs, the SB Charité artificial disc has a "mobile sliding core"

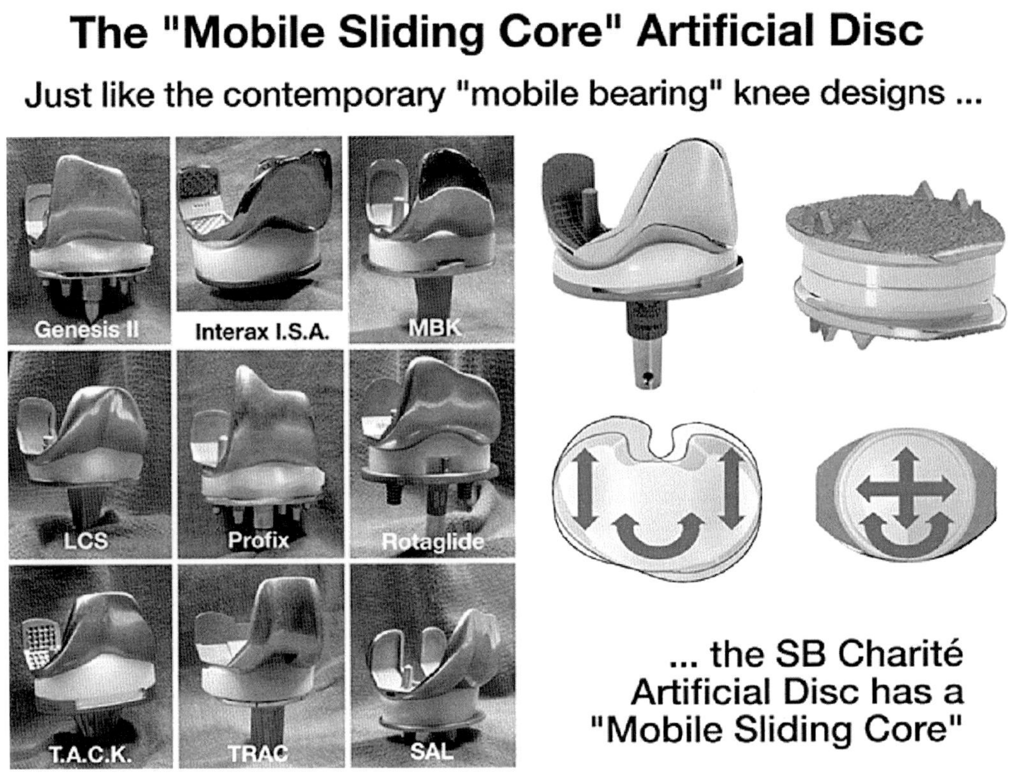

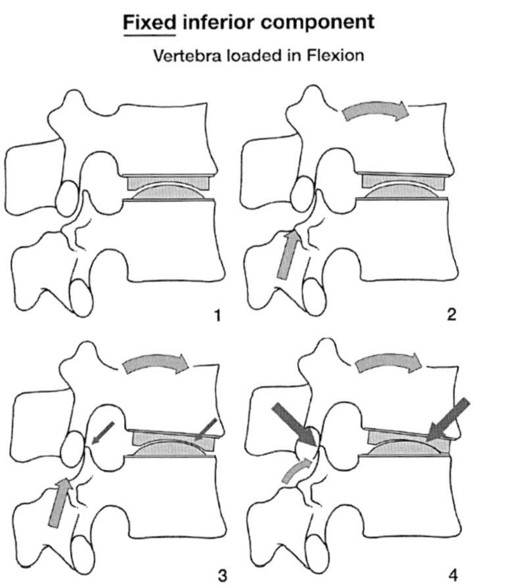

Fig. 10 Fixed inferior component: vertebra loaded in flexion

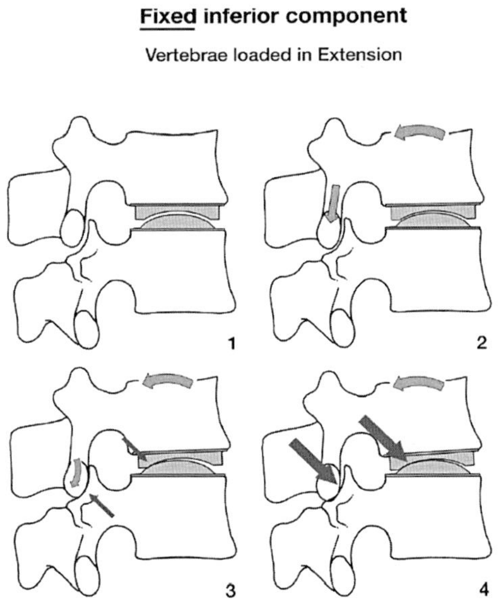

Fig. 11 Fixed inferior component: vertebra loaded in extension

implant geometry, to maintain a stable articulation and thus a physiologic restoration of the lumbar segment.

If the vertebra were loaded in flexion and the artificial disc's components allowed no translational movements, what would happen to the zygapophysial joints? The answer is: impingement and stress rising ... due to the inability of the disc's intermediate components to move posteriorly (Fig. 10).

In extension similar kinematics apply in reverse sequence (Fig. 11).

Nature has used the simple ball and socket joint in the vertebra, but only in species where weight bearing is not important, for example in fish, and just to provide mobility of the vertebral column. Wherever weight bearing is important, intervertebral adjustment is required to compensate for the rocking movements of the vertebrae [7].

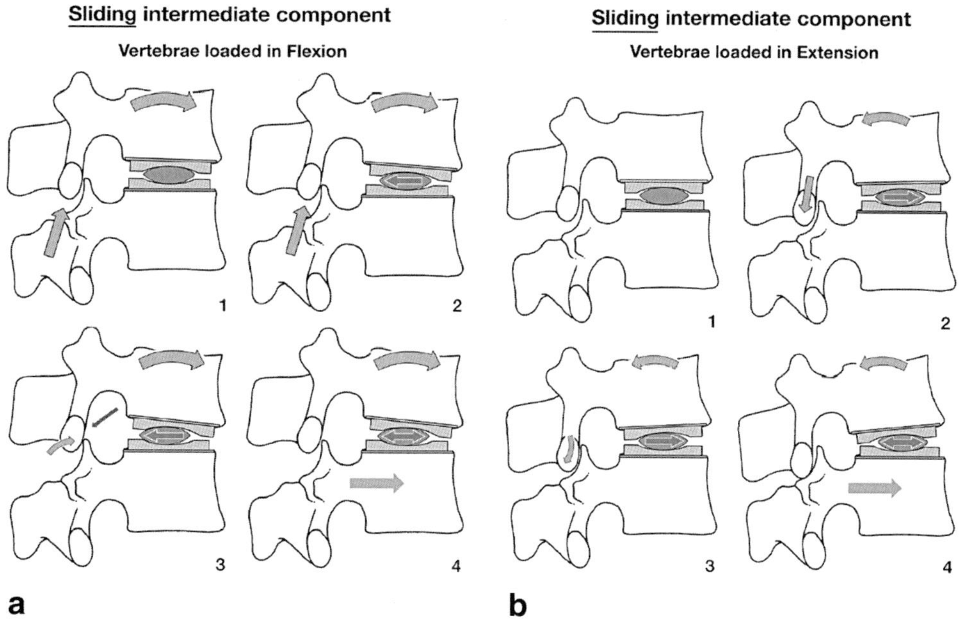

Fig. 12 **A** Sliding intermediate component: vertebrae loaded in flexion. **B** Sliding intermediate component: vertebrae loaded in extension

In a biomechanically sound artificial disc set-up, a sliding component would give way, allowing adjustment of the two adjacent vertebral bodies to each other and avoiding stress risers in the zygapophysial joints (Fig. 12).

Proper biomechanical function and the best possible relationship between anterior (implant loaded) and posterior elements requires, of course, correct implant positioning, which means central positioning in the sagittal and coronal planes. This is one of the basic requirements for successful disc replacement, and is especially necessary to avoid facet problems, as clinical follow-up reports have documented [12, 15, 16, 21, 22].

Biomechanical testing

Several biomechanical tests have been performed with the SB Charité artificial disc. As no mechanical problems with the cobalt-chrome endplates have ever been reported, tests concentrated on the endurance of the UHMWPE sliding core [2, 3, 4].

The University of Kiel as well as the Orthopedic Research Laboratory of the Mt. Sinai Medical Center in Cleveland/Ohio independently performed FDA- (Food and Drug Administration)- required dynamic tests under similar conditions: sliding cores size 2 (second smallest size), 7.5 and 9.5 mm in height were tested with 2.5- and 4.5(!)-kN loads.

Kiel concluded: "None of the specimens tested failed," and "For all testing phases and loads, the creep rates were found to be low" [17]. Cleveland stated: "...under normal in vivo conditions the permanent deformation of the core is not expected to reduce the available articulating surface or result in premature failure of the device due to significant cold-flow or delamination" [28].

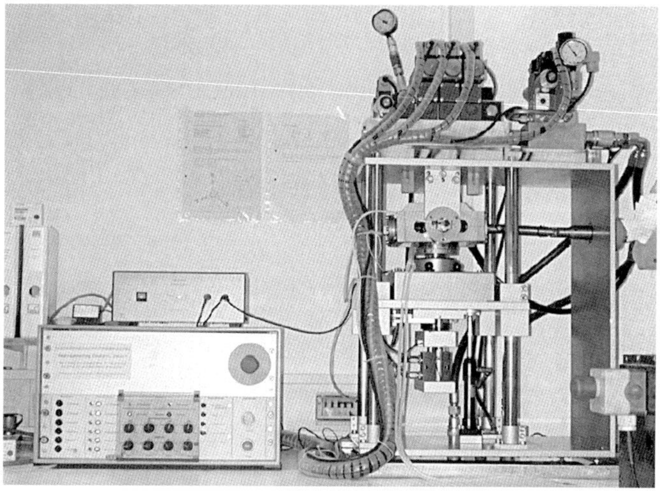

Fig. 13 Simulator test set-up at the Laboratory for Biomechanic Testing, Munich

Most recently, a functional 10 million cycles simulator test was performed at the Laboratory for Biomechanical Testing Grosshadern/Munich (Fig. 13).

The report stated: "An extremely mild abrasive wear was recorded, of negligible volume..." and, "The result of this tribologic investigation is considered to be very positive, especially in light of the 10 million cycles and the demanding test set-up" [20].

Clinical experiences have confirmed the results of such tests. Staudte as well as Zeegers reported that no polyethylene wear particles were detected when surrounding tissues taken during revisions were histomorphologically examined, provided the implants had been properly sized and implanted (personal communications, H-W Staudte/W Zeegers, 1998).

Whether or not wear debris is produced due to improper size or position, progressive bone lysis as seen in patients with aseptic loosening of joint replacements in diarthrodial joints is still unlikely, and has not been reported. This is most probably due to the absence of synovial membrane in the intervertebral joint [29].

Such bone resorbing factors as interleukin-1 (IL-1), interleukin-6 (IL-6), tumor necrosis factor-X (TNF-X), prostaglandin E_2 (PGE_2) and collagenase are produced by activated macrophages and fibroblasts [6, 13, 26]. As the synoviocyte-containing membrane, resembling macrophages and fibroblasts, is not present in amphiarthrosis [A], it can be hypothesized that such synovial absence is the reason for the absence of the "particle disease" in the intervertebral space.

To avoid cold-flow of the polyethylene core, it is important to always choose the largest possible size of implant and to use the appropriately angled endplates, so that the internal surfaces of the endplates encase the UHMWPE sliding core in a parallel fashion, thus distributing the forces evenly.

Conclusion

Biomechanical tests and more than 10 years of clinical experience at various centers have demonstrated that the LINK SB Charité artificial disc is a safe and effective operative treatment for pain of discogenic origin, provided the indications are right, the recommended intervention techniques are followed and implant choice is appropriate.

References

1. Adams MA, Hutton WC, Stott JRR (1980) The resistance to flexion of the lumbar intervertebral joint. Spine 5: 245–253
2. Ahrens J (1997) In vitro evaluation of the LINK SB Charité intervertebral prosthesis: stability biomechanical testing project. Final report. Institute for Spine & Biomedical Research, Plano
3. Ahrens JE (1999) Mechanical evaluation of the SB Charité artificial disc: estimation of permanent deformation. Texas Health Research Institute, Plano
4. Ahrens JE, Phansalkar A (1998) Mechanical evaluation of the SB Charité Artificial Disc static testing, Research Project Report. Texas Health Research Institute, Plano/Texas
5. Ahrens J, Shelokov AP, Carver JL (1998) Normal joint mobilities maintained with an artificial disc prosthesis. Lecture at the International Society for the Study of the Lumbar Spine, Brussels. ISSLS, Toronto
6. Archibeck MJ, Jacobs JJ, Roebuck KA, Glant TT (2000) The basic science of periprosthetic osteolysis. J Bone Joint Surg 82:1478–1489
7. Bogduk N (1999) Clinical anatomy of the lumbar spine and sacrum. Churchill Livingstone, pp 7, 8, 13, 36
8. Bogduk N (2000) Klinische Anatomie von Lendenwirbelsäule und Sakrum: Rehabilitation und Präventation, Chap 57. Springer, Berlin Heidelberg New York, pp 139–143
9. Buckwalter, JA, Einhorn TA, Simon SR (eds) (2000) Orthopaedic Basic Science. Am Acad Orthop Surg pp 769, 772
10. Büttner-Janz K (1992) The development of the artificial disc SB Charité. Hundley & Ass, Dallas, pp 12, 13
11. Büttner-Janz K, Schellnack K (1990) Bandscheibenendoprothetik, Entwicklungsweg und gegenwärtiger Stand. Beitr Orthop Traumatol 3:137–147
12. Büttner-Janz K, Shelokow AP, Hommel H, Ahrens JE, Zeegers W, Lemaire J-P (1997) Langzeiterfahrung mit der LINK-Zwischenwirbelendoprothese SB Charité. Therapie des Bandscheibenvorfalls (Matzen). 5. Symposium Wirbelsäulenchirurgie, Kloster Banz
13. Chiba J, Maloney WJ, Inoue K, Rubash HE (2001) Biomechanical analyses of human macrophages activated by polyethylene particles retrieved from interface membranes after failed total hip arthroplasty. J Arthroplasty 16 [Suppl 1]:101–105
14. David T (1999) Complications and results on 85 patients with a minimum of five years follow-up. EFORT, Brussels
15. David T (2001) Ten years or more follow-up with the LINK SB Charité artificial disc: 17 patients. J Arthroplasty 16 [Suppl 1]:101-105
16. El-Assuity W, Norris H, Hughes D, Persilege C, Ross R (2002) Medium term outcome using Charité III disc prosthesis. Poster presentation, British Spine Society Meeting, Birmingham, UK
17. Es-Souni M (1999) Testing of the polyethylene core; Charité Model III. Test report. Fachhochschule Kiel
18. Gertzbein SD, Seligman J, Holtby R, Chan KW, Ogston N, Kapasouri A, Tile M (1986) Centrode characteristics of the lumbar spine as a function of segmental instability. Clin Orthop 208: 48–51
19. Heim CS, Postak PD, Plaxton NA, Greenwald AS (2001) Classification of mobile bearing knee design: mobility and constraint. Monogr Orthop Res Labs Cleveland, Ohio
20. Huber J (2000) Zwischenwirbel-Endoprothese Modell SB Charité, Simulatorprüfung. Test report. Labor für Biomechanik und Experimentelle Orthopädie, Prüfstelle für Implantate, Ludwig-Maximilians University, Munich
21. Lemaire JP (2000) Intervertebral disc prosthesis: 42 cases with a follow-up over 10 years. Second Annual Meeting of the Spine Society of Europe, October 2000, Antwerp
22. Lemaire JP, Skali W, Lavaste F, Templier A, Mendes F, Dop A, Sauty V, Laloux E (1997) Intervertebral disc prosthesis. Clin Orthop 337:64–76
23. Liefeith K, Hildebrand G, Schade R, Szmukler-Moncler S, Neumann HG (2000) In vitro and in vivo evaluation of a fully resorbable calcium phosphate coating deposited on TPS coated implants. Third International Essen Symposium of the Working Group on Biomaterials and Tissue Compatibility, University of Essen
24. McAfee PC, Cunningham BW, Dmitriev AE, et al (2000) Biologic study of ingrowth-SB Charité. Investigational Device Exemption Investigators meeting, New Orleans
25. McAfee PC, Cunningham BW, Dmitriev AE, Sefter JC, Fedder I L (2001) Analysis of the Link SB Charité Intervertebral Disc Spacer for total disc replacement: a non-human primate model. Eighth International Meeting on Advanced Spine Techniques (IMAST), Atlantis, Bahamas

26. Müller-Ladner U, Gay RE, Gay S (1997) Structure and function of synoviocytes. In: Koopman WJ (ed) Arthritis and allied conditions: a textbook of rheumatology. Williams & Wilkins, Philadelphia, pp 243–254
27. Pearcy MJ, Bogduk N (1988) Instantaneous axes of rotation of the lumbar intervertebral joints. Spine 13:1033–1041
28. Postak DP (1999) Evaluation of the time-dependent displacement of the SB Charité UHMWPE sliding core. Test Report 04–0900–0399, Orthopedic Research Laboratories, Mount Sinai Medical Centre, Cleveland
29. Sibbitt Jr WL (1999) The normal and the diseased joint. In: Bronner F, Worrel RV (eds) Principles of basic and clinical science. CRC Press, Boca Raton, pp 141–163

Stephen H. Hochschuler
Donna D. Ohnmeiss
Richard D. Guyer
Scott L. Blumenthal

Artificial disc: preliminary results of a prospective study in the United States

S.H. Hochschuler (✉) · D.D. Ohnmeiss · R.D. Guyer · S.L. Blumenthal
Texas Back Institute,
Musculoskeletal Research Corporation,
Texas Health Research Institute,
6300 W. Parker Road, Plano, TX 75093, USA
e-mail: shochschuler@texasback.com,
Tel.: +1-972-6085022,
Fax: +1-972-6085020

Abstract Artificial discs have been used in Europe for many years with good results. This technology has recently been available in the United States on a limited, investigational basis. The purpose of this study is to review the preliminary results of one center's experience using the SB Charité III disc replacement. The study group consisted of the series of our first consecutive 56 patients who received the Link SB Charité III artificial disc. There were 25 men and 31 women, with a mean age of 39.9 years. All patients had single-level symptomatic disc disruption at L4-5 or L5-S1. The discs were implanted using the same approach as used for mini-open anterior lumbar interbody fusion procedures. The primary data recorded included visual analog scales (VAS) assessing pain and the Oswestry Disability Questionnaire. Data were collected pre-operatively and at 6 weeks, 3 months, 6 months, and 12 months post-operatively. Peri-operative data as well as complications were recorded. At the time of this preliminary study, 22 patients have reached the 12-month post-operative follow-up period. There was a significant improvement in the VAS and Oswestry scores at the 6-week follow-up period. These improvements were maintained throughout the 12-month follow-up period. The preliminary results of this prospective study indicate that the artificial disc yields significant improvement that is maintained during a 12-month follow-up. Data from more patients and with longer follow-up are needed to determine whether these results can be maintained in the long term.

Keywords Artificial disc · Spinal arthroplasty · Prospective study · Lumbar spine

Introduction

In some areas of orthopedics, implants are commonly used that restore or closely mimic the normal motion of joints. The need for such in spine has long been recognized. There is a great desire to restore the motion of the spinal segment rather than fusing it, which is currently the primary operative treatment for several painful spinal conditions. The first attempts at disc replacement were prompted by a desire to fill the disc space after a discectomy had been performed. This was done to restore the disc height and help avoid problems related to further degeneration of the operated segment. The concept of total disc replacement evolved much later, and is now generally thought of as a replacement for spinal fusion. While total disc replacement and interbody fusion are used to treat the same symptomatic pathology, an artificial disc is used to mimic the loading and motion characteristics of the normal intervertebral disc. Not only does this allow more normal motion of the spine, but it avoids the potential problem of pseudoarthrosis and does not put additional demands on the adjacent segments, particularly with bending. With time, the additional load may lead to breakdown of the disc adjacent to the fusion, requiring further treatment.

Total disc replacements have been used in Europe for more than a decade. The first total disc replacement to emerge into widespread use was the SB Charité (Waldermar Link). The first and second developmental designs of this device were implanted in the mid-1980s, only at the Charité Clinic in East Berlin of the former East Germany, and were not commercially available. With these designs, there were problems with implant migration, damage to a vertebral body, and compression of the implant [1]. The SB Charité III, a third design of the artificial disc, was made commercially available in 1987 and remains in use worldwide today. There have been several studies reporting the clinical results when using this device. Although the outcome measures in the various studies differ, the rate of good to excellent outcome rages from 63% to 75% [2, 3, 6, 8, 9]. The purpose of this study was to describe our preliminary results using the artificial disc in a prospective study with rigid inclusion criteria.

Materials and methods

The data for this study are from one center participating in the FDA (Food and Drug Administration) regulated IDE (investigational device exemption) study being performed to investigate the safety and efficacy of devices prior to their being available for general use. The large-scale IDE study is a prospective, randomized, multicenter study, with an enrollment goal of approximately 300 patients. Patients are randomized to receive either the artificial disc or BAK threaded fusion cages (Sulzer SpineTech). This was selected as a comparison group, since interbody fusion is currently the primary treatment available for disc-related pain unresponsive to non-operative treatment. The randomization is weighted with a 2:1 ratio of artificial disc to fusion cages. Also, each surgeon performed artificial disc operations prior to the randomization, to gain experience with the operative technique. Approval to conduct the study was given by the FDA, and by each participating center's Institutional Review Board (IRB). Due to the relatively small number of BAK patients at our facility, this report is limited to our experience with the artificial disc. Future reports will include comparative data with the fusion group.

Study inclusion criteria are:

1. Age of 18–60 years
2. Symptomatic single-level degenerative disc disease at the L4-5 or L5-S1 level confirmed by plain radiographs, magnetic resonance imaging (MRI), and provocative discography
3. Oswestry score of at least 30, and a pain score on the visual analog scale (VAS) of at least 40
4. Failure to achieve pain relief after at least 6 months of non-operative care
5. Primary complaints of back pain with or without pseudoradicular pain passing into the lower extremities, and
6. Being willing and able to give written informed consent

Exclusion criteria are:

1. Objective evidence of nerve root compression
2. Straight leg raise producing pain below the knee
3. Spinal fracture, bone disease, spondylolysis, spondylolisthesis, scoliosis, spinal tumor, or severe facet joint arthrosis, and
4. Being more than one standard deviation greater than normal body weight

Data were collected prior to surgery, peri-operatively, and at 6 weeks, 3 months, 6 months, and 12 months post-operatively (24-month data are currently being collected). Outcome data were collected, including the visual analog scale (VAS) assessing pain and the Oswestry Disability Questionnaire [5].

This study is based on the consecutive series of our center's first 56 patients who received the SB Charité III prosthesis. The group consisted of 25 men and 31 women. The mean age was 39.9 years, ranging from 19 to 59 years. The prosthesis was used at the L5-S1 level in 44 patients and at the L4-5 level in the remaining 12 patients. Twenty-two patients have reached the 12-month follow-up period.

Operative technique

The approach to the spine for disc replacement surgery is very similar to the mini-open approach we have used for anterior lumbar interbody fusion for many years. The three surgeons participating in this study all had extensive experience with anterior lumbar interbody fusion prior to implanting an artificial disc. In order to achieve proper prosthetic placement, patient positioning is critical. Fluoroscopic imaging is used to ensure that the spinous process is vertical and the pedicles are perpendicular to the spinous process. A general surgeon performs the procedure to gain access to the spine. The incision is approximately 4–5 cm in length. After the general surgeon has achieved access to the spine, disc tissue is removed from the disc space. The spreader instrument is used to distract the disc space. The endplate size is selected with the goal of covering as much of the vertebral body endplate as possible. This aids in avoiding subsidence. Endplate gauges, which are the same sizes as the prosthetic endplates, but without anchoring teeth, are used to determine the desired size of the implant to be used. The obliquities of the prosthetic endplates are selected so that the inner surfaces of the plates are parallel. In some cases, it is necessary to smooth the vertebral body endplates slightly to allow more contact area with the prosthesis. However, care should be taken to avoid damage to the endplates. Ideal positioning of the device is in the center of the disc space when viewed on the anteroposterior image. The ideal position of the device in the lateral view is approximately 2 mm posterior to the sagittal midline of the vertebral body. One must check to confirm that the prosthetic endplates are placed in the insertion device correctly: that is, with the more narrow edge of the prosthesis passing into the posterior section of the disc space, and the thicker, oblique edge being located in the anterior portion of the disc space. It is helpful to use a "breakable" operating table. During the prosthesis implantation, the table should be cracked open to allow easier introduction of the device. The spreading and insertion forceps, loaded with the prosthetic endplates, are maneuvered into the disc space. After assessing the location of the endplates with regard to their location in the lateral view, the forceps are opened and adjusted using a set of spacers. The height of the polyethylene core to be used is determined by using trial cores. After the appropriate size is determined, a core is placed in the core insertion instrument and positioned between the prosthetic endplates. The forceps are gradually released, lowering onto the core. The core insertion instrument is removed and the core position is confirmed with imaging. The forceps are then removed. A final image is obtained to verify correct placement of the endplates and core. The wound is closed in the same fashion as after open anterior fusion.

Patients are discharged from the hospital with a home exercise program. They are encouraged to be cautiously active. They are instructed to walk a few blocks up the street several times a day. Then they are to progress to several miles. After the first few weeks following surgery, patients begin participation in a rehabilitation program incorporating conditioning, motion, and strengthening.

Results

The mean operative blood loss during the disc implantation procedures was 134.3 cc. The mean operative time

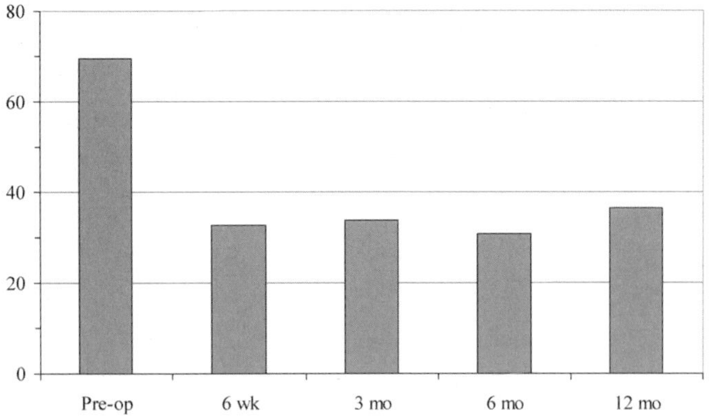

Fig. 1 The mean VAS scores pre-operatively and at the various time periods post-operatively

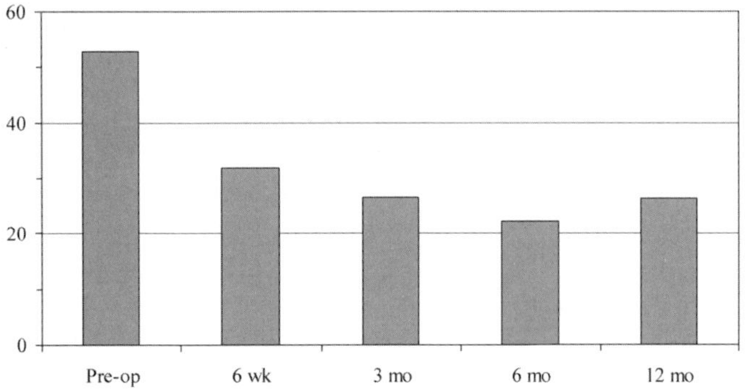

Fig. 2 The mean Oswestry scores pre-operatively and at the various time periods post-operatively

was 78.7 min, ranging from 45 to 165 min. Operative time decreased with the number of cases performed.

As presented in Fig. 1, there was a 52.7% improvement in the mean VAS pain score at the time of the 6-week follow-up. This improvement was statistically significant ($P<0.05$; paired *t*-test) and was maintained throughout the 12-month follow-up period. A similar pattern was noted in the Oswestry disability scores (Fig. 2). There was a 39.6% improvement in Oswestry disability scores at the 6-week follow-up, with slightly more improvement between the 6-week and 3-month follow-up periods. The improvements from the pre-operative values were statistically significant ($P<0.05$; paired *t*-test). In our series, there have been no cases of device fracture or dislocation.

Case report

This patient was a 46-year-old man who presented with a 15-month history of back pain following a severe automobile accident. He did not complain of lower extremity pain. He worked at an Internet business. He had undergone a course of physical therapy and epidural steroid injections that failed to give him adequate pain relief. His physical examination was negative for nerve root compression. Review of his MRI examination showed a degenerated L5-S1 disc with a high-intensity zone posteriorly (Fig. 3). Presented in Fig. 4 are the discogram and the computed tomography (CT)/discogram of the L5-S1 level, showing significant posterior spread of the contrast. The injection provoked pain concordant with the patient's back pain. The artificial disc study was described to the patient and he consented to participate. The operative time was 96 min and the estimated blood loss was 200 cc. Pre-operatively, the patient was working only part time. Post-operatively, he returned to work full time. His pre-operative VAS score was 58 (of 100) and his Oswestry score was 46%. By the 3-month follow-up, both scores had dropped to less than 10. The patient's flexion and extension radiographs made at 12-month follow-up are shown in Fig. 5B, and demonstrate motion at the operated segment.

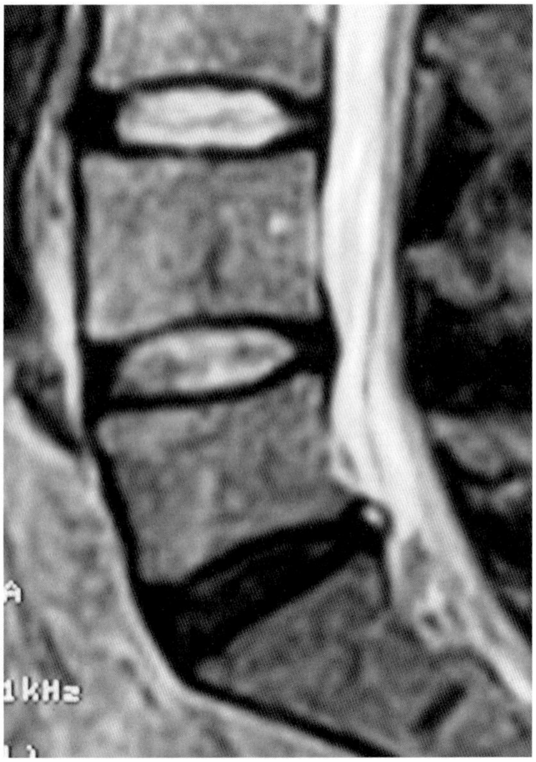

Fig. 3 Magnetic resonance image showing degeneration of the L5-S1 space and a high-intensity zone

Discussion

The results of this study are encouraging and support the artificial disc as a viable treatment option. However, it should be noted that these are the preliminary results on a subgroup of patients participating in a multicenter study. Two-year follow-up data are being collected at all the centers as patients reach that follow-up point. After all the data have been collected, a comparison with the fusion group can be made. The current study is the first prospective report in the literature on a consecutive series of patients undergoing disc replacement. The study design allowed us to make comparisons between the patients' pre-operative and post-operative conditions using standardized

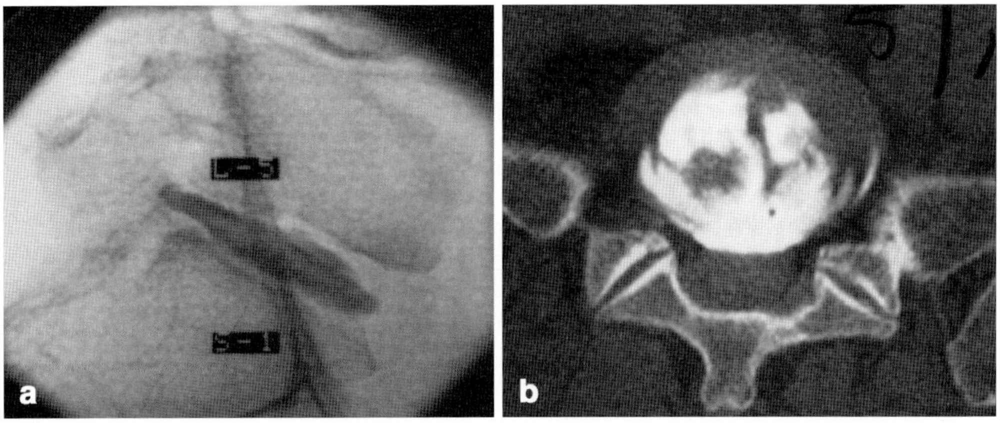

Fig. 4 The pre-operative discogram (**A**) and computed tomography/discogram (**B**) demonstrating significant spread of the contrast posteriorly at the L5-S1 disc level

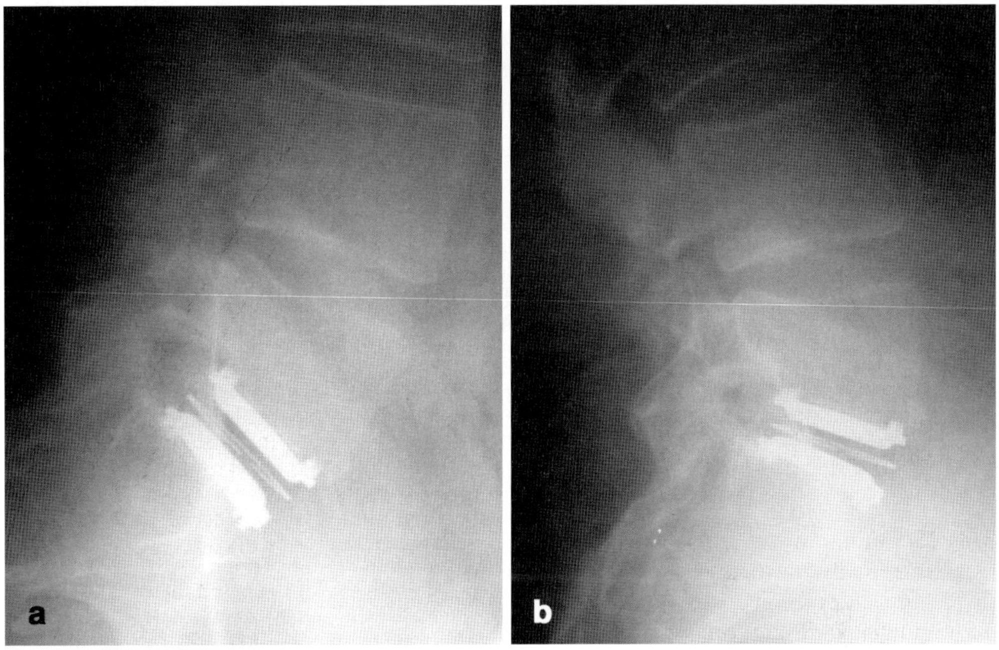

Fig. 5A,B Flexion and extension radiographs made at the patient's 1-year follow-up appointment. There is clear motion at the level with the disc prosthesis

outcome assessments. Significant improvements were seen in these measures at the time of 6-week post-operative follow-up. These improvements were maintained during the 12-month follow-up period. These results support those from earlier retrospective European studies reporting favorable outcomes [2, 3, 6, 8, 9].

The European experience with total disc replacement has provided valuable knowledge concerning the ideal device size and placement, as well as refining the insertion technique for the device. Also, the data supporting early participation in active rehabilitation [2] have been valuable in designing our rehabilitation program for disc replacement patients. Although the indications and approach to the spine are very similar to those used for anterior interbody fusion, the need to restrict motion following surgery is not needed. Instead, patients are taught to engage in gentle bending motions soon after the spinal arthroplasty procedure.

There have been very few reports in the literature for other designs of artificial discs. Enker et al. reported their experience with a disc composed of two titanium endplates with a rubber core fused between them [4]. They implanted the device in six patients. Four of the six patients had satisfactory results, one device failed, and one other patient had no pain relief after surgery. This device was abandoned due to concerns about possible carcinogenic materials in the rubber. A new version of this disc is currently undergoing testing. The ProDisc (Spinal Solutions) has been used in Europe for approximately 10 years. It is composed of two titanium endplates with a fixed polyethylene core between them. The inferior surface of the core is flat, and its edges fit into ridges on the inferior device endplate. Motion occurs by articulation of only the upper plate on the convex superior surface of the constrained core. There has been little published on the results of this device. Marnay reported 8- to 10-year follow-up results on a group of 44 patients who received this prosthesis [7]. A good/excellent result was noted in 78% of these patients.

In our own experience, as well as that reported in the long-term follow-up studies from Europe, the artificial disc designs that allow motion by articulation of bi-convex surfaces have not had technical failures [2, 3, 6, 7, 8, 9]. No problems with wear debris have been identified in clinical or biomechanical studies [1, 2, 3, 6, 7, 8, 9].

Traditional factors dealing with patient selection and surgical skills remain true for disc replacement. Surgery should only be considered after the patient has failed an appropriate course of non-operative treatment including medication, activity modification, and active rehabilitation. Patients with poor psychological profiles are poor candidates for disc replacement. Surgeons must be trained appropriately in the indications and contraindications for disc replacement. Also, surgeons must undergo appropriate training in the operative technique and use of the instrumentation.

The results of this study support the European experience that disc replacement surgery is a promising treatment. Patients on whom this report was based will be followed for a longer period of time. Also, these data will be combined with those from the other centers participating in the multicenter trial. The final results from that large-scale study will provide more information about the performance of the disc compared to spinal fusion.

Acknowledgements The authors would like to recognize our fellow investigators for their collaborative work in this multicenter study: Paul McAfee, MD; Richard Holt, MD; Rolando Garcia, MD; Jorge Isaza, MD; Doug Wong, MD; Bradford Mullin, MD; Michael McNamara, MD; James Maxwell, MD; Fabien Bitan, MD; Fred Geisler, MD; Ted Goldstein, MD; Andy Cappuccino, MD; and Robert Banco, MD.

References

1. Büttner-Janz K (1992) The development of the artificial disc: SB Charité. Hundley & Associates, Dallas
2. Cinotti G, David T, Postacchini F (1996) Results of disc prosthesis after a minimum follow-up period of 2 years. Spine 21:995–1000
3. David TJ (2000) Lumbar disc prosthesis: five years follow-up study on 96 patients. Presented at the Annual Meeting of the North American Spine Society, New Orleans
4. Enker P, Steffee A, McMillin C, Keppler L, Biscup R, Miller S (1993) Artificial disc replacement. Preliminary report with a 3-year minimum follow-up. Spine 18:1061–1070
5. Fairbank JCT, Couper J, Davies JB, O'Brien JP (1980) The Oswestry Low Back Pain Disability Questionnaire. Physiotherapy 66:271–273
6. Lemaire JP, Skalli W, Lavaste F, Templier A, Mendes F, Diop A, Sauty V, Laloux E (1997) Intervertebral disc prosthesis. Results and prospects for the year 2000. Clin Orthop 337:64–76
7. Marnay T (2001) Lumbar disc arthroplasty, 8–10 year results using titanium plates with a polyethylene inlay component. Presented at the Spine Arthroplasty conference, Munich
8. Sott AH, Harrison DJ (2000) Increasing age does not affect good outcome after lumbar disc replacement. Int Orthop 24: 50–53
9. Zeegers WS, Bohnen LM, Laaper M, Verhaegen MJ (1999) Artificial disc replacement with the modular type SB Charite III: 2-year results in 50 prospectively studied patients. Eur Spine J 8: 210–217

Karin Büttner-Janz

Optimal minimally traumatic approach for the SB Charité™ Artificial Disc

K. Büttner-Janz (✉)
VIVANTES Klinikum Hellersdorf,
Orthopädische Klinik,
Myslowitzer Straße 45,
12621 Berlin, Germany
e-mail: orthopaedie@kh-hellersdorf.de,
Tel.: +49-30-56512180,
Fax: +49-30-56512678

Abstract The skin incisions and minimally traumatic approaches required for the optimal dissection of the intervertebral space and thereby for the correct implantation of the LINK® SB Charité™ Artificial Disc are described.

Keywords Skin incision · Approach · Double level

Introduction

Modern surgery aims at minimally traumatic approaches that bear the smallest possible risks. Patients expect surgery to exclude complications and produce a cosmetically acceptable scar. These objectives for surgery also apply to the minimally invasive approach used during implantation of the LINK® SB Charité™ Artificial Disc, which is described in this paper.

Preparation for surgery

The SB Charité™ Disc is implanted via an anterior retroperitoneal approach. The patient is placed supine on a level operating table. An operating table that can be adjusted during the operation to place the patient in hyper- or hypolordosis is preferred. Where the intervertebral space is extremely narrow or where bisegmental implantation is planned, such a table ensures that there is sufficient space for impacting the prosthesis.

Before antimicrobial preparation of the patient's skin, one should determine whether placing the C-arm at the appropriate angle will later permit intraoperative radiographs of the affected segment in a true anteroposterior (AP) projection. The surgeon consults the AP radiograph to determine the topography of the affected disc in relation to the iliac crest, which usually is partially imaged. On the sagittal and transverse magnetic resonance (MR) images, the surgeon evaluates the abnormal findings that correlate with the patient's complaints and clinical symptoms, and inspects the level that will undergo surgery.

Variations of skin incisions

The LINK® SB Charité™ Artificial Disc can replace the entire lumbar disc in any of the segments from L2-3 through to the pre-sacral motion segment. The prosthesis with the greatest possible surface area should always be implanted. First and foremost, this requires choosing the optimum site for the skin incision. The incision for monosegmental implantation normally ranges between 5 cm and 7 cm, depending on the patient's body size and the thickness of the subcutaneous layer. For bisegmental implantation in two adjacent segments, the skin incision is approximately 8–9 cm long.

The surgeon traces the planned incision from the AP radiograph directly onto the patient and, after palpating the iliac crest, places this incision so that the affected L4-5

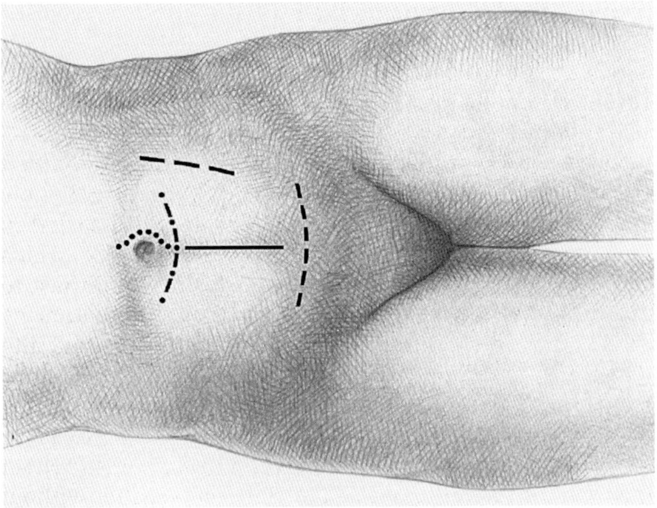

Fig. 1 Variations of the skin incisions. The *solid line* indicates the preferred incision

or L5-S1 segment lies directly in the middle of a skin incision carried from superior to inferior. When operating on the L2-3 or L3-4 segments, the skin incision is extended distally to gain distal access to the retroperitoneal space. Alternatively, when operating on the L2-3 or L3-4 segments or in patients who have undergone previous surgery, one may follow a modified procedure after exposing the posterior rectus sheath (see below). Of course, the position of the skin incision may also be determined on a lateral fluoroscopic image, where the surgeon simultaneously marks the skin.

Figure 1 shows the various options for making the skin incision. Pfannenstiel's incision is only suitable for the pre-sacral segment. We favour a median longitudinal incision along the linea alba inferior to the umbilicus. Depending on the affected level, the incision may be extended superiorly around the umbilicus. Alternatively, one may choose to make a straight or slightly curved transverse incision inferior to the umbilicus and directly anterior to the affected segment. The curved incision more closely follows the skin cleavage lines and may be expected to produce the most inconspicuous, cosmetically acceptable scar.

Surgical approach

After the skin incision is made, the subcutaneous tissue superficial to the linea alba is dissected longitudinally. In patients undergoing their first anterior spinal procedure, we expose the linea alba and then continue with a left lateral blunt dissection to expose the medial region of the anterior rectus sheath. This sheath is then incised longitudinally, approximately along the medial margin of the muscle belly of the left rectus. Now the entire muscle belly is bluntly dissected laterally to the left as far as the junction between the anterior rectus sheath and posterior rectus sheath. Mobilizing the muscle belly may occasionally require dividing some of the medial tendinous intersections of the rectus abdominis.

The inferior margin of the posterior rectus sheath is exposed with the finger near its lateral junction with the anterior sheath. Then the peritoneum and visceral sac are carefully bluntly dissected medially and slightly superiorly away from the posterior aspect of the posterior rectus sheath. Taking care to protect the peritoneum, a longitudinal incision is made in the posterior sheath. The length of this incision depends on the affected segment. It is often not necessary to incise the posterior sheath for an implantation at L5-S1.

When implanting a prosthesis at L2-3 or L3-4, it is not necessary to expose the inferior margin of the posterior sheath. The posterior sheath can be slightly lifted directly adjacent to the lateral junction of the two sheaths with two blunt forceps and then carefully incised longitudinally. This immediately exposes the peritoneum, which, together with the visceral sac, is then mobilized off the posterior sheath and retracted medially. Now it is possible to gradually incise the posterior sheath longitudinally and continue on through the retroperitoneal fat tissue. This dissection is also successful where previous retroperitoneal surgery makes it impossible to expose the inferior margin of the posterior sheath and gain access to the retroperitoneum.

Further dissection in the deeper posterior planes is performed directly through the retroperitoneal fat tissue using blunt swabs or finger dissection. One should not dissect too far left and lateral through the retroperitoneal fat and connective tissue, as this increases the distance to the affected segment. To reach the affected segment directly, it is advisable to palpate the patient's iliac crest from time to time for better orientation and to avoid carrying the dissection too far inferiorly. After penetrating the retroperitoneal tissue, one can use the psoas muscle as a landmark. After it is reached, blunt dissection is continued to the right as far as the lumbar spine. Occasionally, the ureter will be visible (it typically will contract when palpated); it is always retracted to the right with the peritoneum.

In patients who have had previous retroperitoneal surgery in the left lower abdomen, the retroperitoneal approach may be made through the right lower abdomen. A transperitoneal approach can be chosen when a retroperitoneal approach in a previous procedure has caused adherence of fascial planes. In men, one should be aware of the risk of injury to the superior hypogastric plexus in the approach to the pre-sacral disc space, which could result in retrograde ejaculation.

Approach to L5-S1

After the sacral promontory has been identified by palpation, the dissection is continued with small swabs as far as the bifurcation of the major vessels. The tissue immediately superficial to the L5-S1 intervertebral disc is dissected off the disc toward both sides and superiorly to expose the median sacral artery and vein that course longitudinally across the L5-S1 disc. The number, position, and diameter of these vessels are highly variable. After sufficient exposure has been obtained, the medial sacral vessels are ligated and divided. Do not use cauterization in this area in male patients.

Further dissection is carried first to the left and then to the right to achieve the maximum possible lateral exposure of the disc. Special care should be taken to preserve the left and right common iliac vessels. Therefore, blunt dissection is performed with small swabs, beginning on the superior sacrum and extending to about 2 cm distal to the inferior margin of the intervertebral disc, and then laterally to the left and right. This makes it easier to mobilize the major vessels at the level of and superior to the intervertebral disc.

The surgeon begins the vascular dissection by bluntly mobilizing the left common iliac vein with small swabs and then the right common iliac artery together with the right common iliac vein that lies deep to it. All of these vessels are retracted laterally and occasionally slightly superiorly. The dissection should be carried to where the anterior surface merges with the lateral surface of the last lumbar vertebral body. Now four sharp Hohmann retractors or 3-mm Steinmann pins can be impacted into the adjacent vertebral bodies at a distance of approximately 1 cm to the superior and inferior margins of the disc. These retractors or pins are impacted nearly parallel to the vertebral endplates.

Each of the Hohmann retractors is placed such that its broad surface lies parallel to the course of the adjacent major vessels, taking care to ensure a broad area of contact between instrument and vessel to reduce the risk of thrombosis. If it hasn't been verified yet, the surgeon should check that the vertebral level is correct by fluoroscopy in the lateral view. If Hohmann retractors or Steinmann pins have not been impacted, a needle should be inserted into intervertebral disc L5 S1 to mark the site.

The intervertebral disc and anterior longitudinal ligament are vertically incised in the centre, and superior and inferior horizontal incisions are made close to the respective vertebral bodies. The two parts of the incised "H" shape of the annulus fibrosus are reflected laterally to the left and right like French windows to protect the vascular structures, and retaining sutures are passed through the raised flaps. Alternatively the flaps may be held with mosquito clamps. When the annulus fibrosus is later closed, the suture knot should lie between the major vessels.

Approach to L4-5 through L2-3

When implanting a prosthesis at L4-5, the surgeon, after first exposing the psoas muscle and digitally palpating the sacral promontory, exposes the lateral region of the L4-5 intervertebral disc directly at the medial margin of the left psoas by blunt dissection using small swabs. Usually, the sympathetic trunk is mobilized and partially dissected in the process. After identifying the intervertebral disc, which will appear as a prominent white structure in contrast to the vertebral body, one should verify proper location by fluoroscopy in the lateral view with a needle inserted into the disc.

The purpose of further dissection is to mobilize the major vessels, especially the left common iliac vein as far as its junction with the inferior vena cava, and to retract them as far laterally and to the right as possible without inducing vascular injury. Therefore, one first attempts to identify the left ascending lumbar vein, which lies directly on the vertebral body and communicates directly with the left common iliac vein. However, it is not possible to identify this vessel in every patient.

Where indicated, the left ascending lumbar vein is ligated and divided at a sufficient distance from the left common iliac vein. Ligation of this vein will be necessary where the surgeon finds the left ascending lumbar vein in the superior third of the L5 vertebral body or even at the level of the L4-5 disc. Occasionally, several small lumbar veins communicating with the left common iliac vein will be found in the superior portion of the L5 vertebral body. To prevent avulsion of these vessels from the left common iliac vein when that vessel is mobilized, they should be ligated and divided.

Then the soft tissue on the L4 vertebral body is mobilized from left to right, laterally, by blunt dissection in order to mobilize the major vessels for placement of retractors superior to the L4-5 disc space. Occasionally the lumbar vein and artery coursing transversely close to the vertebral body will have to be ligated and divided to allow sufficient mobilization of the major vessels to the right and lateral at the level of the disc. Using small swabs, one now carefully dissects the left common iliac vein anterior to the L5 vertebral body, proceeding laterally from left to right to where the anterior aspect of the L5 vertebral body and the L4-5 disc merges with the lateral aspect. Occasionally, venous bleeding from a small vessel in the L5 vertebral body will occur. This bleeding should be controlled by electrocautery or bone wax, taking care to protect the major vessels. Once the vessels have been sufficiently mobilized, a sharp Hohmann retractor or a 3-mm Steinmann pin is impacted into the L5 vertebra on the right. Then additional retractors or pins are impacted into L4 on the right, L4 on the left, and finally into L5 on the left if desired.

Dissection at the L3-4 and L2-3 intervertebral discs is performed in a similar manner. Our experience has shown that no problems are to be expected with the left renal vessels, which lie further superiorly. Compared with the L4-5 and L5-S1 segments, the vascular anatomy and dissection at L3-4 or L2-3 are usually far easier to master. In most cases, it will only be necessary to ligate and divide segmental lumbar arteries and veins.

The intervertebral disc and the anterior longitudinal ligament at the L4-5, L3-4, and L2-3 levels are incised vertically at a left lateral location, and superior and inferior horizontal incisions are made close to the respective vertebral bodies. When the annulus fibrosus is later closed, the suture knot should lie in a left lateral position to avoid contact with a major blood vessel.

Double-level approach

In a bisegmental operation with implantation of prostheses in segments L4-5 and L5-S1, it is best to dissect L5-S1 and implant the prosthesis at this level first. However, where the L4-5 intervertebral space is particularly narrow in comparison to L5-S1, the prosthesis should be implanted at the L4-5 level first. Where both affected levels are narrow and bisegmental implantation appears difficult, we recommend first completing the entire dissection of both levels before deciding which level should be treated first. The surgeon should implant the first prosthesis at the level that is narrower or more difficult due to the vascular anatomy. Usually the Hohmann retractors or Steinmann pins can be easily reinserted into the existing holes in the vertebral bodies after changing levels.

When levels L3-4 (or L2-3) and L4-5 are to receive implants, we recommend first implanting the prosthesis at L4-5, as the vascular dissection is usually more difficult at this level. When implants are to be placed at levels L3-4 (or L2-3) and L5-S1, one may complete the dissection of the disc spaces at both levels with the Hohmann retractors or Steinmann pins left in place and then decide where to implant the first prosthesis on the basis of how easily the respective intervertebral spaces can be distracted. Adjusting the operating table to induce lumbar hyperlordosis will facilitate initial insertion of the prosthesis. Final insertion should, however, be performed with the operating table level, to ensure that the prosthesis is implanted in a sufficiently posterior position.

The described skin incisions and minimally traumatic approaches are a prerequisite for the optimal dissection of the intervertebral space and thereby for the correct implantation of the LINK® SB Charité™ Artificial Disc.

J. C. Le Huec
S. Aunoble
T. Friesem
H. Mathews
T. Zdeblick

Maverick total lumbar disk prosthesis: biomechanics and preliminary clinical results

J. C. Le Huec (✉) · S. Aunoble
Départment orthopédie Pr D Chauveaux,
spine unit, CHU Pellegrin Tripode,
33076 Bordeaux cedex, France
Tel.: +33-556794956,
Fax: +33-556796089,
e-mail: j-c.lehuec@chu-bordeaux.fr

T. Friesem
University Hospital of North Tees,
Nardwick, Stockton on Tees,
TS 19 8PE, UK

H. Mathews
Mid-Atlantic Spine Specialists,
7650 Parham Road, Suite 200,
Richmond, VA 23294-4309

T. Zdeblick
Madison school of medecine,
Wisconsin, USA

Abstract The treatment of chronic low back pain due to advanced disk degeneration requires restabilization of the lumbar column, mainly by restoring disk function. Disk restabilization involves restoration and stabilization of the ligaments and annulus. Such restabilization represents a new concept [14, 29] in treating disk pathologies without the definitive loss of disk function [11, 13, 26]. Unlike fusion [20], the procedure is not definitive and makes it possible to restore function and mobility. Two prosthetic devices have now been on the market for about 10 years: the SB Charité [6, 8, 12, 15, 18, 27, 35], produced by Link, and the Prodisc [3, 30], manufactured by Spine Solution. This chapter looks at a new device, the Maverick disk prosthesis, which was developed according to biomechanical principles [21] and in the light of the biomechanical results obtained with the SB Charité and Prodisc. Preliminary results are promising.

Keywords Spine · Disc arthroplasty · Degenerative disc disease

The Maverick total lumbar disk device

The Maverick is a device with two metal parts that rub together according to the principle of a ball and socket. One part is therefore fixed inside the other (Fig. 1). The device rotates on a posterior center, in agreement with the biomechanical data reported by Dooris et al. [10]. According to that report [10], the posterior rotational center limits stress to the posterior facets during flexion, extension and lateral inclination. The center of the ball is situated below the vertebral endplate, allowing controlled automatic translation during flexion and extension (Fig. 2). This sort of controlled translation is not possible in the SB Charité [27] device, where a mobile core floats between two metal plates. The Maverick is anchored to the bone by a hydroxyapatite coating and a connector press-fitted into the vertebral body (Fig. 3).

Biomechanical analysis

Mobility and stiffness

Re-establishing disk mobility is one of the aims when using a disk prosthesis. Many authors have demonstrated the mobility of such devices 10 years after insertion, including Lemaire et al. [27] and Griffith et al. [15] with the SB Charité prosthesis, and Bertagnoli and Kumar [3] with the Prodisc. The mobility obtained is about 6° in flexion and extension at the L5-S1 level and 8° at L4-L5 [27]. Mobility in lateral inclination has also been analyzed, and found to be about 3°–4°. Lemaire et al. [27] analyzed rotational mobility with the SB Charité by investigating torsion on normal cadaver spines compared to others fitted with the SB Charité. The results were very interesting, because they demonstrated that a spine fitted with the SB Charité had a degree of mobility in torsion that was more than 140% that found in normal spines [27]. Rotational hypermobility may therefore be obtained. Such a finding

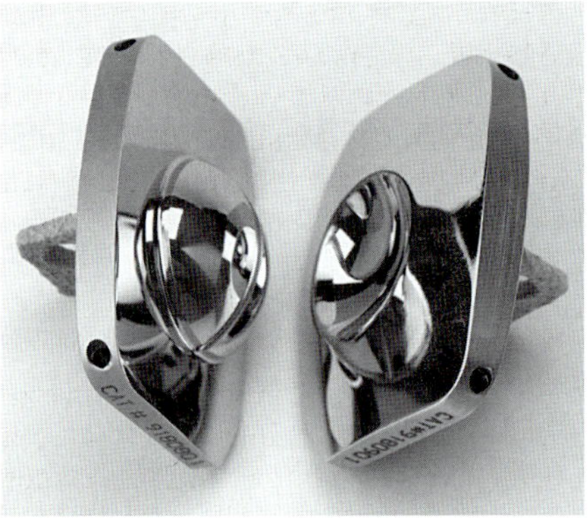

Fig. 1 The Maverick implant

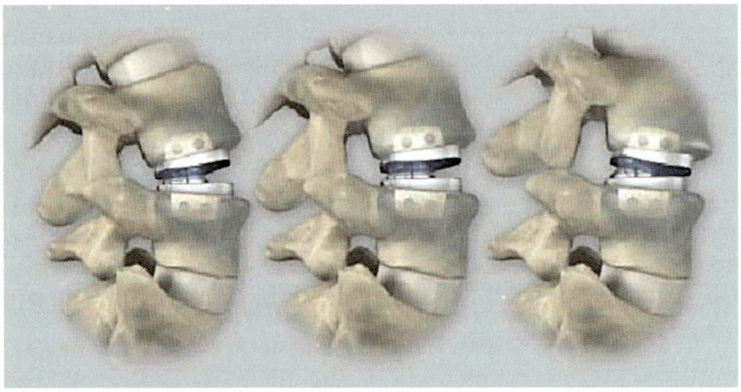

Fig. 2 Controlled translation during flexion/extension

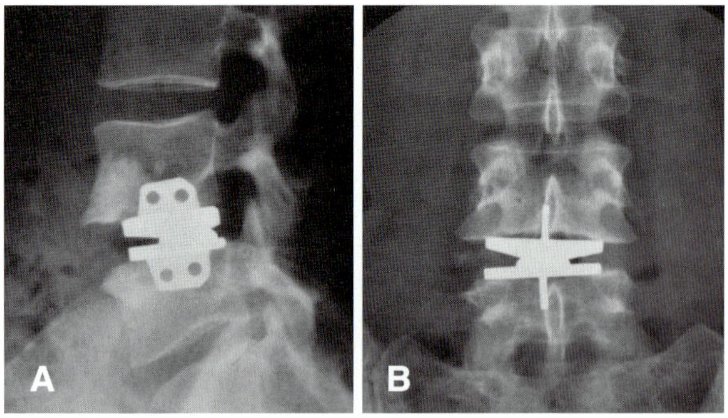

Fig. 3 **A** Antero-posterior view of a Maverick (Medtronic USA); **B** lateral view of a prosthesis at level L4-L5

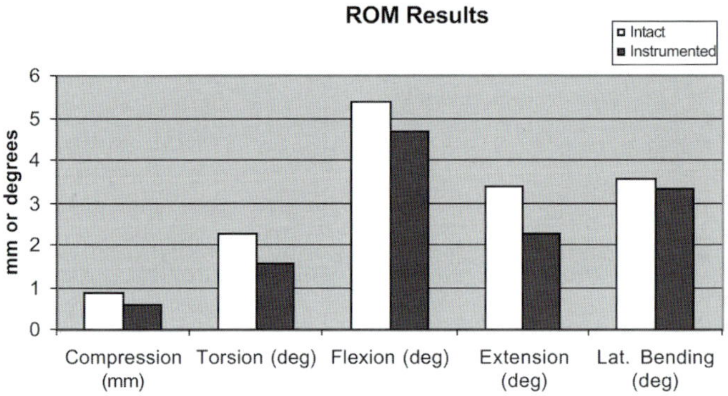

Fig. 4 Bar graph showing range of motion after Maverick prosthesis insertion compared to the intact spine. Cadaver study [28]

has not yet been reported with the Prodisc. The Maverick device has also been tested with the same torsion mobility protocol, and compared with a healthy spine [28]. The results were slightly inferior to those obtained in a normal spine, i.e., a certain stiffness was found in segments fitted with the device (Fig. 4). These findings are important to bear in mind because, although the aim of restoring disk function is to obtain a degree of flexion, extension and lateral inclination close to normal values, it is not desirable to end up with a degree of torsion greater than normal. Such hypermobility might induce an overload on the posterior facets, risking early degeneration. Moreover, the posterior structures of patients treated in this way are not fully intact [5, 7], owing to the disk degeneration, so any hypersolicitation of the posterior facets may induce pain.

Stability

The SB Charité device is composed of three parts: two metallic plates and a polyethylene insert. This biomechanical concept provides scope for five degrees of freedom, but it also involves the risk of dislocation to the polyethylene core. There have been very few reports of such dislocation in the literature [33], but wear to the polyethylene may favor this risk because the device is not intrinsically stable owing to the polyethylene implant. The Prodisc device is also composed of three parts, but the polyethylene insert is fixed to the lower endplate, thereby normally avoiding the risk of dislocation. However, the latter may occur and has been reported by Aunoble et al. [1]. The Maverick device comprises only two metal parts, according to the ball and socket principle. No dislocation is therefore possible. The anchoring of the device to the vertebral endplates is also a very important feature. When it was first introduced, the SB Charité prosthesis was not solidly anchored, and this led to several cases of early expulsion of the device [6, 33] (Fig. 5). Subsequently, the technique was modified to include a hydroxyapatite coating, and the resulting bony growth around the vertebral endplates seems to have greatly reduced this risk. However, isolated cases of early expulsion have still been reported for the SB Charité, particularly by Van Ooij [33]. It would therefore seem that hydroxyapatite coating around the endplates is not in itself sufficient to stabilize the implant. The Prodisc, in contrast, has had not a single reported case of expulsion due to an anchoring defect over the 10 years it has been in use [3, 30], which would seem to indicate that the system of anchoring by fins, used by the Prodisc, is much more reliable over time. This is the anchoring system used by the Maverick.

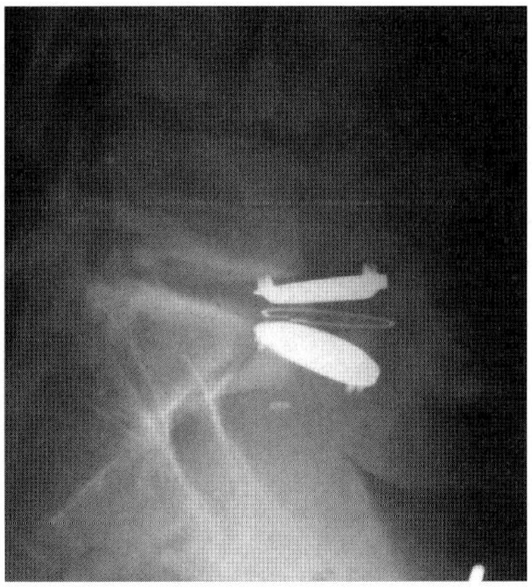

Fig. 5 Radiograph of a dislocated SB Charité disk prosthesis (courtesy of A. Van Ooij)

Wear tests

No data regarding polyethylene wear in the SB Charité and Prodisc devices have yet been published. Both devices use a combination of polyethylene and metal, and the only comparative data available are those concerning polyethylene-metal devices for hip replacement [32]. According to Hedman et al. [17], the lumbosacral spine undergoes about 125,000 significant flexions per year. A significant flexion can be considered to correspond to the forward flexion of the spine when raising a 20-kg load. On the basis of this finding, it is possible to test disk prostheses. It may therefore be considered that 10 million cycles of flexion, extension, lateral inclination and rotation correspond to clinical use of about 31.5 years [28]. Such tests have been performed with hip prostheses, and it has been reported that metal-polyethylene prostheses produce between 1,354 and 4,500 mm^3 of debris [32], and that metal-metal hip prostheses produce about 157.5 mm^3 [16, 34]. Under the same conditions of use, the Maverick device produced between 12 and 14 mm^3 of debris [28], so the amount of debris produced by the metal-polyethylene hip prosthesis was greater than that produced by the Maverick metal-metal disc prosthesis by a factor of between 97 and 322 [19, 31]. The risk of the Maverick device wearing out is therefore extremely low. However, it is important to assess the toxic potential of metallic debris on the surrounding structures [31]. Allen et al. [2] analyzed the toxicity of metallic debris in vitro on cell cultures of osteoblasts at concentrations of 0.01, 0.1 and 1 g/cm^3. They showed that at a concentration of 1 g/cm^3, the expression of alkaline phosphatase and osteocalcin was inhibited. Since the production of metal debris by the Maverick device is about 0.1 g/cm^3 after 61 years of use [28], its toxic potential is ten-fold lower than the toxic threshold on the cells after this period of time. Therefore, the metal-metal combination seems perfectly suited to obtaining the optimal longevity of the device. An epidural toxicity of the wear debris of the Maverick was conducted on rabbits and reported by Le Huec [25]. The results showed that there was no difference between controls and tested animals. In cases of total hip replacement, the polyethylene wear debris is responsible for prosthesis loosening over time, due to the macrophagic reaction induced by the macro particles [32].

Capacity to absorb shocks

It is essential to understand the shock-absorbing potential of a disk prosthesis. In fact, this sixth degree of freedom has not yet been analyzed for any of the devices discussed so far. Only the Acroflex device [9], a metal-polyethylene prosthesis, has been reported to possess this capacity, but it is not commercially available, and, so far, studies have only been performed in animals [9]. Metal-polyethylene devices could therefore have a better capacity to absorb shocks, and this might be an advantage. In order to establish whether this is the case, the Prodisc metal-polyethylene prosthesis and the Maverick metal-metal device were compared in terms of their shock absorption and transmission of vibrations, in a study conducted by Le Huec et al. [23]. The preload applied was 350 N, and a 100-N overload was applied with a frequency varying from 0 to 100 Hz. The data showed that at the sensitivity threshold of the measuring devices used, there was no difference between the implants regarding shock absorption or the transmission of vibrations. The two implants would therefore seem to have similar dynamics, with neither having any detectable shock absorbing effects.

Technique for inserting total lumbar disk prosthesis

The aim of a total lumbar disk prosthesis is to recover the mobility of the segment concerned and its stability. Given the indications [22], such as discopathy with loss of disk height and inflammation of Modic type I or II in vertebral endplates eventually associated with osteophytic involvement, it is essential before inserting the prosthesis to prepare the disk space.

The prosthesis is introduced by an anterior approach [24]. We prefer the video-assisted retroperitoneal approach, which is much less invasive and does not destroy the muscle structures, thus helping to maintain the stability of the lumbar column [24]. The prosthesis is implanted anteriorly, and it is essential to establish a minimum width of 35 mm on the anterior part of the disk to perform the implantation safely. After opening the anterior annulus, which is retained at the end of the intervention for protective purposes, the disk is removed as far as the posterior annulus, while the lateral annulus is conserved on both sides. The posterior longitudinal ligament is not sectioned, but a posterior release is performed in order to mobilize the vertebral segment. In fact, owing to the frequent presence of osteophytes, there may be very considerable posterior adhesions and very low posterior mobility of the vertebral segment. It is therefore essential to perform posterior release with ablation of these osteophytes and partial release of the posterior longitudinal ligament on both sides of the vertebrae. This release must be checked during the intervention with intra-operative control during parallel distraction of the vertebral endplates. If this release is not performed, then the disk will have an anterior opening that could lead to a prosthesis being inserted in an excessively oblique position, which would not be physiological. It is also important to remove the fragments of the annulus or osteophytes at the entry to each foramen, in order to avoid pushing them into the foramen during implantation.

The vertebral endplates must be prepared, but the subchondral bone must not be removed in order not to weaken the plates, so guarding against any risk of subsidence. Pre-operative bone densitometry in subjects aged over 55 years is therefore essential in order to ensure the bone quality is good. The instruments used must make it possible to determine the angle of the prosthesis, the height to be implanted, and the width and depth of the implant. For this purpose, templates may be used to assess the optimal size of implant to be used on pre-operative computed tomography (CT) scan or magnetic resonance imaging (MR) cuts. Intraoperatively, it is possible to assess the obliquity of the disk after release and its height. The choice can then be made with the instrument provided. For this, the Maverick prosthesis uses an instrument known as a "4 in 1," which gives information about the obliquity of the disk, its height, and the width of the implant to be used. The anchoring pins are prepared with chisels guided by the 4 in 1 device. Sectioning is very precise, so it is possible to implant the definitive prosthesis on bone rails according to the press-fit technique. Unlike devices requiring the secondary insertion of a central core, the Maverick prosthesis is inserted en bloc, obviating the need for distraction on the annulus during implantation, and thus avoiding any iatrogenic lesions to the annulus caused by such distraction.

Preliminary results with a prospective series of 30 patients implanted with the Maverick prosthesis

Method

A prospective study was performed using the Maverick total lumbar disk prosthesis (Medtronic, USA) to treat 30 patients with a highly degenerative lumbar discopathy at one level. All patients had been suffering chronic back pain that had resisted conservative treatment for at least 1 year, with medical and rheumatological follow-up, and all the patients had received rehabilitation physiotherapy. All had received radiologic, static, dynamic and load-bearing evaluation, in addition to magnetic resonance imaging (MRI). The devices are inserted by a mini-invasive anterior approach with complete discectomy and release of the discal space. The patient is positioned supine in the so-called "French position," with legs bent and open laterally (Fig. 6).

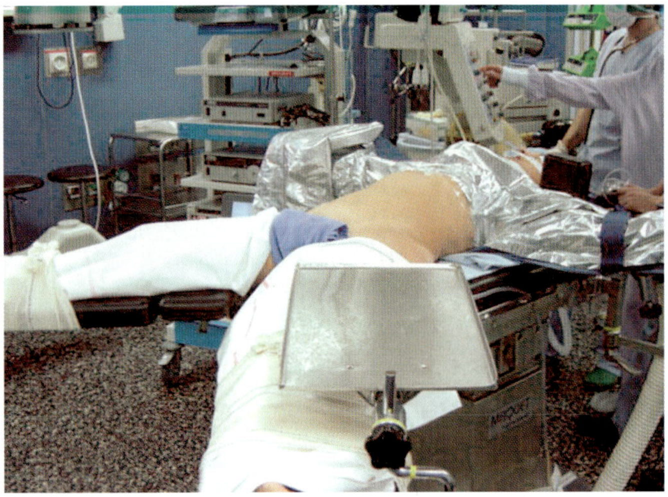

Fig. 6 "French position" on the operation table

The surgeon stands between the legs facing the lumbar spine in the cephalad-caudal direction, which is ergonomic for checking the midline of the spine when approaching the L5-S1 and L4-L5 levels. The assistant stands on the right or left side of the patient. The incision is longitudinal, 7–8 cm long and 3 cm parallel to the midline. A Pfannenstiel incision is more cosmetic for the L5-S1 level. After vertical incision of the rectus abdominis sheath, the muscle is detached laterally to reach the common fascia of the external oblique muscles. This fascia is opened in order to enter the retroperitoneal space and retract the peritoneal sac. The peritoneal sac is pushed to the contralateral side with the ureter and the hypogastric plexus. The vessel bifurcation is now exposed and analyzed. To reach L5-S1, the left iliac vein must be carefully retracted and the medial sacral vessels ligated. An opening to the anterior part of the L5-S1 disc of least 32 mm must be exposed. At the L4-L5 level, the left approach is commonly used. The surgeon must pay attention to the ascending lumbar vein, which is located at the corner of the psoas belly and the left iliac vein. This important collateral must be ligated. The segmental vessels at L4 and L5 must also be ligated to allow retraction of the aorta and vena cava. Traction on the left iliac vein must be controlled throughout the procedure. Specific blade retractors are used to keep the operating field free. The anterior part of the spine is exposed and disc surgery can start.

The anterior part of the disc is opened according to the size of the templates. The anterior annulus and nucleus are removed using disc rongeur, kerisson, curettes and a scraper. The posterior annulus must be opened to free the disc space and to allow good restoration of the disc height. It is not necessary to open the posterior longitudinal ligament, but it must be detached from the posterior border of the endplates using the specific instruments. This is very important to avoid anterior opening of the disc space with abnormal obliquity of the disc space. The mobility of the disc space is tested with a spreader under C-arm control. The midline is checked with antero-posterior (AP) fluoroscopy. The 4-in-1 instrument is inserted into the disc space, making sure of the alignment of the instrument with the midline marker. The T-handle of the 4-in-1 is then turned to create a parallel distraction of the disc, thus restoring the disk height. The upper or the lower keel cutter is slid onto the 4-in-1 and impacted into the vertebral body to prepare the bed for the anchoring fin of the prosthesis. The corner cutting process helps to remove the prominent bony irregularities on the endplates, thereby considerably facilitating insertion of the implant. The cutters and the 4-in-1 are then removed and the endplates are cleaned. The prosthesis is impacted into the prepared disc space under fluoroscopic control. The blade retractors are carefully removed and bleeding is controlled. The rectus abdominis fascia and subcutaneous fat are closed with drainage.

All patients were seen at 1, 3, and 6 months and 1 year, with assessment of pain, according to a visual analog scale, neurologic function, Oswestry scores, and the SF36 [18]. Clinical success was taken to be a 30% improvement on the Oswestry score, i.e., the success rate defined by the US Food and Drug Administration (FDA) in a randomized prospective study concerning anterior lumbar fusion with cage and bone morphogenic protein [4]. Radiologic assessment of mobility at the implanted levels and analysis of frontal and sagittal equilibrium were performed. Measurements performed by the independent radiologist on AP and lateral radiographs were accurate to 3° for angles and 3 mm for distances.

Results

All the patients underwent follow-up examinations. They had been operated either at L4-L5 [13] or at L5-S1 [17]. Clinical success according to the Oswestry scale at 6 months and 1 year was 82 and 86%, respectively. Low back pain improved from a mean VAS of 7.5±1.7 pre-operatively to 3±1.8 post-operatively. At 1 year, there was no measurable prosthetic subsidence except in a 57-year-old woman who had early depression of the posterior part at the level of the superior endplate. The subsidence was measured to be 3 mm and was stable at 1-year follow-up. Her outcome was very good, with an Oswestry score of 8, a pain score on VAS of 2, and pain-free resumption of work after 3 months.

There was no case of anterior or posterior prosthetic migration. There was no calcification or bone bridging around the prostheses or in the disc spaces. Mobility in flexion and extension was 4° and 8°, respectively, with a mean value of 6°±4°. No implant had to be removed or surgically revised. There was one complication, which was not due to the implant: a ureter suffering damage during the surgical approach. The lesion was repaired and outcome was uneventful. The mean SF36 score improved from 40 (±20.1) to 72 (±18.6) at one year.

Table 1 Classification for total disc arthroplasty insertion (Le Huec, SAS Montpellier 2002)

	Back pain	X ray	HIZ or Black disk on MRI	MODIC I or II	Disk height
Stage 0	yes	normal	no	no	normal
Stage 1	yes	normal	yes	no	normal
Stage 2	yes	Spurr +	yes	partial	Loss < 30%
Stage 3	yes	Spurr + knutssen+	yes	complete	Loss > 30%

	Posterior facets	Muscle fatty degeneration	Ligamentum flavum, interspinous	Bone density	Adjacent level	Spinal balance
O	intact	< 50%	intact	< 2 DS	intact	normal
1	damaged	> 50%	damaged	> 2 DS	damaged	scoliosis

Discussion

Discectomy with insertion of a total disk prosthesis has been widely reported to improve the clinical symptoms of chronic back pain [8, 12, 15, 18, 27, 35]. The degree of improvement is equivalent to that obtained with anterior fusion cages using the mini-invasive technique [4]. Radiographic follow-up in our series showed a degree of mobility close to normal, and confirms the results obtained with other devices such as the SB Charité, as reported by many authors [8, 12, 15, 18, 27, 35], and with the Prodisc, as reported by Bertagnoli and Kumar [3] and Mayer et al. [30]. The technique is safe because the intra- and post-operative complication rate is very low [3, 27]. The patients recover rapidly and the mean hospital stay in Europe is 3–5 days [3, 27], compared with 8–12 days for an arthrodesis [20]. Disk prostheses offer the prospect of earlier treatment of certain recalcitrant chronic back pain without having recourse to an arthrodesis. It is always possible to revert to an arthrodesis if results are poor or if there is progressive degeneration of the posterior structures. A few cases of arthrodesis with posterior fixation and a posterolateral graft have been reported by Lemaire et al. [27] for treating patients whose pain is recalcitrant. The failure may be due to a technical error or to an erroneous indication, so patients should be selected according to very rigorous criteria. Le Huec et al. [22] has proposed a classification to help in making this choice, which takes into account the characteristics not only of the pathologic level (disk and posterior elements) but also of the adjacent levels (Table 1). The spontaneous fusion of certain prostheses has been reported by Lemaire et al. [27] – a problem that is always accompanied by intra-prosthetic calcification. One solution is to prescribe post-operative non-steroidal anti-inflammatory drugs, as in lower member prostheses [16]. Another is to limit the bleeding of the vertebral endplates by applying a hemostatic agent on the bony tissue not covered by the prosthesis.

Conclusion

The metal-metal Maverick device with a posterior center of rotation and controlled translation is a promising therapeutic technique. Its mechanical characteristics and resistance to wear make it an interesting option in terms of its life cycle. Only long-term follow-up exceeding 5 years will make it possible to confirm these very favorable preliminary results and to analyze the effects on the segments adjacent to the levels operated.

References

1. Aunoble S, Donkersloot P, Le Huec JC (2003) Dislocations with intervertebral disc prosthesis: two case reports. Eur Spine J (in press)
2. Allen et al (1997) The effects of particulate cobalt, chromium, and cobalt-chromium alloy on human osteoblast-like cells in vitro. J Bone Joint Surg Br 79:475–482
3. Bertagnoli R, Kumar S (2002) Indications for full prosthetic disc arthroplasty: a correlation of clinical outcome against a variety of indications. Eur Spine J [Suppl 2]:131–136
4. Burkus JK, Heim SE, Gornet MF, Zdeblick TA (2003) Is INFUSE bone graft superior to autograft bone? An integrated analysis of clinical trials using the LT-CAGE lumbar tapered fusion device. J Spinal Disord Tech 16:113–122
5. Butler D, Trafimow JH, Andersson GB, et al (1990) Discs degenerate before facets. Spine 15:111–113
6. Buttner-Janz K, Schellnack K, Zippel H (1989) Biomechanics of the SB Charité lumbar intervertebral disc endoprosthesis. Int Orthop 13:173–176
7. Cavanaugh JM, Ozaktay AC, Yamashita HT, et al (1996) Lumbar facet pain: biomechanics, neuroanatomy and neurophysiology. J Biomech 29:1117–1129
8. Cinotti G, David T, Postacchini F (1996) Results of disc prosthesis after a minimum follow-up period of 2 years. Spine 21:995–1000
9. Cunningham BW, Lowery GL, Serhan HA, Dmitriev AE, Orbegoso CM, McAfee PC, Fraser RD, Ross RE, Kulkarni SS (2002) Total disc replacement arthroplasty using the acroflex lumbar disc: a non human primate model. Eur Spine J 11 [Suppl 2]:115–123
10. Dooris AP, Goel VK, Grosland NM, Gilbertson LG, Wilder DG (2001) Load sharing between anterior and posterior elements in a lumbar motion segment implanted with an artificial disc. Spine 26:122–129
11. Eck JC, Humphreys SC, Hodges SD (1999) Adjacent-segment degeneration after lumbar fusion: a review of clinical, biomechanical, and radiologic studies. Am J Orthop 28:336–340
12. Enker P, Steffee A, McMillin C, et al (1993) Artificial disc replacement: preliminary report with a 3-year minimum follow-up. Spine 18:1061–1070
13. Ferstrom U (1996) Arthroplasty with intercorporal endoprosthesis in herniated disc and painful disc. Acta Orthop Scand 10 [Suppl]:287–289
14. Frymoyer JW (1992) Indications for consideration of the artificial disc. In: Weinstein JN (ed) Clinical efficacy and outcome in the diagnosis and treatment of low back pain. Raven Press, New York, pp 227–236
15. Griffith SL, Shelokov AP, Buttner-Janz K, et al (1994) A multicenter retrospective study of the clinical results of the LINK SB Charité intervertebral prosthesis: the initial European experience. Spine 19:1842–1849
16. Haynes D, Rogers S, Hay S, Pearcy M, Howie D (1993) The differences in toxicity and release of bone resorbing mediators induced by titanium and cobalt-chromium alloy wear particles. J Bone Joint Surg Am 75:825–834
17. Hedman TP, Kostuik JP, Fernie GR, et al (1991) Design of an intervertebral disc prosthesis. Spine 16 [Suppl]:256–260
18. Hochschuler SH, Ohnmeiss DD, Guyer RD, Blumenthal SL (2002) Artificial disc: preliminary results of a prospective study in the United States. Eur Spine J [Suppl 2]:106–110
19. Jacobs JJ, Skipor AK, Doorn PF, et al (1996) Cobalt and chromium concentrations in patients with metal on metal total hip replacements. Clin Orthop [Suppl]:256–263
20. Katz JN (1995) Lumbar spinal fusion: surgical rates, costs, and complications. Spine 20 [Suppl]:78–83
21. Kostuik JP (1997) Intervertebral disc replacement: experimental study. Clin Orthop 27–41
22. Le Huec JC, Friesem T, Bertagnoli R, Mathews H (2002) Choice criteria for lumbar disc replacement indications. Presentation at the meeting of the Spine Arthroplasty Society, Montpellier
23. Le Huec JC, Kiaer T, Friesem T, Mathews H, Liu M, Eisermann L (2003) Shock absorption in lumbar disc prostheses, a preliminary mechanical study. J Spinal Disord Tech 16:346–351
24. Le Huec, Aunoble S, Magendie J, Hadidane R (2003) Video-assisted anterior approach to the spine. In: Surgical techniques in orthopaedics and traumatology. Editions scientifiques et médicales Elsevier SAS, Paris, 55-060-D-10
25. Le Huec JC, Friesem T, Mathews H et al (2003) Histological analysis of effects of wear debris toxicity of chrome cobalt molybdenum alloy in epidural space in rabbit. Presentation at the meeting of the Spine Srthroplasty Society, Phoenix
26. Lee CK (1988) Accelerated degeneration of the segment adjacent to a lumbar fusion. Spine 13:375–377
27. Lemaire JP, Skalli W, Lavaste F, et al (1997) Intervertebral disc prosthesis: results and prospects for the year 2000. Clin Orthop 337:64–76
28. Mathews H, Le Huec JC, Bertagnoli R, Friesem T, Eisermann L (2002) Design rationale and early multicenter evaluation of Maverick total disk arthroplasty. Presented at the International Meeting on Advanced Spine Technologies, Montreux
29. Mayer HM, Korge A (2002) Non fusion tehnology in degenerative lumbar spinal disorders: facts, questions, challenges. Eur Spine J 11 [Suppl 2]:85–91
30. Mayer HM, Wiechert K, Korge A, Qose I (2002) Minimally invasive total disc replacement: surgical technique and preliminary results. Eur Spine J 11 [Suppl 2]:124–130
31. Merritt K, Brown SA (1996) Distribution of cobalt chromium wear and corrosion products and biologic reactions. Clin Orthop [Suppl]:233–243.
32. Schmalzried TP, Jasty M, Harris WH (1992) Periprosthetic bone loss in total hip arthroplasty. Polyethylene wear debris and the concept of the effective joint space. J Bone Joint Surg Am 74: 849–863
33. Van Ooij A (2002) Analysis of 21 patients with clinically failed Charité disc prosthesis. Eur Spine J [Suppl 1] Abstract 47
34. Willert H, Buchhorn G, Gobel D, et al (1996) Wear behavior and histopathology of classic cemented metal on metal hip endoprotheses. Clin Orthop 329 [Suppl]:160–186
35. Zeegers WS (1999) Bohnen LMLJ, Laaper M, et al (1999) Artificial disc replacement with the modular type SB Charité III: 2-year results in 50 prospectively studied patients. Eur Spine J 8:210–217

Bryan W. Cunningham
Gary L. Lowery
Hassan A. Serhan
Anton E. Dmitriev
Carlos M. Orbegoso
Paul C. McAfee
Robert D. Fraser
Raymond E. Ross
Samir S. Kulkarni

Total disc replacement arthroplasty using the AcroFlex lumbar disc: a non-human primate model

Abstract Using a non-human primate model, the current study was undertaken to investigate the efficacy of the AcroFlex lumbar disc as an intervertebral disc prosthesis, based on biomechanical, histopathologic and histomorphometric analyses. A total of 20 mature male baboons (Papio cynocephalus, mean weight 30 kg) were randomized into two equal groups based on post-operative time periods of 6 (n=10) and 12 months (n=10). Each animal underwent an anterior transperitoneal surgical approach to the lumbar spine, with intervertebral reconstructions performed at L3-L4 and L5-L6 using the following techniques: (1) tricortical iliac autograft and (2) AcroFlex lumbar disc. The two treatments were equally randomized between the non-contiguous operative lumbar levels. Post-mortem analysis included histopathologic assessment of the systemic reticuloendothelial tissues, multi-directional flexibility testing of the operative functional spinal units and quantitative histological analysis of trabecular bone coverage at the prosthesis endplates. Data were statistically compared using a one-way ANOVA with the Student-Newman-Keuls test. All animals survived the operative procedure and post-operative interval without significant intra- or peri-operative complications. Histopathologic analysis of the paraffin-embedded systemic reticuloendothelial tissues indicated no significant pathologic changes at the 6- or 12-month intervals. Plain film radiographic analysis showed no lucencies or loosening of any prosthetic vertebral endplate. Biomechanical testing of the 6-month autograft, reconstructions with AcroFlex lumbar disc and non-operative control (n=10) intact motion segments indicated no significant differences in peak range of motion (ROM) in axial compression. However, axial rotation produced significantly lower ROM for the autograft treatment compared to the intact and AcroFlex groups ($P<0.05$). The most significant differences in peak ROM were noted between all treatment groups under flexion/extension and lateral bending loading modalities ($P<0.05$). By 12 months, the intact condition indicated significantly more motion in all bending modes compared to the AcroFlex and autograft treatments, which were not statistically different from each other ($P>0.05$). Gross histopathologic analysis of the AcroFlex disc prosthesis demonstrated excellent ingrowth at the level of the implant-bone interface, without evidence of fibrous tissue or synovium. BioQuant histomorphometric analysis at the metal-bone interface (bone contact area/total endplate area) indicated the mean ingrowth was 54.59± 13.24% at 6 months and 56.79± 5.85% at 12 months. Radiographic analysis showed no lucencies or loosening of the AcroFlex vertebral

B.W. Cunningham (✉) · A.E. Dmitriev
P.C. McAfee
Orthopedic Biomechanics Laboratory,
Department of Orthopaedic Surgery,
Union Memorial Hospital,
201 East University Pkwy,
Baltimore, MD 21218, USA
e-mail: bcspine@aol.com,
Tel.: +1-410-5542914,
Fax: +1-410-5542408

G.L. Lowery · S.S. Kulkarni
Research Institute International,
Phoenix, Arizona, USA

H.A. Serhan
DePuy-Acromed Inc.,
Raynham, Massachusetts, USA

C.M. Orbegoso
Department of Pathology,
Union Memorial Hospital,
Baltimore, Maryland, USA

R.D. Fraser
The University of Adelaide,
South Australia, Australia

R.E. Ross
Hope Hospital, Manchester, UK

endplate. Based on multi-directional flexibility testing, motion was preserved in axial rotation, but significantly diminished in the other bending modalities, particularly at the 12-month interval. This effect may be secondary to the limited surface area of device-vertebral endplate contact. Histomorphometric analysis of porous ingrowth coverage at the vertebral bone-metal interface was more favorable for total disc arthroplasty compared to historical reports of cementless femoral components. This project serves as the first comprehensive in vivo investigation into the AcroFlex disc prosthesis, and establishes an excellent research model in the evaluation of total disc replacement arthroplasty.

Keywords Total disc replacement arthroplasty · Animal model · Biomechanics · Histomorphometry · Porous ingrowth

Introduction

Total disc replacement arthroplasty is the next frontier in the surgical management of intervertebral disc pathology. As an alternative to interbody arthrodesis, an artificial disc serves to replace the symptomatic degenerated disc, restore the functional biomechanical properties of the motion segment, and protect neurovascular structures. To this end, the implanted device should encourage osseointegration at the bone-metal interface, re-establish normal kinematics to the functional spinal unit and promote an anterior/posterior column load-sharing environment.

To date, disc replacement technology has focused on two fundamental design strategies with regard to spinal kinematics: (1) unconstrained (mobile bearing core) prosthesis, and (2) constrained (fixed axis of rotation) prosthesis. Unconstrained devices (e.g. SB Charité III) are consistent with the principles of a mobile bearing arthroplasty [3], as the ultra-high molecular weight polyethylene core is able to translate between the vertebral endplates [34]. This design strategy allows for six-degrees-of-freedom segmental motion, with translations and rotations about three independent axes, and markedly diminishes the stress concentration at specific points on the polyethylene core, reducing the incidence of "cold flow" [4]. Constrained devices, in contra-distinction, typically permit rotation in all planes; however, they include a fixed axis of rotation, which limits segmental translation under flexion-extension and lateral bending conditions (e.g. ProDisc). This constrained design concept is thought to minimize anteroposterior shear forces at the operative facet level, while permitting unconstrained rotational motion of the operative segment.

The AcroFlex lumbar disc (Depuy-AcroMed, Inc, Raynham, Mass.) – an unconstrained design – is composed of porous coated titanium endplates and a polyolefin rubber core. Using an in vivo non-human primate model, the current study was undertaken to investigate the nature and magnitude of porous osseointegration following total disc replacement arthroplasty using the AcroFlex lumbar disc, with success criteria based on biomechanical, histopathologic and histomorphometric analyses.

Materials and methods

Animal research permission

The Institutional Animal Care and Use Committee (IACUC) at the Southwest Foundation for Biomedical Research (SFBR), San Antonio, Texas granted approval for this 20-animal project.

Animal model and surgical preparation

A total of twenty skeletally mature male baboons (Papio cynocephalus, 8–10 years old, mean weight 35 kg) were included in this study and followed for a period of 6 (n=10) and 12 (n=10) months post-operatively. Following normal health status determination, each animal was sedated with intravenous (IV) injection of ketamine (10 mg/kg) and diazepam (0.15 mg/kg) anesthetic medications, followed by endotracheal intubation and general anesthesia using 1.5–2.0% isoflurane. With the animal positioned supine, the anterior abdominal lumbar region was shaved, aseptically prepared and draped in sterile fashion. Prophylactic antibiotics (cefazolin sodium 1 g, IV) and analgesics (Butorphenol 125 mg/kg, IV) were administered pre- and post-operatively.

Surgical technique and treatment groups

Tricortical iliac crest bone graft was obtained from each animal using standard technique. Surgical exposure consisted of a 10- to

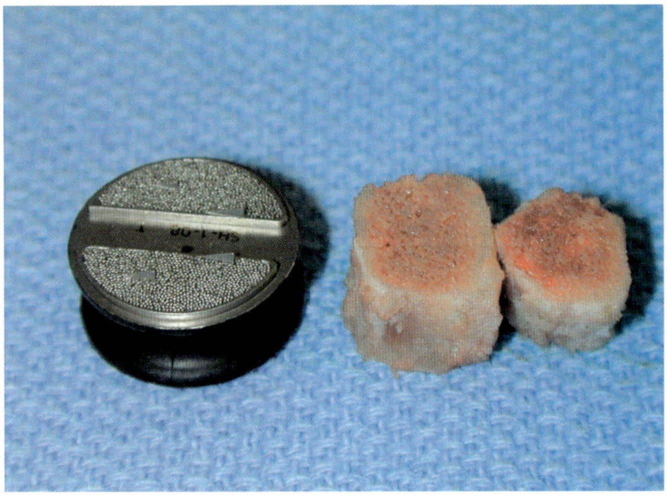

Fig. 1 View of the AcroFlex lumbar disc prosthesis (11 mm height × 20 mm diameter) and tricortical autogenous graft used for intervertebral reconstructions

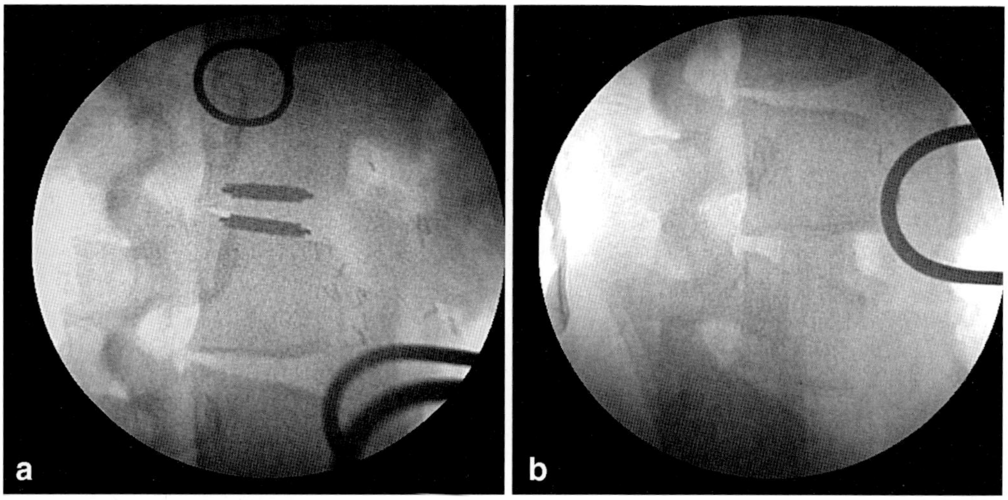

Fig. 2 Lateral fluoroscopic view confirming proper placement of an autograft treatment at L5-L6 (**b**) and AcroFlex disc at L3-L4 (**a**)

15-cm incision along the abdominal midline, followed by soft tissue dissection to permit transperitoneal exposure of the anterior lumbar spine. Blunt dissection using ligatures, Cobb elevator and electrocautery were performed as needed to expose the anterior aspects of the L3-L4 and L5-L6 intervertebral disc spaces. The anterior longitudinal ligament and anterior annulus were incised, followed by complete discectomy including the inner annulus and nucleus pulposus. A special box chisel was used to partially decorticate the vertebral endplates and ensure optimal contact at the bone-implant interface. The two randomized implant treatments were: (1) AcroFlex lumbar disc and (2) tricortical iliac crest (Fig. 1).

A custom distractor was utilized to insert the specially manufactured AcroFlex disc according to the manufacturer's guidelines, while implantation of the iliac crest graft was performed at the other non-contiguous level, using similar technique. The treatments were equally randomized between the two non-contiguous levels, with final positions verified with anteroposterior and lateral fluoroscopic images (Fig. 2).

Following the surgical procedure, the fascia and underlying muscle were closed in an interrupted fashion using 1.0 Vicryl, and the skin approximated using 2.0 Vicryl. Blood loss, operative times and intra- and peri-operative complications were quantified. Ambulatory activities and wound healing were monitored daily and all animals received analgesics and prophylactic antibiotics for the first 10 days post-operatively. Animals were humanely euthanized at the appropriate post-operative time interval, using an overdose (150 mg/kg, IV) of concentrated pentobarbital sodium (concentration=390 mg/ml). Systemic tissues – inguinal, periaortic and mesenteric lymph nodes, lungs, heart, liver, kidneys, spleen and pancreas – and spinal column were then carefully dissected for subsequent histopathologic examination.

Material specifications

The AcroFlex lumbar disc itself (11 mm height × 20 mm diameter) consists of three primary components: two ASTM F-136 implant-grade titanium endplates (Ti-6Al-4V ELI alloy) with sintered titanium beaded ingrowth surfaces, bound together by a hexene-based polyolefin rubber core (Fig. 1). The process of manufacturing of the custom AcroFlex disc was challenging, due to the diminution in size as compared to one that would be implanted in the human intervertebral disc.

Multi-directional flexibility testing

For flexibility assessment, the frozen lumbar specimens were thawed at room temperature, and the surrounding soft tissue and musculature carefully removed to obtain the operative ligamentous functional spinal units (AcroFlex n=20, autograft n=20). Ten intact lumbar motion segments from baboon cadaver spines were evaluated and served as non-operative controls (n=10). For fixation, the superior half of the proximal vertebral body and inferior half of the distal body were secured into rectangular tubing foundations using four, four-point compression screws. Two Plexiglas motion detection markers, each containing three non-co-linear light-emitting diodes designed for detection by an optoelectronic motion measurement system (3020 Optotrak System, Northern Digital Inc, Waterloo, Ontario) were placed on the anterior aspects of the superior and inferior vertebral elements. Using an MTS 858 testing device (MTS Systems, Minneapolis, Minn.) configured with a six-degrees-of-freedom spine simulator, six non-destructive pure moments of flexion/extension ($\pm x$ axis, 4 Nm), lateral bending ($\pm z$ axis, 4 Nm) and axial rotation ($\pm y$ axis, 4 Nm) were applied to the superior end of the vertically oriented specimen, while the caudal portion remained fixed to a testing platform. A total of three load/unload cycles were performed for each motion, with data analysis based on the final cycle. For the six main motions – corresponding to the moments applied – the operative level vertebral rotations (degrees) were quantified in terms of peak range of motion (ROM). To prevent desiccation during assessment, specimens were moistened with 0.9% NaCl sterile irrigation solution.

Histopathologic and histomorphometric analyses

Undecalcified tissue analysis

Following biomechanical analysis, the operative motion segments were processed using undecalcified histologic technique. The motion segments were sectioned in the mid-sagittal plane along the geometric centerline of the intervertebral disc spacer using a Beuhler Isomet saw (Beuhler Inc., Lake Bluff, Ill.). Histologic preparation of the sections included dehydration in 100% ethanol, staining using the Villanueva Osteochrome Bone Stain, undecalcified solution processing and embedding in polymethyl-methacrylate (PMMA). Using the EXAKT Microgrinding Device (EXAKT Technologies, Oklahoma City, Okla.), the embedded specimens were cut to 250- to 300-µm-thick sections, and then ground and polished to 120 µm. Microradiographs were obtained using a Faxitron X-ray Unit and Konica Graphic Arts Film. The slide-

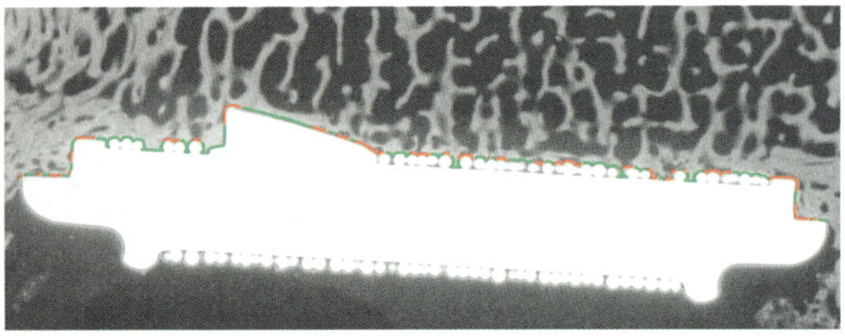

Fig. 3 Microradiograph of the AcroFlex disc prosthesis 6 months post-operatively, demonstrating the histomorphometric method of trabecular ingrowth calculation (% trabecular area/total endplate area)

mounted specimens were placed 12 in. (approx. 30.5 cm) from the beam and exposed for 2 min., using a technique of 45 kV and 3 mA while in direct contact with the single emulsion high-resolution graphics arts film. The resulting high-resolution microradiographs were used for histomorphometric quantification of trabecular bone area at the implant interface. Histopathologic assessment of the slide-mounted undecalcified sections and systemic reticuloendothelial tissues included assessment of particulate wear debris, as well as any signs of inflammatory giant cell reactions, degenerative changes or autolysis.

Using a BioQuant Image Analysis System (R&M Biometrics, Nashville, Tenn.), the high-resolution microradiographs permitted quantification of percentage trabecular ingrowth at the prosthesis-bone interface. The prosthesis surface was manually traced and expressed as a total endplate area pixel count. The regions of trabecular contact were subsequently traced, quantified in pixels and expressed as a percentage of the total endplate area (% ingrowth = apparent bone contact area/gross total endplate area) (Fig. 3).

Data and statistical analysis

For the non-destructive biomechanical analysis, peak ROM for each loading mode was calculated as the sum of motions [displacement (mm) for axial compression or maximum rotation (degrees) for torsion, flexion-extension and lateral bending] occurring in the neutral and elastic zones at the fourth loading cycle. Histomorphometric data represent the percentage of trabecular bone in contact with the AcroFlex (titanium endplates). All data are shown as mean plus/minus one standard deviation and were statistically compared using an analysis of variance (ANOVA) with the Student-Newman-Keuls comparison between groups. Significance was indicated at $P<0.05$.

Results

Surgical procedures

All 20 animals survived the surgery and post-operative time period without incidence of neurologic or infectious complications. The average operative time required was 156±40 min. Average blood loss was 235±35 cc. Assessments of general appearance, ambulation and wound healing were performed for each animal. All animals were characterized as having a normal recovery throughout the post-operative periods. Based on plain film radiographic evaluation and gross histology, all 20 AcroFlex prostheses were solidly fixed – there was no evidence of radiolucency or loosing at a single implant-bone interface (Fig. 4).

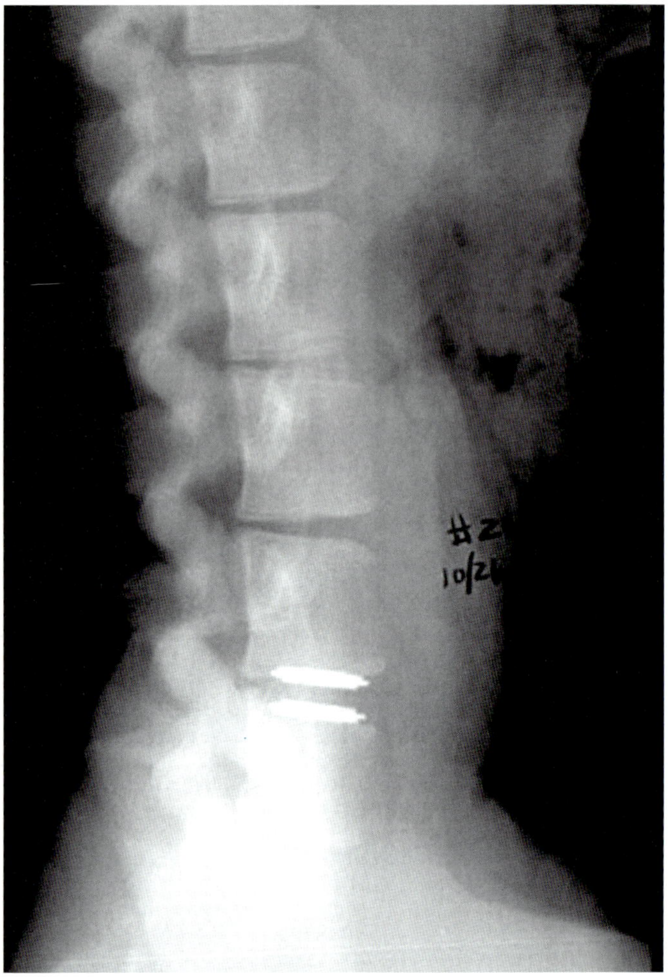

Fig. 4 Lateral plain film radiograph obtained 6 months post-operatively, demonstrating position of the AcroFlex device at L5-L6 and autogenous fusion control at L3-L4. Six and 12 months post-operatively, none of the prostheses were subluxed anteriorly or exhibited radiolucencies at the implant-bone interface

Radiographically, seven of the ten autograft levels showed evidence of fusion at 6 months and eight of the ten at 12 months, thus yielding an 80% fusion rate for the autograft group. One animal from the 12-month group was noted to have extravasation of the polyolefin core at the AcroFlex disc level, which was localized in the immediate soft tissue structures. No histopathologic effects were noted in the distant reticuloendothelial/systemic tissues. Implant failure was considered secondary to insufficient curing of the polyolefin core.

Fig. 5 Multidirectional flexibility testing of the operative functional spinal units was performed 6 (**A**) and 12 (**B**) months post-operatively. At 6 months (**A**), the intact spine and AcroFlex treatments were significantly different from autogenous controls in all loading modes except axial compression ($P<0.05$). Moreover, the intact condition was different from the AcroFlex in flexion/extension and lateral bending ($P<0.05$). At 12 months (**B**), the intact spine was different from the AcroFlex and autograft treatments in all rotational modes ($P<0.05$). Significance is indicated at $P<0.05$ and error bars represent standard deviation

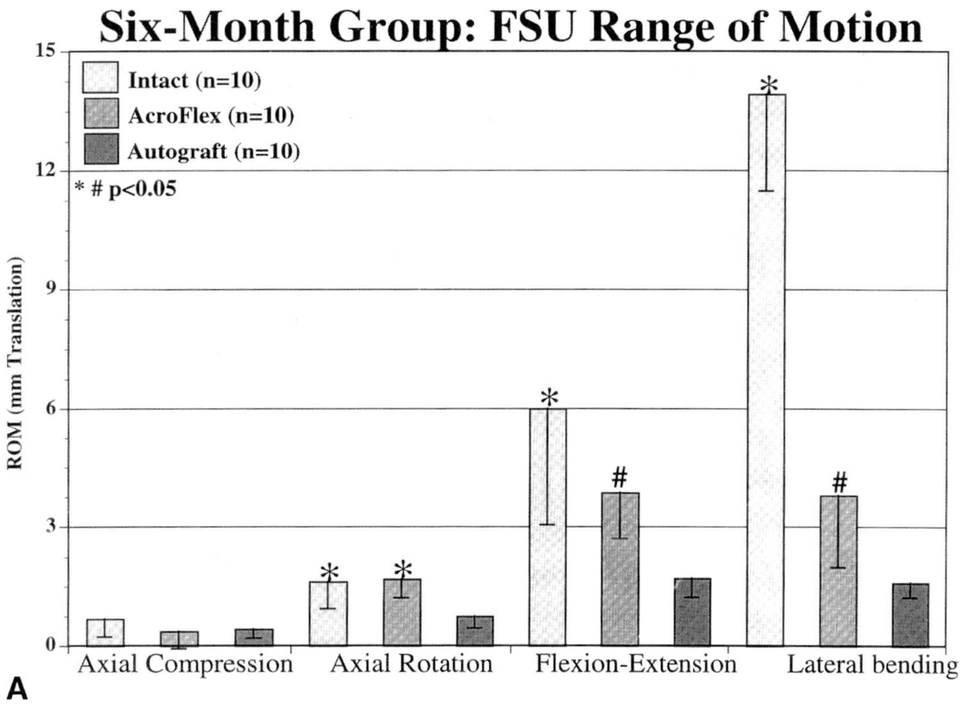

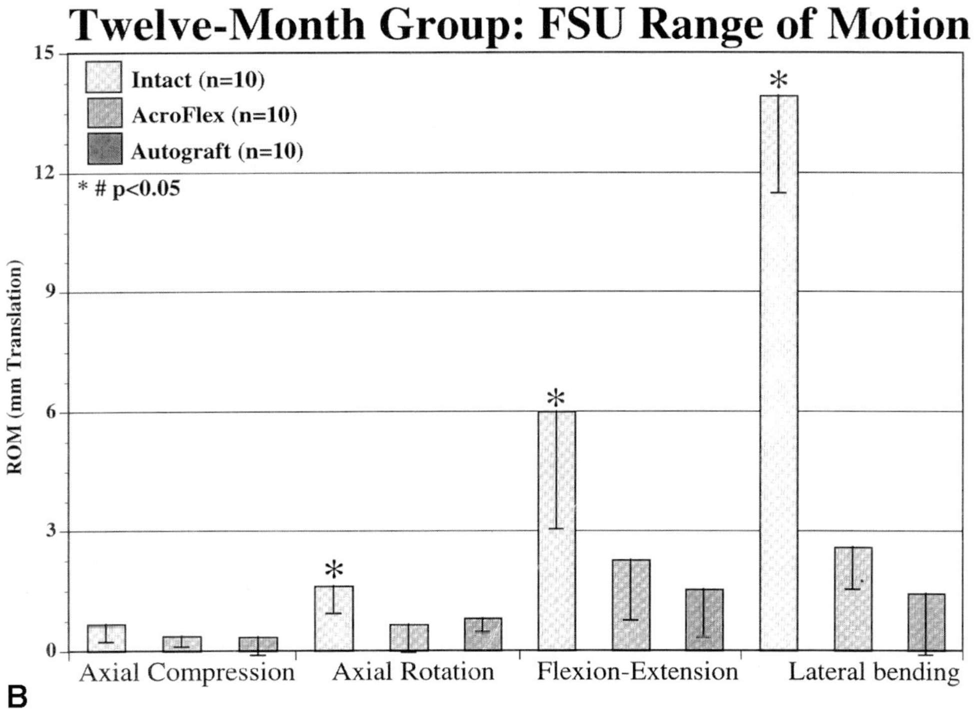

Multi-directional flexibility testing

Six-month treatment groups

Peak ROM comparisons of the 6-month post-operative anterior lumbar interbody fusions, reconstructions with AcroFlex lumbar disc, and non-operative intact motion segments indicated no significant differences in axial compression ($P>0.05$). Axial rotation testing results showed significantly lower ROM for the autograft specimens compared to the AcroFlex and intact treatments ($P<0.05$). The most significant differences in peak ROM were noted between all three treatment groups under flexion/extension and lateral bending loading modalities.

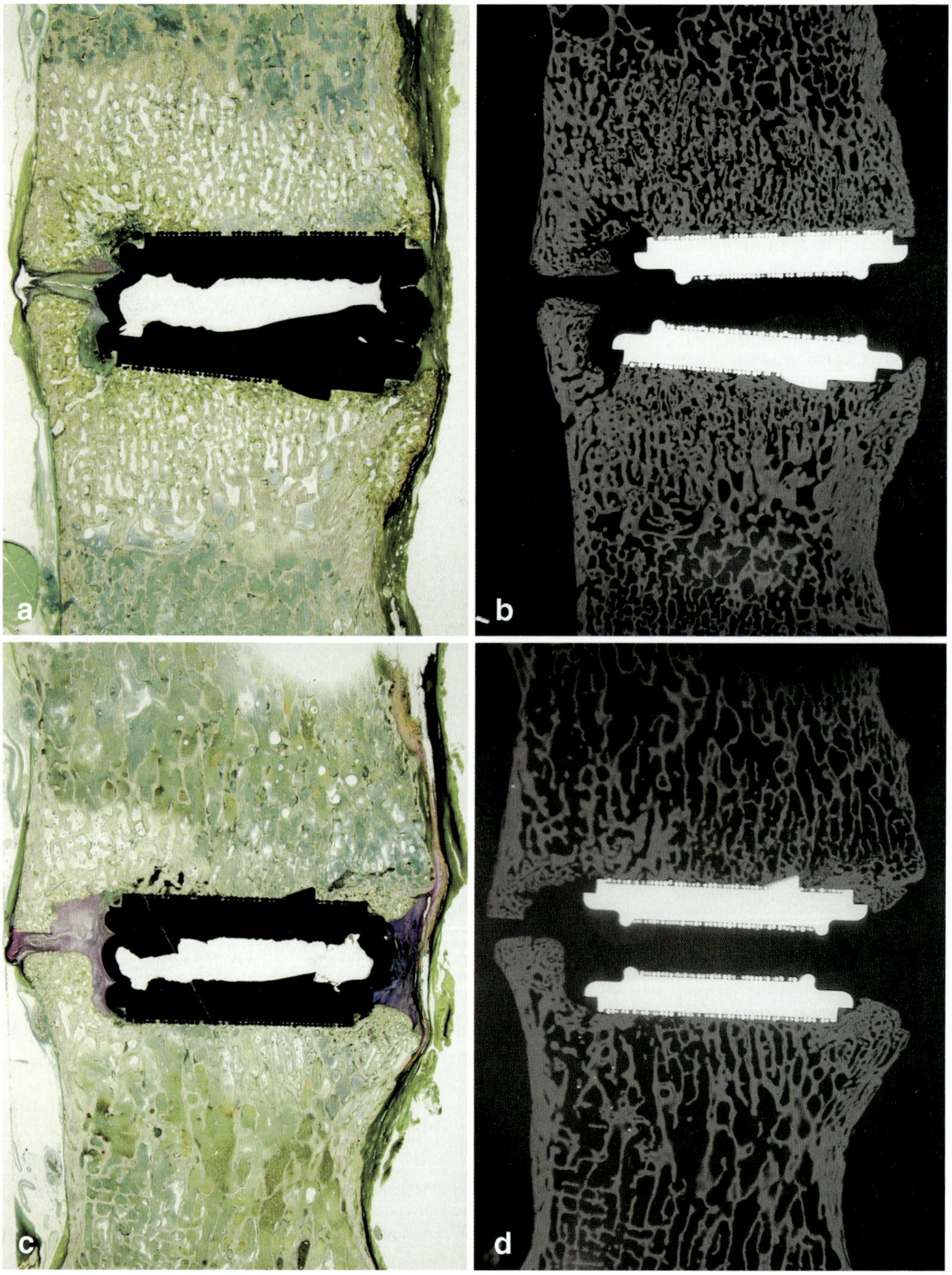

Fig. 6 Undecalcified histologic sagittal sections and corresponding microradiographs obtained from 6-month (**A,B**) and 12-month (**C,D**) treatments. The extent of osseointegration at the bone-metal interface is well demonstrated in these treatments. The absence of the black core is secondary to the cutting and grinding histologic processes necessary for histologic slide production (anterior is to the *right* and posterior *left*; Osteochrome Villanueva Bone Stain)

Specifically, the intact motion segment afforded greater ROM than the AcroFlex treatment, which was significantly different from the autograft fusions (Fig. 5A) (one way ANOVA results: axial compression F=1.10, P= 0.350; axial rotation F=7.64, P=0.003; flexion/extension F=10.36, P=0.000; lateral bending F=105.21, P=0.000).

Twelve-month treatment groups

By the 12-month time interval, the differences in range of motion between the intact spine and AcroFlex treatments had significantly increased. In axial compression, no differences were observed (P>0.05). However, in rotation, flexion-extension and lateral bending the intact spine ROM was significantly greater than the autograft and AcroFlex treatments (P<0.05), which were not statistically different from each other (Fig. 5B) (one way

ANOVA results: axial compression F=1.42, P=0.262; axial rotation F=7.36, P=0.004; flexion/extension F=15.74, P=0.000; lateral bending F=115.36, P=0.000).

Undecalcified bone histomorphology

Histopathologic interpretation of the slide-mounted undecalcified specimens indicated no evidence of significant pathologic changes in tissues within or surrounding the AcroFlex lumbar disc prosthesis. Based on plain- and polarized-light microscopic review of the slide-mounted vertebral specimens, there was no evidence of a fibrous or collagenous tissue interface at the prosthesis-bone interface. The trabecular bone in direct contact with the implant was lamellar in structure, without any evidence of sclerosis. Interstitial marrow cavities, devoid of fibrosis, account for the remainder of the implant-bone interface. Histopathologic interpretation of the microradiographs indicated confluent inter-digitization of trabeculae at the prosthetic endplate-bone interface, without evidence of radiolucent lines or gaps (Fig. 6).

The incidence of heterotopic ossification (peri-annular calcification) is observed in many specimens at the 12-month time period and most likely accounts for the decreased ROM observed in multi-directional flexibility testing. The one AcroFlex case demonstrating extravasation of the polyolefin core indicated black wear particles and a localized histiocytic foreign body reaction, without evidence of polymorphonuclear cells. In all remaining cases, there was no incidence of prosthetic endplate migration or evidence of particulate wear debris. Moreover, all histologic specimens were characterized as undergoing a normal healing process, with normal marrow cellularity, osteocyte distribution, osteoid seam widths and without evidence of bone necrosis, inflammatory/giant cell reaction or other significant histopathologic changes.

Histomorphometry

Light microscopic analysis of the 6- and 12-month AcroFlex specimens demonstrated excellent osseointegration at the level of the bone-implant interface (Fig. 3). BioQuant histomorphometric analysis at the metal-bone interface (bone contact area/total endplate area) indicated the mean ingrowth was 54.59±13.24% at 6 months and 56.79±5.85% at 12 months.

Histopathology: systemic/reticuloendothelial tissues

Histologic analysis of the local and systemic tissues at the 6-month interval indicated no significant pathologic changes induced by either AcroFlex disc prosthesis or surgical manipulations. Although no pathology was recorded that could be associated with the AcroFlex lumbar disc device, pre-existing conditions in the animals most likely account for the mild pathologic changes in some tissue structures. For example, the axillary, inguinal, periaortic and mesenteric lymph nodes were characterized as showing mild reactive changes with sinus histiocytosis. In two cases, the presence of eosinophils was noted in axillary nodes. Lungs of all animals with the exception of one showed histiocytic granulomas with tiny polarized particles. These lymph node and lung findings were considered secondary to the environmental housing conditions and unrelated to the implant procedures or materials. The spinal cord sections, based on H&E and Kluver-Barrera (Luxol Blue with PAS) staining methods did not reveal any variations from normal histologic appearance of myelin and nerve cells.

Discussion

The logical progression in the management of joint pathology has been from an immobilizing arthrodesis towards replacement arthroplasty. In the spinal column too, the concept of total disc replacement arthroplasty in order to restore structure and function to the operative motion segment is gaining popular support. A variety of disc designs have been described over the past 35 years, based on the principle of replacing either the nucleus pulposus or the entire disc utilizing a wide assortment of materials in an attempt to replicate the properties of a healthy functional spinal unit [1, 5, 19, 27, 34]. Only a few of these designs have been used in human clinical trials, with varied success [10, 13, 29, 34].

In the current study, radiographic analysis showed no lucencies or loosening of the prosthetic vertebral endplates. A significant decrease in the operative level ROM was observed for the AcroFlex group at 12 months versus the 6-month time period. This was considered secondary to the peri-annular calcification noted in six of ten levels containing the AcroFlex implant at the longer time interval. This anterior ossification is attributed to the custom-made implant having a significantly smaller endplate footprint as compared to the vertebral endplate dimensions (<50%) and limited intrinsic flexibility of the device in the acute post-operative timeframe. Moreover, based on previous studies with the Link Charité III in the same animal model, there was no incidence of peri-annular calcification noted, with operative level ROM equivalent to or greater than intact non-operative controls [20]. Despite the decreased flexibility at the operative levels, there were no issues of debonding of the rubber-titanium interface appreciated radiographically or upon gross inspection. However, extravasation of the polyolefin core did occur in one of the 12-month cases.

Based on the histomorphometry data, definitive trabecular osseointegration of the prosthetic vertebral endplates appears complete by the 6-month timeframe (54.59%), with only slight increases by the 12-month interval (56.79%). It is important to note that previous studies using hydroxyapatite- (HA)-coated porous ingrowth surfaces (SB Charité III) [20] did not demonstrate an inordinately higher percentage ingrowth (47.9±8.12%) at corresponding time periods versus the sintered titanium beaded surface used in the AcroFlex prosthesis. To put these osseointegration values in perspective, it is useful to look at animal models of porous ingrowth in total hip and total knee arthroplasty. Harvey et al. [14] found the mean ingrowth for femoral stems in a canine model was 9.7± 5.38% for a composite stem and 28.1±5.31% for a titanium alloy stem. Jasty et al. [8, 15] retrieved five femoral stems from patients, and the ingrowth ranged from 4 to 44% (mean 24%). Sumner et al. [31, 33] reported mean ingrowth of bone at 2 years in a canine cementless total hip arthroplasty model. The amount of ingrowth of bone averaged 32.7±4.7% (range 19.7–47.5%) with fiber metal coatings and 24.1±1.8% (range 19.0–31.2%) using bead coatings. Pidhorz et al. [26] retrieved cementless acetabular components in humans, 5 weeks to 75 months post-operatively (mean 41 months) (n=11), and found a mean ingrowth of 12.1±8.2%.

With regard to the quantification methods for osseointegration, there is controversy regarding the most accurate method of measurement of porous ingrowth of cementless prostheses [2, 3, 4, 6]. The three most widely used methods are microradiography, stained histology, and backscattered electron imaging scanning electron microscopy (BEI-SEM) [3]. Turner and co-workers' [32] canine study of femoral component ingrowth most directly approximates our study, as both used microradiography, 6 months post-operative follow-up, and the BioQuant image analysis system. Turner et al.'s microradiographs were made from 100-µm-thick sections, whereas our study utilized 120-µm-thick histology sections. At 6 months, the fiber metal Ti-coated femoral stem in their study showed a 37.3±3% ingrowth of bone, while the figure for the Ti beaded surface femoral stems was 23.3±3.3%.

One potential reason for variability in the quantification of bony ingrowth in total hip replacements is the mismatch between the geometry of the total hip stems and the shape of the surrounding bony cortex – the likelihood of bone ingrowth increases with the proximity of the porous coating to the cortical bone.[9] Other confounding variables include the fact that the porous coating extends different lengths and across different portions of the bone-metal surface in joint components in the extremities [2, 6, 9, 14]. In the SB III Charité and AcroFlex disc replacements studied in our laboratory [7, 20], the porous coating extended across the entire bone-metal interface. Furthermore, in the spine, with total disc replacements there was consistent bony architecture throughout the width and depth of the vertebral body, and the surface was completely flat.

As with joint replacement in the appendicular skeleton, there are a number of clear-cut anatomical and biomechanical considerations in total disc replacement arthroplasty. Foremost, the human functional spine represents a three-joint complex, with segmental rotations and translations occurring along three axes – x, y, z [25]. Moreover, the centers of intervertebral rotation change under flexion/extension and lateral bending conditions, and produce an elliptical instantaneous axis of rotation (IAR) localized in the posterior half and along the inferior endplate of the intervertebral disc [11, 12, 28]. To this end, the device should allow normal, unconstrained physiologic motions; permitting the spine to regulate the device, as opposed to spinal motion adapting to the implant. Additionally, the device must adequately address the in vivo loading conditions [17, 18, 21, 22, 23, 24, 30], must function as a stand-alone implant in the presence of an intact posterior column, and must resist wear, cold flow and material delamination. Most importantly and most challenging is for the device to encourage osseointegration at the bone-metal interface while preserving the biomechanical properties of motion.

The baboon model illustrates a "worst case" scenario, as the animals are not braced or immobilized post-operatively, are rapid to ambulate and perform their natural gymnastics, trapeze utilization and cage rocking within the 1st post-operative week. Moreover, the disc space dimensions (9 mm height, 25 mm depth and 30 mm width) are more accommodating to the smaller human-sized prosthetic implants, with minimal endplate resection required compared to other animal models – sheep, goats or canines [16, 17]. These models can also be used for defining the anatomical feasibility of the surgical approach and instrument design strategies.

This concept of total disc replacement arthroplasty represents a new paradigm in the surgical management of discogenic pathology. As we move from an era of interbody spinal arthrodesis to one in which segmental motion is preserved, this promising new technology offers increasing challenges in the research areas of implant design, spinal kinematics and histologic osseointegration. In the current study, we postulate that the reason for the improved degree of porous osseointegration in total disc replacement prosthesis is due to ligamentotaxis causing sustained compression across the metal-bone interface. Moreover, there were no specific pathologic changes in the local, systemic or reticuloendothelial system to suggest any toxicity or bio-incompatibility issues with regard to implant materials. However, the observed mechanical failure pattern should be considered in future design strategies for total disc replacements. The decreased flexibility properties observed at the 12-month time period appear secondary to implant size, design and implantation technique. This project serves as the first comprehensive in-vivo investigation of the AcroFlex disc prosthesis and establishes an excellent research model in the evaluation of total disc replacement arthroplasty.

References

1. Bao QB, McCullen GM, Higham PA, Dumbleton JH, Yuan HA (1996) The artificial disc: theory, design and materials biomaterials. 17:1157–1167
2. Bloebaum RD, Bachus KN, Jensen JW, Scott DF, Hofman AA (1998) Porous-coated metal backed patellar components in total knee replacement. A postmortem retrieval analysis. J Bone Joint Surg Am 80:518–528
3. Bloebaum RD, Rhodes DM, Rubman MH, Hofman AA (1991) Bilateral tibial components of cementless designs and materials. Microradiographic, backscattered imaging, and histologic analysis. Clin Orthop 268:179–187
4. Buechel FF Sr, Buechel FF Jr, Pappas MJ, D'Alessio J (2001) Twenty-year evaluation of meniscal bearing and rotating platform knee replacements. Clin Orthop 388:41–50
5. Cinotti G, David T, Postacchini F (1996) Results of disc prosthesis after a minimum follow-up period of 2 years. Spine 21:995–1000
6. Collier JP, Mayor MB, Chac JC, Surprenant VA, Surprenant HP, Dauphinais LA (1988) Macroscopic and microscopic evidence of prosthetic fixation with porous-coated materials. Clin Orthop 235:173–180
7. Cunningham BW, Lowery GL, Gonzales V, Orbegoso CM (2001) An analysis of the AcroFlex lumbar disk prosthesis. A non-human primate model. Proceedings of the North American Spine Society. Seattle, Washington, 3 November, pp 74,75
8. Engh CA, Zettl-Schaffer KF, Kukita Y, Sweet D, Jasty M, Bragdon C (1993) Histological and radiographic assessment of well functioning porous-coated acetabular components. A human postmortem study. J Bone Joint Surg Am 75:814–824
9. Engh CA, Hooten JP, Zettl-Shaffer KF, Ghaffarpour M, McGovern TF, Bobyn JD (1995) Evaluation of bone ingrowth in proximally and extensively porous-coated anatomic medullary locking prostheses retrieved at autopsy. J Bone Joint Surg Am 77:903–910
10. Enker P, Steffee A, Mcmillin C, Keppler L, Biscup R, Miller S (1993) Artificial disc replacement. Preliminary report with a 3-year minimum follow-up. Spine 18:1061–1070
11. Gertzbein SD, Chan KH, Tile M, Seligman J, Kapasouri A (1985) Moire patterns: an accurate technique for determination of the locus of the centres of rotation. J Biomech 18:501–509
12. Gertzbein SD, Seligman J, Holtby R, Chan KH, Kapasouri A, Tile M, Cruickshank B (1985) Centrode patterns and segmental instability in degenerative disc disease. Spine 10:257–261
13. Griffith SL, Shelokov AP, Buttner-Janz K, LeMaire JP, Zeegers WS (1994) A multicenter retrospective study of the clinical results of the LINK SB Charite intervertebral prosthesis. The initial European experience. Spine 19:1842–1849
14. Harvey EJ, Bobyn JD, Tanzer M, Stackpool GJ, Krygier JJ, Hacking SA (1999) Effect of flexibility of the femoral stem on bone-remodeling and fixation of the stem in a canine total hip arthroplasty model without cement. J Bone Joint Surg 81:93–107
15. Jasty M, Bragdon CR, Maloney WJ, Haire T, Harris WH (1991) Ingrowth of bone in failed fixation of porous-coated femoral components. J Bone Joint Surg Am 73:1331–1337
16. Kostuik JP (1997) Intervertebral disc replacement. Experimental study. Clin Orthop 337:27–41
17. Kotani Y, Abumi K, Shikinami Y, Takada T, Kadoya K, Shimamoto N, Ito M, Kadosawa T, Fujinaga T, Kaneda K (2002) Artificial intervertebral disc replacement using bioactive three-dimensional fabric: design, development, and preliminary animal study. Spine 27:929–935; discussion 935,936
18. Langrana NA, Parsons JR, Lee CK, Vuono-Hawkins M, Yang SW, Alexander H (1994) Materials and design concepts for an intervertebral disc spacer. I. Fiber-reinforced composite design. J Appl Biomater 5:125–132
19. Lee CK, Langrana NA, Parsons JR, Zimmerman MC (1991) Development of a prosthetic intervertebral disc. Spine 16:S253–S255
20. McAfee PC, Cunningham BW, Orbegoso CM, Sefter JC, Dmitriev AE, Fedder IL. Analysis of porous ingrowth in intervertebral disc prostheses: a non-human primate model. Spine (in press)
21. Nachemson A (1959) Measurement of intradiscal pressure. Acta Orthop Scand Suppl 28:269–289
22. Nachemson A (1960) Lumbar intradiscal pressure. Acta Orthop Scand Suppl 43:1–104
23. Nachemson A (1965) The effect of forward leaning on lumbar intradiscal pressure. Acta Orthop Scand 35:314–328
24. Nachemson A (1966) The load on lumbar disks in different positions of the body. Clin Orthop 45:107–122
25. Panjabi MM (1988) Biomechanical evaluation of spinal fixation devices. I. A conceptual framework. Spine 13:1129–1133
26. Pidhorz LE, Urban RM, Jacobs JJ, Sumner DR, Galante JO (1993) A quantitative study of bone and soft tissues in cementless porous-coated acetabular components retrieved at autopsy. J Arthroplasty 8:213–225
27. Ray CD, Schonmayr R, Kliniken HS (1997) A prosthetic lumbar nucleus "artificial disc". NASS Proceedings 12th Annual Meeting, October 22–25, New York
28. Rolander SD (1966) Motion of the lumbar spine with special reference to the stabilizing effect of posterior fusion. An experimental study on autopsy specimens. Acta Orthop Scand Suppl 90:1–144
29. Ross ESR (1997) A prospective cohort study of the Charite disc replacement. NASS, Proceedings, 12th Annual Meeting, October 22–25, New York
30. Schultz A, Andersson G, Ortengren R, Haderspeck K, Nachemson A (1982) Loads on the lumbar spine. Validation of a biomechanical analysis by measurements. J Bone Joint Surg Am 64: 713–720
31. Sumner DR, Bryan JM, Urban RM, Kuzak JR (1990) Measuring the volume fraction of bone ingrowth: a comparison of three techniques. J Orthop Res 8:448–452
32. Turner TM, Sumner DR, Urban RM, Rivero DP, Galante JO (1986) A comparative study of porous coatings in weight-bearing total hip-arthroplasty model. J Bone Joint Surg Am 68: 1396–1409
33. Urban RM, Jacobs JJ, Sumner DR, Peters CL, Voss FR, Galante JO (1996) The bone- implant interface of femoral stems with non-circumferential porous coating. A study of specimens retrieved at autopsy. J Bone Joint Surg Am 78:1068–1081
34. Zeegers WS, Bohnen LM, Laaper M, Verhaegen MJ (1999) Artificial disc replacement with the modular type SB Charite III: 2-year results in 50 prospectively studied patients Eur Spine J 8:210–217

H. M. Mayer
K. Wiechert
A. Korge
I. Qose

Minimally invasive total disc replacement: surgical technique and preliminary clinical results

Abstract Total disc replacement has become an option for the treatment of degenerative disc disease of the lumbar spine. A new generation of implants has been developed that can be implanted through minimally invasive anterior approaches to the lumbar levels L2/3, L3/4, L4/5 and L5/S1. However mid- and long-term data are still lacking. This paper describes the minimally invasive surgical approach – techniques as well as the preliminary results of our first 34 consecutive patients. The intervertebral spaces L5/S1, L4/5, L3/4 and L2/3 were each approached through slightly different, but standardized, mini-laparotomies either through a retroperitoneal or a transperitoneal route. The clinical results with a follow-up of up to 1 year show satisfactory outcomes in about 80% of the patients. Oswestry score as well as VAS values show significant changes during the postoperative course. There have been three complications (8.8%), two of which were specific to the implantation process, but were resolved with a good clinical outcome in both patients. The preliminary results suggest that total disc replacement may become a reasonable alternative to spinal fusion under the selection criteria used in this study.

Keywords Artificial disc · Degenerative disc disease · Lumbar spine · Total disc replacement · Low-back pain

H.M. Mayer (✉) · K. Wiechert · A. Korge
Spine Center,
Orthopedic Clinic Munich-Harlaching,
Harlachinger Strasse 51,
81547 Munich, Germany
e-mail: MMayer@schoen-kliniken.de,
Tel.: +49-89-62112011,
Fax: +49-89-62112012

I. Qose
Ancona University, Italy

Introduction

Degenerative disc disease remains a therapeutic challenge. The therapeutic gap that existed between conventional non-surgical treatment and spinal fusion surgery has been closed by a variety of so-called 'semi-invasive' techniques. Epidural catheter treatments, intradiscal electrothermal therapy (IDET), and partial (nucleus pulposus) or total disc replacement techniques have been developed and are being used more and more frequently in clinical studies, although safety and efficacy are not yet evidence based [1, 2, 3, 4, 5, 10, 11, 12]. This is also true for total disc replacement in the therapeutic regime of chronic discogenic low back pain. The clinical and radiological results thus have to be monitored closely. A new generation of implants for total disc replacement has been developed, designed especially for application through a minimally invasive anterior approach (Prodisc, Spine Solutions, Tuttlingen). It has been in clinical use since 1999. We report on the results of our own series of patients, which formed part of an international prospective clinical multicenter trial.

Implant and minimally invasive surgical technique

The clinical study was performed with a new generation implant (ProDisc). The modular implant technology allows a stepwise implantation, which fulfils all necessary criteria for a minimally invasive surgical access (Fig. 1). Preparation as well as application instruments play a key role in minimally invasive approaches for total disc replacement. Thus, all instruments for preparation of the implantation (probe implant, distractor, chisels) as well as

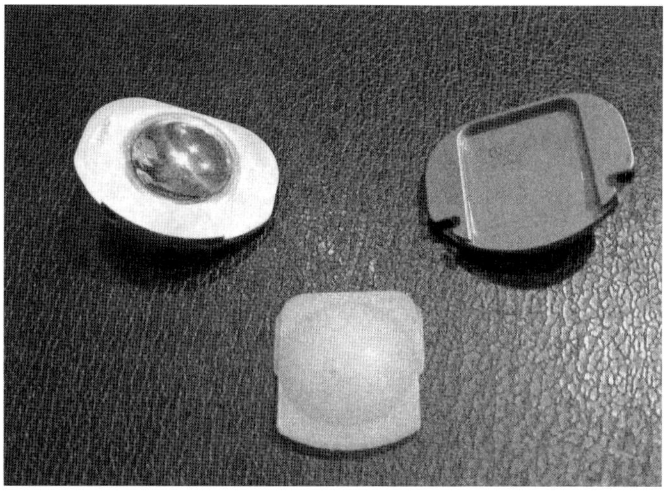

Fig. 1 ProDisc implant: modular design for minimally invasive step-by-step implantation

instruments for performing the implantation (applicator, distractor, inlay insertion, etc.) have been designed following microsurgical criteria (Table 1).

Surgical approaches

General remarks

Total disc replacement requires an anterior midline approach. Due to the designs of the implant, insertion into the intervertebral space must be performed strictly in the midline. This requires meticulous preoperative planning as well as a modification of the surgical technique, especially at L4/5 and higher levels.

Preoperative planning includes magnetic resonance imaging (MRI) investigation of the lumbar spine, as well as three-dimensional computed tomography (3D CT) angiography, to evaluate the size, shape and topography of the retroperitoneal blood vessels (Fig. 2). This technique makes it possible to clearly visualize the venous and arterial bifurcation and also shows the topographical relation between the arterial and venous branches. With these preoperative data, surgical planning can be performed in detail. The knowledge of the individual vascular situation of the patient influences the surgical technique and, in rare cases, might lead to a contraindication for disc replacement (e.g. venous bifurcation covering completely the anterior circumference of the target disc space). All other preoperative planning criteria correspond to the ones that have been described for minimally invasive anterior interbody fusion (MiniALIF) [6, 7, 8, 9].

All implantations can be performed through a midline mini-laparotomy. The patients are placed in a neutral mini-ALIF position (*cave*: hyperextension of the lumbar spine increases segmental lordosis) (Fig. 3). The target level is localized under antero-posterior and lateral fluoroscopic control and marked on the skin. All implantations are performed through small 4- to 5-cm transverse skin incisions (Fig. 4). Because of anatomical and topographical details, each level has very specific technical demands.

Technique for the L5/S1 level

This is the easiest segment to approach. After exposure of the rectus fascial sheet, the linea alba is split in the midline, and the peritoneum is exposed. There are three options for exposing the L5/S1 disc space from anterior: retroperitoneal from the right side, retroperitoneal from the left side or transperitoneal. The 'approach decision' should follow the following guidelines.

Retroperitoneal approach from the right side

This approach should be the first choice. The peritoneum is bluntly detached from the inner abdominal wall on the right side. The transverse fascia has to be incised to mobilize the abdominal contents adequately. The psoas muscle as well as the common iliac artery with the urether are identified. Preparation is continued towards the midline between the urether (displaced medially) and the artery. Medial to the common iliac artery, the lateral circumference of L5/S1 can be exposed. In this area, the superior hypogastric plexus is very thin with rare and small branches, which decreases the risk of damaging this plexus. Blunt dissection of the prevertebral fat tissue including the plexus exposes the medial sacral artery and vein, which can then be clipped or coagulated and dissected. Thus L5/S1 can be exposed easily. The left common iliac vein

Table 1 Instrument and implant properties for minimally invasive implantation

Instrument	Properties
Distractor	Slim instrument design for small approach corridors
Probe implant	Same size as implant, fits through small corridor easy, coupling mechanism guides chisel
Chisel	Guided by probe implant, no additional space required
Implant applicator/distractor	Same width as implant, no additional space required, easy coupling/uncoupling, easy distraction and inlay insertion

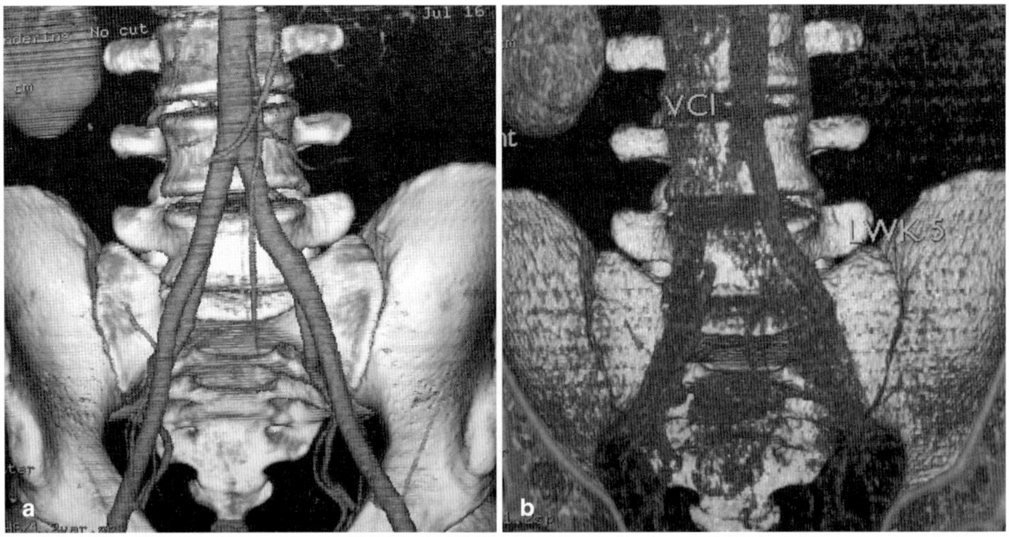

Fig. 2a, b Three-dimensional computed tomography (3D CT) angiography of the retroperitoneal blood vessels of the lumbar spine: **a** arterial branch, **b** venous branch

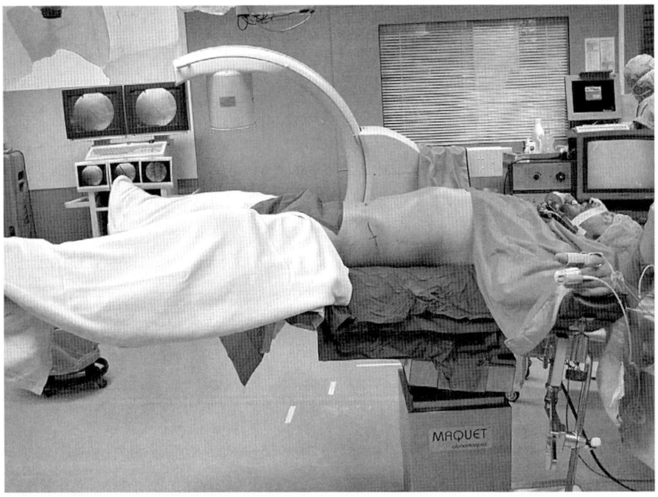

Fig. 3 Positioning of the patient (*nb* hyperextension must be avoided!)

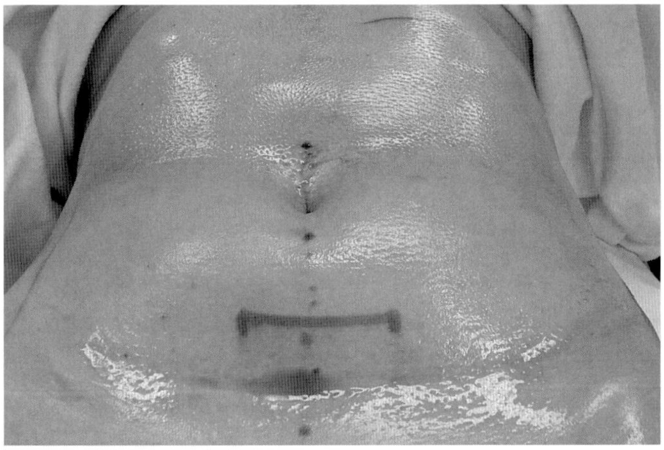

Fig. 4 Skin incision for mini-laparatomy

can be retracted carefully to the left (Fig. 5). This is the safest and easiest approach to L5/S1.

Retroperitoneal approach from the left side

This approach is chosen in cases with previous abdominal surgery in the lower right quadrant (e.g. appendectomy, gynecological operations, operation for abdominal hernia). The dissection process is the same as on the right side. Dissection is performed across the common iliac vein to the disc space L5/S1, which is sometimes difficult, especially if the vein has a large diameter. The plexus hypogastricus superior has to be pushed medially with care, avoiding any coagulation. These two factors make this approach the 'second-choice approach'; however, exposure of L5/S1 can be achieved as completely as from the right side.

Transperitoneal approach

In very obese patients, in patients who have had conventional abdominal surgery and in revision cases, the transperitoneal minimally invasive approach is the appropriate technique. It is the most direct way to L5/S1, and can be performed easily even in obese and previously operated patients [7].

Technique for the L4/5 level

Vascular anatomy determines the approach to L4/5 (see Fig. 2B). Due to the venous anatomy, the retroperitoneal approach from the left side is preferred in conventional surgery. Dissection can be performed across the aorta or the common iliac artery first. The arcuate line has to be incised in order to get adequate mobilization.

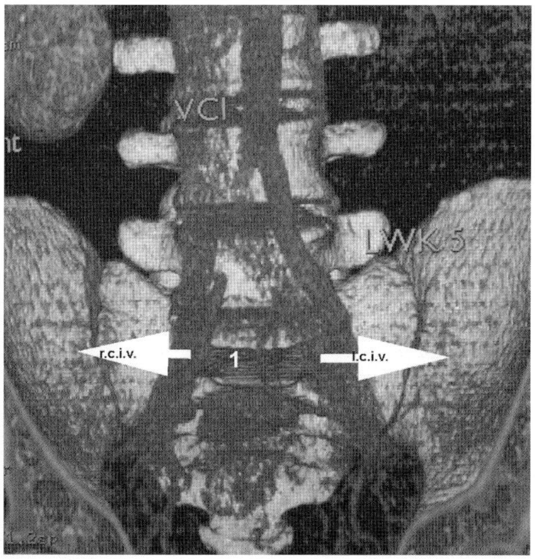

Fig. 5 Three-dimensional CT angiography: direction of vascular mobilization and retraction at L5/S1 (*r.c.i.v.* right common iliac vein, *l.c.i.v.* left common vein, *1* ligation of medial sacral artery and vein)

However, retroperitoneal exposure of L4/5 has its limitations in a minimally invasive approach. Mobilization of the abdominal contents is more difficult through a 4- to 5-cm skin incision. The same is true for preparation and retraction of the blood vessels. Due to the lordotic curve of the lumbar spine, the distance between the L4/5 disc space and the anterior abdominal wall is quite short. This makes a direct transperitoneal approach reasonable. Easy orientation and dissection of the superior hypogastric plexus and the perivascular tissues are further advantages. Exposure of the disc space follows the vascular situation (Fig. 6). Care has to be taken to ligate and dissect all segmental arterial and venous branches as well as the ascending lumbar vein on the left side to prevent indirect injury to these structures.

Technique for the L2/3/4 levels

The approach to L3/4 and L2/3 needs modifications on the skin-to-spine-route. The skin incision is usually at the level of, or above, the umbilicus. If it is at the umbilical level, a small, longitudinal paramedian incision on the left side is preferred. Retroperitoneal exposure is much more difficult at these levels, since the peritoneum is adherent to the posterior rectus sheet. Innervation of the rectus muscle must be preserved and the integrity of the fascial indentations at these levels must be respected. It is thus recommended to expose the retroperitoneal space in two steps: (1) longitudinal midline incision of the anterior rectus sheet 5 mm lateral to the linea alba and exposure of the left rectus muscle, and (2) dissection anterior to the muscle to its lateral border and opening of the retroperitoneal space. Thus, the peritoneum can be detached from the posterior rectus sheet from left lateral to the midline. The exposure is then continued by opening of the posterior rectus sheet close to the midline and retroperitoneal dissection from the left to the right. In obese patients, again, a transperitoneal route is recommended. The various options of vascular preparation are shown in Fig. 7.

After removal of the nucleus pulposus and after endplate preparation, the implant is positioned according to manufacturer's guidelines.

Materials and methods

Study design

This was a prospective, non-randomized clinical multicenter study. All patients had to give written informed consent. Study documen-

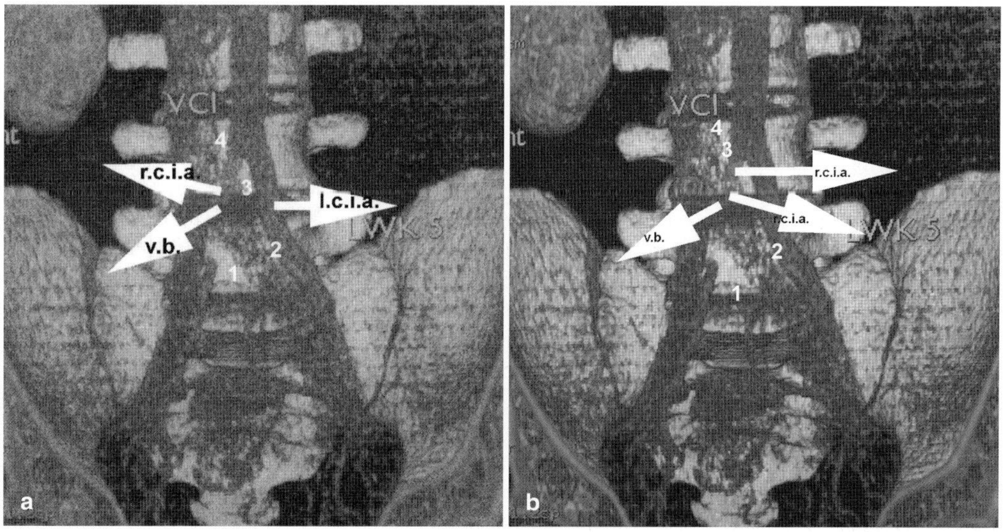

Fig. 6a, b Three-dimensional CT angiography: direction of vascular mobilization, retraction and branches to be ligated – most common variants at L4/5. **a** Approach between arterial bifurcation, lateral to venous bifurcation (*v.b.* venous bifurcation, *r.c.i.a.* right common iliac artery, *l.c.i.a.* left common iliac artery; ligations of *1* medial sacral vein, *2* ascending lumbar vein, *3* medial sacral artery, *4* segmental vein L5 left). **b** Approach between venous and arterial bifurcation (*v.b.* venous bifurcation, *r.c.i.a.* right common iliac artery; ligation of *1* medial sacral vein and artery, *2* ascending lumbar vein, *3* right segmental artery L4, *4* left segmental vein L4)

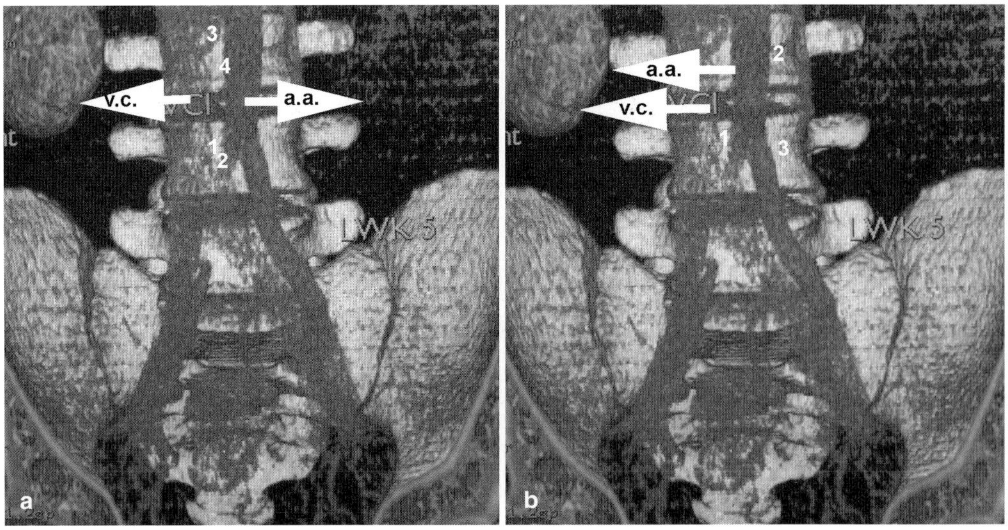

Fig. 7a, b Three-dimensional CT angiography: direction of vascular mobilization, retraction and branches to be ligated – most common variants at L2/3/4. **a** Approach between the vena cava and the abdominal aorta (*v.c.* vena cava, *a.a.* abdominal aorta; ligation of *1* segmental vein L4 left, *2* segmental artery L4 right, *3* segmental vein L3 left, *4* segmental artery L3 right). **b** Approach from the left side. (*v.c.* vena cava, *a.a.* abdominal aorta; ligation of *1* segmental vein L4 left, *2* segmental artery L3 left, *3* segmental artery L4 left)

tation was standardized, and included the visual analog scale (VAS), the Oswestry Disability Score, the SF36 Health Questionnaire and numerous clinical and radiological parameters. Data acquisition was performed preoperatively and at 3, 6, 12 and 24 months postoperatively. For each follow-up visit, radiographs of the lumbar spine in antero-posterior and lateral projection plus functional views in flexion and extension were acquired.

Patient selection

The indications were mono- or bisegmental lumbar disc degeneration and postoperative disc degeneration, as well as osteochondrosis and degeneration of levels adjacent to a former lumbar fusion. In all patients, symptoms had not responded to an extensive course of outpatient and inpatient physiotherapy including fluoroscopy-guided infiltrations as part of the preoperative workup. Conservative treatments were performed for more than 6 months in all patients. The symptoms of the patients had to be concordant with the results of preoperative imaging.

Contraindications were all kinds of translational instability (e.g. spondylolisthesis), spinal stenosis, significant osteoarthritis of the facet joints, deformities, infection or tumor, unwillingness to comply with study requirements regarding follow-up visits and radiological controls, previous fusion attempts in the affected levels, pregnancy and incomplete worker's compensation procedures.

All patients were operated according to the surgical philosophy described above. Postoperatively, the patients were mobilized on the day after surgery. With physiotherapeutic advice, most patients were able to be discharged a few days postoperatively.

Results

Patient population

Between June 2000 and March 2002, 34 patients were operated. Gender distribution was 12 males and 22 females. Average age was 44.0 years, ranging from 25.2 to 65.4 years. The predominant diagnosis was degenerative disc disease in 61.8% (21 patients), while disc degeneration in combination with a median nucleus pulposus herniation was found in 11.8% (four patients). Five patients (14.7%) had a postoperative osteochondrosis following disc surgery, three patients (8.8%) had a disc degeneration adjacent to a spinal fusion, and one patient had a dislocated nucleus replacement device at the affected level (Table 2). The lumbosacral motion segment, L5/S1, was affected in most cases (24 patients; 70.6%). In three patients (8.8%) it was L5/6, in a further three patients L4/5 was symptomatic, and in three patients we found a bisegmental affection in L4/5 and L5/S1. One patient (2.9%) had an affection of L2/3.

Table 2 Diagnosis for total disc replacement (*FBS* failed back syndrome)

Degenerative disc disease	61.8% (21/34)
Degenerative disc disease + disc herniation	11.8% (4/34)
FBS/postop. osteochondrosis	14.7% (5/34)
Adjacent level degeneration	8.8% (3/34)
Degenerative following nucleus replacement	2.9% (1/34)

Intra-operative data

In 54.8% a transperitoneal approach was used and in 45.2% a retroperitoneal midline approach was used. Mean operating time was 130.9 min, ranging from 88 to 300 min, with a standard deviation of 45.9 min. Average blood loss was 117 ml per level (range 30–350 ml).

The Prodisc implant is available in two sizes. The "medium" size was used in 36 of 37 affected segments, and "large" was used at one level. The implant with 6° lordosis angle was used in 65.4%; the 11° angle was used in 34.6%. The polyethylene inlay of 10 mm height was used in 34 segments, the 12-mm inlay in two segments and the 14-mm inlay in one segment.

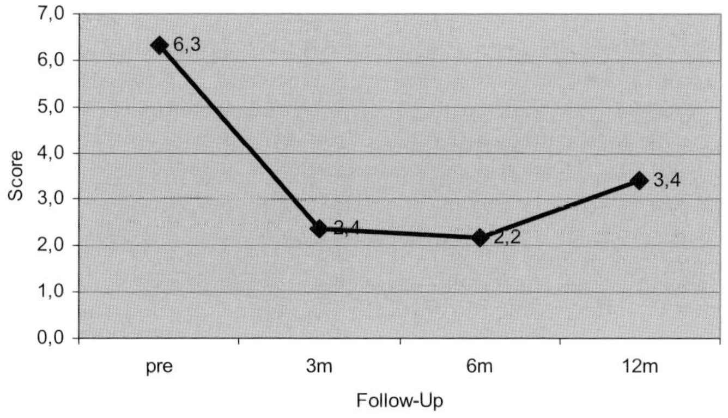

Fig. 8 Visual analog scale (VAS) pre-operatively and after total disc replacement

Clinical results

Twenty-six of 34 patients (76.5%) attended at least one follow-up visit for evaluation. The remaining patients had not yet finished the first 3-month interval postoperatively. Average follow-up was 5.8 months, with a standard deviation of 3.0 months.

The VAS scale averaged 6.3 points preoperatively. It was reduced by 3.9 points on average, ranging from 8.4 points reduction to 7.5 points increase (Fig. 8).

The Oswestry score ranged from 1 to 32 points before surgery, with an average of 19.1 points (standard deviation 7.4 points). It was reduced postoperatively by an average of 11.5 points. The change in the postoperative score ranged from 27 points reduction to an increase of 12 points (standard deviation 9.6 points) (Fig. 9).

While all patients had low-back pain before surgery, 76% had no low-back pain at the time of their latest follow-up.

Presently, we do not see any difference in clinical outcome between the subgroups of those patients previously operated or between the patients with a bisegmental versus those with a unisegmental implantation.

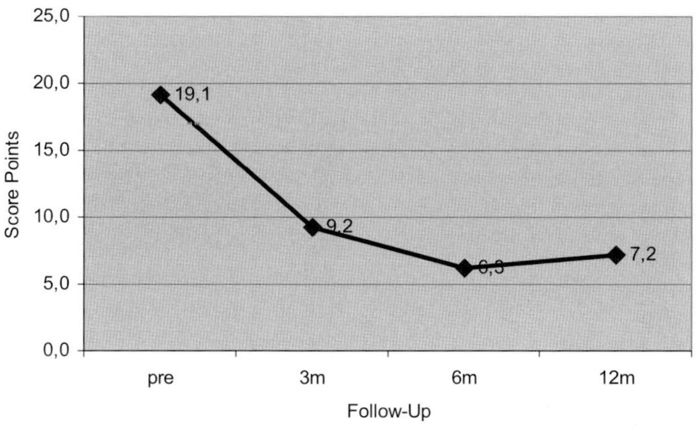

Fig. 9 Oswestry Low Back Disability Index pre-operatively and following total disc replacement

The duration of the postoperative hospital stay averaged 12.0 days (range 4–25 days).

At the time of the latest follow-up, 60.9% of all patients were "completely satisfied", while 21.7% were "satisfied", which gives an overall success rate according to the subjective rating of 82.6%. However, all of the 17.4% who were not satisfied with the clinical result stated that they would undergo the operation again if they were again faced with that choice.

Radiological results

Regarding all 37 devices implanted, we saw no loosening of the implant and no migration. Follow-up radiographs showed no change in the function of the implant over time. Endplates of the adjacent vertebrae did not show any subsidence.

Complications

In 91.2% of all patients, we did not see any complications. We have seen three complications related to the surgical procedure. There were no intra-operative complications, no general complications and no deaths. No patient in our series had to be fused in a re-operation of the affected segment. We did not see any superficial or deep infections.

One patient experienced a nerve root irritation of the L5 nerve root several days postoperatively. Computed tomography revealed an extra-foraminal protrusion of nucleus material compromising the L5 nerve root on the left side. Neurological examination was normal. A 3-week outpatient course of conservative treatment and perineural infiltrations led to complete and permanent pain reduction.

One other case showed substantial pain reduction in the immediate postoperative course. Five weeks later, an increase of pain was noted with no notable trauma. Radiographs showed an inlay dislocation anteriorly. The surgical revision revealed an intact polyethylene inlay. The endplates were solidly fixed and showed no signs of loosening. They were removed and the whole device was replaced by a new implant. We believe that this case was a technical failure at the time of the first implantation, when the polyethylene inlay obviously was not completely snapped into the inferior endplate. The ongoing clinical course was uneventful, pain reduction was achieved, and radiographic controls were normal. One patient complained of a retrograde ejaculation at 3 months follow-up.

Conclusions

These are preliminary results with a new implant for total disc replacement. As compared to a first-generation competing implant system, which has been in clinical use since 1984, there are striking differences with respect to the design and implantation technique [1, 4]. The major advantage of this kind of implant is that removal of the disc, distraction of the intervertebral space and insertion of the device can be performed through standardized minimally invasive approaches, which have already been used successfully for anterior lumbar interbody fusion with slight modifications. Minimally invasive approaches are possible even in difficult anatomical regions such as L4/5 and higher lumbar levels. The perioperative results show that iatrogenic morbidity is very low. All patients could get out of bed the day after the operation. For study and academic reasons, we kept most of the patients in hospital for more than 1 week; however, our data suggest that the majority of the patients will be able to leave the hospital after a few days where there is an uneventful perioperative course. Intra-operative data are virtually the same as with anterior interbody fusion, except for the fact that there is no co-morbidity at the donor site for bone grafts [6]. Although this was not a randomised study, the early clinical results are promising. There were two "specific" complications, which were resolved and ended up with a favorable clinical result. The postoperative L5 root irritation in one patient was most probably the result of inadequate removal of the nucleus pulposus. Since the implant is space-occupying, there might be a certain risk that remaining disc tissue is pushed towards the spinal canal or the foramen while the implant is impacted into the disc space. The second complication (anterior dislocation of the polyethylene inlay) was definitely a technical error during the implantation. The snap-locking mechanism of the inlay prevents dislocation, but requires precision during the insertion. The anterior border of the inlay must be in line with the anterior border of the inferior endplate. Even slight "steps" of less than 1 mm should not be tolerated.

In summary, although preliminary, the results suggest, that total disc replacement for the indications mentioned above might be a reasonable alternative to lumbar fusion.

References

1. Büttner-Janz K, Schellnack K, Zippel H (1989) Biomechanics of the SB Charite lumbar intervertebral disc endoprosthesis. Int Orthop 13:173–176
2. Cinotti G, David T, Postacchini F (1996) Results of disc prosthesis after a minimum follow-up peroid of 2 years. Spine 21:995–1000
3. Danish Institute for Health Technology Assessment (1999) Low-back-pain – frequency, management and prevention from an HTA perspective. Danish Institute for Health Technology Assessment series, vol. 1(1)
4. David T (1993) Lumbar disc prosthesis: surgical technique, indications and clinical results in 22 patients with a minimum of 12 months follow-up. Eur Spine J 1:254–259
5. Enker P, Steffee A, McMillin C, Keppler L, Biscup R, Miller S (1993) Artificial disc replacement. Spine 18:1061–1070
6. Mayer HM (1997) A new, microsurgical technique for minimal invasive anterior lumbar interbody fusion (MINIALIF). Spine 22:691–700
7. Mayer HM (2000) Microsurgical anterior interbody fusion: the transperitoneal approach to L5/S1. In: Mayer HM (ed) Minimally invasive spine surgery. Springer, Berlin Heidelberg New York, pp 133–144
8. Mayer HM (2000) The ALIF concept. Eur Spine J 9:S35-S43
9. Mayer HM (2000) Minimally invasive anterior arthrodesis of the lumbar spine. In: Duparc J (ed) Surgical Techniques in Orthopaedics and Traumatology, 55–070-E-10. Elsevier, Paris
10. Saal JS, Saal JA (2000) Management of chronic discogenic low back pain with a thermal intradiscal catheter. Spine 25:382–388
11. Scott AH, Harrison DJ (2000) Increasing age does not affect good outcome after lumbar disc replacement. Int Orthop 24:50–53
12. Zeegers WS, Bohnen LMLJ, Laaper M, Verhaegen MJA (1999) Artificial disc replacement with the modular type SB Charite III: 2-year results in 50 prospectively studied patients. Eur Spine J 8:210–217

Rudolf Bertagnoli
Selva Kumar

Indications for full prosthetic disc arthroplasty: a correlation of clinical outcome against a variety of indications

R. Bertagnoli (✉) · S. Kumar
Klinikum St. Elisabeth,
Kay 2a, 94315, Straubing, Germany
e-mail: bertagnoli@ogp.de,
Tel.: +49-9421-7101816,
Fax: +49-9421-530475

Abstract In this prospective study, a total of 134 prosthetic discs were replaced in 108 patients undergoing total disc replacement surgeries for degenerative disc disease. It was the aim of this study to correlate the clinical findings and the outcome of our patients treated with Prodisc II prostheses for various indications and to formulate indication criteria for disc replacement surgeries. The discs were implanted at L5/S1 in 61 patients, L5/L6 in 3 patients, L4/L5 in 31 patients, L3/L4 in 7 patients, and L2/L3 in 3 patients. There were 12 patients with two-level implants: from L4 to S1 in 11 of them and from L2 to L5 in the remaining one. Two patients also had three-level implants, from L3 to S1. Follow-up evaluation included plain radiographs, physical evaluation, and subjective evaluation by the patient using the Oswestry scale, the visual analog pain scale, and the SF-36V2 well-being questionnaire. The evaluation exercise showed that 90.8% of patients had excellent results, 7.4% had good results and 1.8% had fair results, with no poor results seen. Postoperatively, the average vertebral motion was increased in all patients at the operated level. Progression of disc degeneration at the adjacent levels was noted in ten patients. The average time to resuming activities of daily living unaided was 2.3 weeks. No implant failures or complications due to surgery were encountered in this study. Total prosthesis disc replacement for degenerative disc disease was found to be a good treatment modality, provided proper patient selection and criteria are adhered to. We were able to formulate indication criteria based on this.

Keywords Total prosthetic disc replacement · Disc arthroplasty · Degenerative disc disease · Lumbar spine

Introduction

Chronic back pain and degenerative disc disease are among the most common ailments affecting the population worldwide. Seventy to eighty percent [28] of the population of the Western world experiences low-back pain at one time or another. Although many of these complaints can be treated conservatively, there have been a growing number of cases that have failed conservative management, and treatment for these cases usually entails surgical intervention. There are numerous surgical options available for degenerative disc disease, ranging from standard discectomies (open or microsurgical) to percutaneous nucleotomies, chemical and thermal nucleolysis and spinal fusion modalities. Although they may give symptomatic relief initially, long-term reviews of these treatment modalities have shown them to be less favorable [11, 13, 14]. Even the fusion modalities that were once thought to be the answer to these problems have, in the long term, proved to have their own pertinent problems in the forms of accelerated degeneration of the adjacent lumbar segments, pseudoarthrosis, spinal stenosis and low-back pain, to name a few [4, 16, 21, 24]. It is these problems, coupled with the need for a better treatment modality, that have brought about the idea of a total prosthetic replacement as a treatment for degenerative disc disease.

Though a few studies involving clinical trials have been done [6, 10, 15, 30], they have all included very few study subjects, and none gives a clear picture as regards indications for such operative treatments. It was hence the aim of this study to correlate the clinical findings and outcomes of our patients treated with full prosthetic disc replacement with the various indications, to formulate an indication pattern as a guideline for full prosthetic disc replacement surgeries.

Materials and methods

A total of 134 discs were replaced in 108 patients, operated by a single surgeon, and all patients were available for evaluation The follow-up period ranged from 3 months to 2 years.

There were 58 men and 50 women, with an average age of 41.5 years (range 34–65 years). Preoperative diagnosis included disc degeneration (vertical instability) in 67 patients, failed disc surgery syndrome in 35, and 6 patients were diagnosed with transition zone syndrome (TZS). The operated levels were L5/S1 (61 patients), L5/L6 (3 patients), L4/L5 (31 patients), L3/L4 (7 patients), L2/L3 (3 patients), L4/L5 and L5/S1 (10 patients), L2/L3 and L4/L5 (1 patient), and L3/L4, L4/L5 and L5/S1 (2 patients).

All patients were evaluated with plain radiographs, which were standardized, and also with magnetic resonance imaging (MRI), which showed disc degeneration at one or more levels and the status of the facet joints. Plain radiographs were also used to assess the spinal range of motion on flexion and extension at the operated levels and the adjacent levels, and status of the implant. The preoperative status of the discs and facet joints at the adjacent levels was evaluated. Clinical evaluation included physical examination, which included spinal range of movements, motor strength, peripheral nerve assessment and patients' subjective response to the Oswestry questionnaire, the SF-36V2 well-being questionnaire and the visual analog pain scale (VAS). On follow-up, patients' response to pain sensation, their need of analgesics and duration of analgesic use were also recorded. All patients undergoing surgery had previously been treated with conservative management for a minimum period of 6 months, and all had shown a positive preoperative response to discography. All operations were performed using an anterior approach, approaching the disc space retroperitoneally whenever possible. The patients were all positioned supine in the "French position". As is our practice, all operations were performed using less invasive techniques. Postoperatively, all patients underwent physiotherapy within 1 week of operation. They were also required to wear a lumbar corset for a maximum of 3 months.

Severe osteoporosis, physiological dysfunction, history of previous disc infection, severe posterior element pathologies, fracture of the vertebra, and tumor were deemed to be contraindications, and formed the basis for exclusion criteria.

Statistical analysis was performed using the *t*-test and chi-squared test.

Results

From the analysis obtained preoperatively and during the follow-up period, the overall clinical outcome was deemed to be excellent in 98 patients (90.8%), good in 8 patients

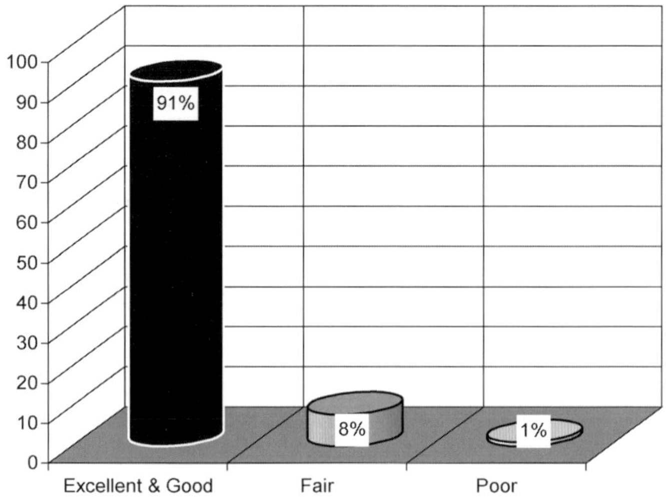

Fig. 1 Clinical outcome: overall results

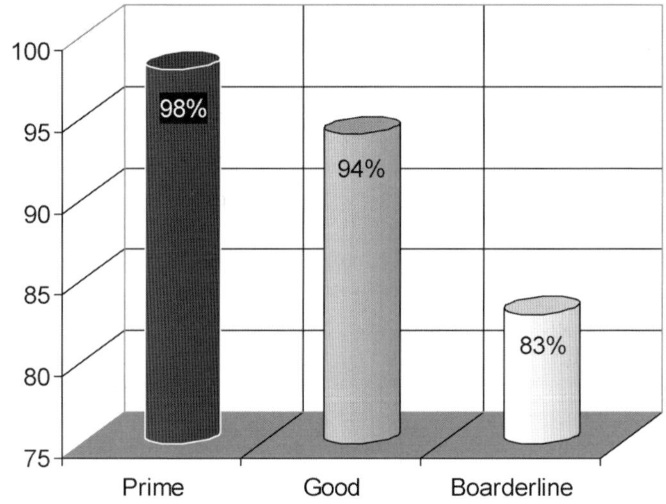

Fig. 2 Average patient satisfaction with outcome correlated with "prime", "good", and "borderline" indications

(7.4%), fair in 2 patients (1.8%), and poor in none (0%). Of the two patients who had fair results, both had advanced disc degeneration also involving the adjacent levels and secondary osteoarthrosis of the facet joints.

Postoperatively, nine patients had residual leg pain or back pain including facet joint pain. There were 45 patients who required analgesics for more than 2 weeks, 12 of whom required regular analgesics for a period ranging from 6 months to 1 year, and 33 patients required analgesics only occasionally. Immediate postoperative complications were noted in only one patient, in the form of systemic septicemia, which resolved with a course of antibiotics. This was not, however, related to the surgery. The patients were able to resume their activities of daily living unaided after an average of 2.3 weeks (range 1.5–3.2 weeks) ($P<0.001$).

Table 1 Indication criteria of categories for full disc replacement (*OA* osteoarthritic)

Indications	Disc levels	Accompanying features
Prime	Single level	>4 mm remaining disc height No OA changes to facet joints No adjacent level degeneration Intact posterior elements
Good	Single level/ double level	>4 mm remaining disc height No primary OA changes to facet joints Minimum degeneration of adjacent discs Minimum posterior segment instability, e.g. post microdiscectomy
Borderline	Single/double/ triple level	<4 mm remaining disc height Primary OA changes to facet joints Minimum adjacent level degeneration Minimum posterior segment instability Adjacent to fusions
Poor	Single/double/ triple level	Gross degeneration of the spine Secondary OA changes to the facet joints <4 mm disc height remaining at the adjacent levels Posterior segment instability

There were 54 patients who were on follow-up for more than 1 year, 35 of whom were able to resume work at the same level as prior to surgery, 17 were able to resume work at a lower level than prior to surgery, and 2 patients were unable to return to work due to residual back or leg pain ($P>0.005$). The average range of vertebral motion at the L5/S1 operated levels was 9° (range 2°–13°), at the L4/L5 levels it was 10° (range 9°–13°, at L3/L4 it was 10° (range 8°–15°) and at L2/L3 it was 12° (range 9°–15°). The average range of vertebral motion at the adjacent segments compared to the preoperative range of motion was: decreased range 5° (range 3°–8°) (6 patients), increased range 6° (range 3°–8°) (86 patients), and it was unchanged in 16 patients. Analysis also showed that, postoperatively, all patients had an increase in the average range of motion at the operated levels. Twelve of those who showed no change in the average range of motion at the adjacent levels had presented with advanced degenerative disc disease prior to surgery, and four had secondary changes of the facet joints in addition to advanced degenerative disc disease prior to surgery. In these patients, the average preoperative range of motion at the operated segment was 4° (range 2°–6°), and postoperatively, the range of motion averaged 7° (range 5°–10°). Progression of disc degeneration at the adjacent levels was noted in five patients (4.6%); at L5/S1 levels in three of them and at L4/L5 levels in two ($P=0.003$). It was also noted that all the patients who had progression of disc degeneration had presented with an anterior disc height of less than 7 mm prior to surgery. We correlated the outcome of the surgery with the indications (number of degenerate discs and the accompanying features), and then categorised the indications from "prime", which correlated with the best outcomes, to "borderline" and "poor", which were associated with the least satisfactory results (Fig. 1, Fig. 2, Table 1).

The average level of patient satisfaction with outcome in the prime category was 98% (range 96%–99%); it was

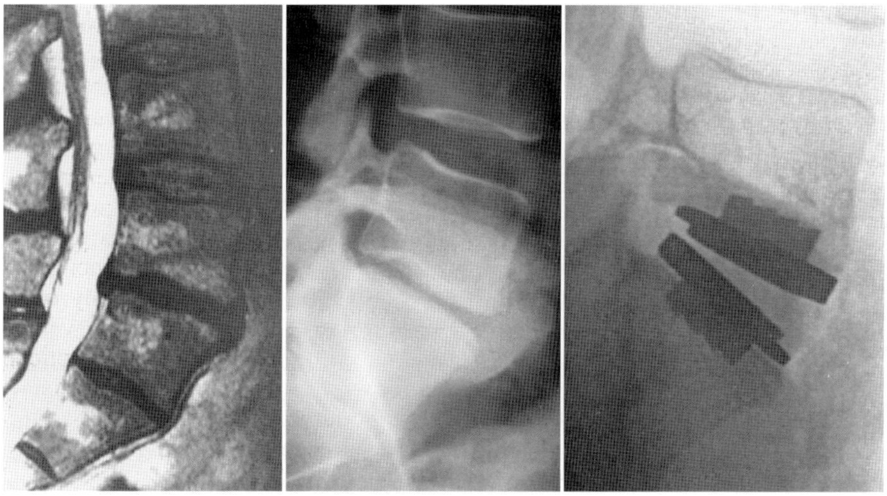

Fig. 3 Case 1 (prime indication): a 44-year-old woman with vertical instability and severe low-back pain, who had previously undergone unsuccessful conservative treatment

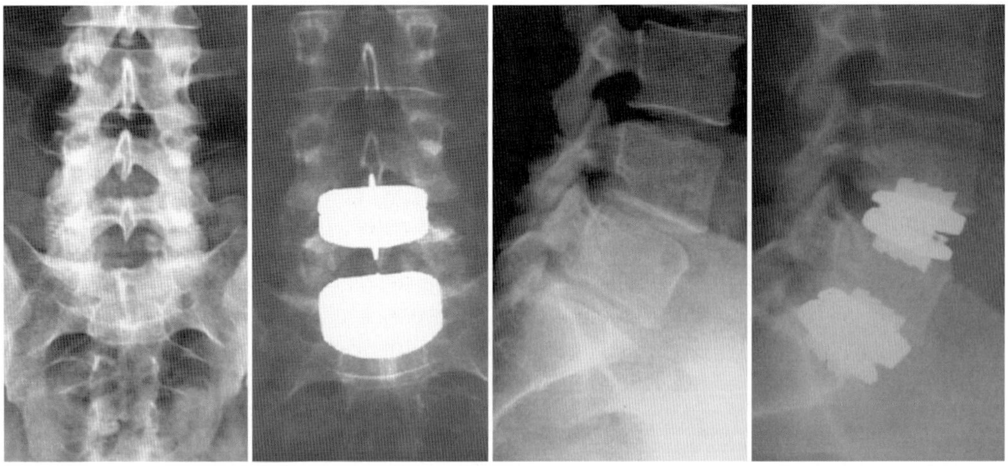

Fig. 4 Case 2 (good indication): a 30-year-old man with radicular symptoms at L4, L5, and severe low-back pain. He had previously undergone unsuccessful percutaneous nucleotomy treatment at L5/S1, as well as unsuccessful conservative treatment

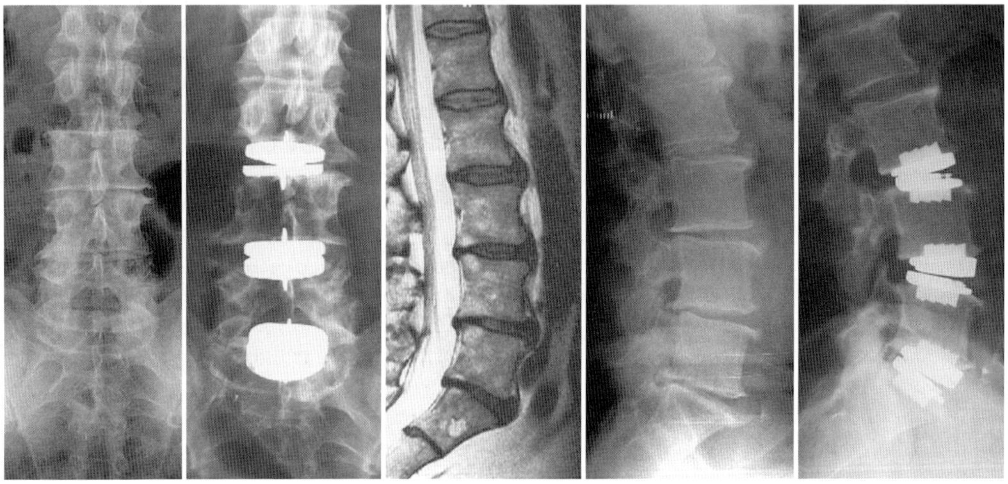

Fig. 5 Case 3 (borderline indication): 53-year-old man with vertical segmental instabilities at L3-S1, radicular symptoms at L4, L5, and severe low-back pain. He had previously undergone unsuccessful conservative treatment

93% in the good category (range 89%–97%) and 83% in the borderline category (range 79%–88%).

Radiographic evaluation during follow-up did not show any implant loosening or subsidence of the prosthesis, nor was there any structural failure of the implants, such as rupture of the plate or expulsion of the polyethylene. Examples of cases in various categories are given in Fig. 3, Fig. 4 and Fig. 5.

Discussion

This prospective study was carried out in order to analyze the effectiveness of a prosthetic disc replacement in degenerative discs of various indications and stages of degeneration, so as to formulate indication criteria for total disc replacement surgeries for degenerative disc disease.

Since the early work of Fernström in the late 1960s, who explored the possibility of replacing the diseased intervertebral disc with a prosthetic device, much work has been done in this field in terms of research and development of designs [1, 3, 9, 17, 20, 22]. Early clinical trials on humans [5, 6, 8, 10, 15, 26, 29] have shown varying degrees of optimism. Nevertheless, the need for a better treatment modality has been emphasized by studies showing the unwarranted sequelae of present treatment modalities, especially those following spinal fusion [4, 16, 21]. It has been postulated that an ideally performed total disc replacement would eliminate untoward results of disc surgery, such as instability pain, stenosis, pseudoarthrosis, accelerated degeneration of the adjacent segment and spondylosis, to name a few that may be encountered in other treatment modalities [23, 25, 27, 30]. In addition, it has also been postulated that such a device may have a protective role on the facet joints, as suggested by Hedman et al. [17]. Overcoming the long-term unwarranted outcomes, while at the same time restoring the lumbar motion segment would be most welcome.

In 1991, in his series using the SB Charité artificial disc prosthesis, Zippel reported 54% very good results, 29% improved, 15% unchanged and 2% poor results. Further studies done by Zippel and also by Fernström have all failed to address the status of the posterior elements, particularly the facet joints [12, 30]. This is an important point, not to be overlooked when performing a total disc replacement, especially when the posterior elements have been shown to carry at least 18% of the compressive loads and resist one-third of the shear forces of the functional motion segment. As the facet joints also serve the kinematics function of guiding segmental spinal motion, better results would naturally be obtained in cases that have less facet joint degeneration or before secondary osteoarthritic changes of the facets are noted. In the same context, preserving the posterior longitudinal ligament is also desired, as this adds to the load sharing device in concert with the posterior elements [2, 7, 18]. From the results obtained in our series, we concur with the study by Kilkardy-Willis [19], that the best results of a prosthetic disc replacement are obtained in patients with disc degeneration before secondary changes in the facet joints are seen, otherwise progression of the degenerative process of the facet joints leads to instability. Though advanced disc degeneration may pose a challenge in total disc replacement, we have found that in such cases alone, resection of the posterior longitudinal ligament facilitates the mobilization of the segment. The analysis of our results, with varying follow-up periods and scenarios, has shed some light on the indications for a total disc replacement with a prosthesis in degenerative disc disease. This has helped us in formulating an indication criterion for total disc replacement surgeries, which we have subdivided into four categories (Table 1).

In accordance with this, the contraindications for a total disc replacement surgery would be: osteoporosis or other osteopathy that results in a reduced load-bearing capacity of the vertebral body endplates, and generally all severe dorsal pathologies, e.g. spondylolisthesis or hypertrophic facet joints with secondary spinal stenosis, fractures, infection and tumors. Using these basic guidelines, we believe that a more favorable outcome may be obtained for total disc replacement surgeries, putting emphasis on better patient selection and indications.

Conclusion

In conclusion, from the overall favorable results obtained in our series, we strongly believe that total disc replacement with a prosthetic disc is a good treatment option for degenerative disc disease of the spine, provided the proper criteria are adhered to in patient selection. The early results presented here, which were obtained under study conditions, though lacking in the duration of follow-up of for a portion of the patients, nevertheless allow a great deal of optimism regarding this mode of therapy. However, it should be emphasized that not all patients with degenerative disc disease will be ideal candidates for disc replacement. As we encountered in our series, the best results were seen in the prime and good indications. The overall outcome of disc replacement surgeries may be compromised by the inclusion of patients with borderline and poor indications. Hence, great emphasis should be placed on the indications, especially for surgeons who are new to such operations. It is also pertinent to continue to critically judge and closely follow the progress of this treatment modality, in order to ascertain whether the good short-term results are also demonstrated in the long term. More prospective multicenter studies would be helpful in order to better evaluate the outcome of total disc replacement surgeries for degenerative disc disease.

References

1. Aharinejad S, Bertagnoli R, Wicke K, Schneider B (1990) Morphometric analysis of vertebra and intervertebral discs as a basis of disc replacement. Am J Anat 189:69–76
2. Bertagnoli R (1992) Ergebnisse der dorsoventralen Stabilisierungsverfahren beim Postnucleotomiesyndrom und bieausgeprägten osteochondrotischen Veränderungen im Lumbalbereich. In: Matzen KA (ed) Wirbelsäulenchirurgie, vol II. Thieme, Stuttgart, pp 234–248
3. Bertagnoli R (2001) Continuum of care in degenerative disc disease. Back Up 1:4–8
4. Brodsky AE (1976) Post-laminectomy and post-fusion stenosis of the lumbar spine. Clin Orthop 115:130
5. Büttner-Janz K, Schellnack K, Zippel H, Conrad P (1988) Experience and results with the SB-Charité lumbar intervertebral endoprosthesis. Z Klin Med 43:1785–1789
6. Cinotti G, David T, Postacchini F (1996) Results of disc prosthesis after a minimum follow-up of 2 years. Spine 21:995–1000
7. Cryon BW, Hutton WC (1980) Artificial tropism and stability of the lumbar spine. Spine 5:168–172
8. David T (1993) Lumbar disc prosthesis: surgical technique, indications and clinical results in 22 patients with a minimum of 12 months follow-up. Eur Spine J 1:254–259
9. Eljkelkamp MF, Dankelaar Van CC, Veldhuizen AG, Horn Van J R, Huyghe JM, Verkerke GJ (2000) Requirements for an artificial intervertebral disc. Int J Artif Organs 24:311–321
10. Enker P, Steffee A, Mcmillin C, Keppler L, Biscup R, Miller S (1993) Artificial disc replacement. Preliminary report with a 3-year minimum follow-up. Spine 18:1061–1070
11. Etsuro Y, Kasuhiro C, Yoshiaki T, Kiyoshi H (2001) Long-term study of standard discectomy for lumbar disc herniation. A follow-up study of more than 10 years. Spine 26:652–657
12. Fernström U (1996) Arthroplasty with intercorporal endoprosthesis in herniated disc and painful disc. Acta Chir Scand 357 [Suppl]:154–159
13. Feymore JW, Hanley EN Jr, Howe J, Kuhlmann D, Matteri RE (1979) A comparison on radiographic findings in fusion and non-fusion patients 10 or more years following lumbar discal surgery. Spine 4:435–440
14. George AL, Konstandinos S, Paul GK, George S, Dimitrios SK, George H (1999) Seven to 20-year outcome of lumbar discectomy. Spine 24:2313–2317

15. Griffith FL, Shelokof AP, Buttner-Janz K, LeMrie JP, Zeegers WS (1994) A multicenter retrospective study of the clinical results of the link SB Charité intervetebral prosthesis. Spine 19: 1842–1849
16. Harris RI, Wiley JJ (1963) Acquired spondylolysis as a sequel to spine fusion. J Bone Joint Surg Am 45:1159
17. Hedman TP, Kostuik JP, Fernie GR, Hellier WG (1991) Design of an intervertebral disc prosthesis. Spine 16 [Supp1]:256–260
18. King AL, Prasad P, Ewing CL (1975) Mechanism of spinal injury due to cephalocaudal acceleration. Orthop Clin North Am 6:19–31
19. Kirkaldy-Willis WH, Burton CV (1992) Managing low back pain, 3rd edn. Churchill Livingstone, New York, pp105–119
20. Langrana LA, Lee CK, Yang SW (1991) Finite element modeling of the synthetic intervertebral disc. Spine 16 [Suppl 6]:245–252
21. Lee CK (1988) Accelerated degeneration of the segment adjacent to a lumbar fusion. Spine 13:375–377
22. Lee CK, Langrana LA, Parsons JR, Zimmerman MC (1991) Development of a prosthetic intervertebral disc. Spine 16 [Suppl 6]:253–255
23. Lee CK, Parsons JR, Langrana LA, Zimmerman MC (1992) Relative efficacy of the artificial disc versus spinal fusion. In: Weinstein JN (ed) Clinical efficacy and outcome in the diagnosis and treatment of low back pain. Raven Press, New York, pp 237–244
24. Lehman TR, Spratt KF, Tozzi JE, et al (1987) Long-term follow-up of lumbar fusion patients. Spine 12:97–104
25. Ray CD (1992) The artificial disc: introduction, history and socioeconomics. In: Weinstein JN (ed) Clinical efficacy and outcome in the diagnosis and treatment of low back pain. Raven Press, New York, pp 205–226
26. Sott AT, Harrison DJ (2000) Increasing age does not affect good outcome after lumbar disc replacement. Int Orthop 24:50–53
27. Steffee AD (1992) The Steffee artificial disc. In: Weinstein JN (ed) Clinical efficacy and the outcome in the diagnosis and treatment of low back pain. Raven Press, New York, pp 245–258
28. Vijay KG, Nishiama K, Weinstein JN, King YL (1986) Mechanical properties of the lumbar spinal motion segments as affected by partial disc removal. Spine 11:1008–1012
29. Zeegers WS, Bohnen LM, Laaper M, Veerhaegen MJ (1999) Artificial disc replacement with modular type SB Charité. III. 2-year results in 50 prospectively studied patients. Eur Spine J 8:375–377
30. Zippel H (1991) 'Charité modular': conception, experience and results. In: Weinstein JN, Mayer HM, Weigel K (eds) The artificial disc. Springer, Berlin Heidelberg Nw York, pp 69–78

Charles D. Ray

The PDN® prosthetic disc-nucleus device

Disclosure: The author initially conceived and patented the prosthetic disc nucleus and much of its associated instrumentation. He is a consultant to and owns shares in Raymedica, Inc., the manufacturer of the devices and instruments. The devices are not yet approved for implantation in the United States, although the CE mark has been obtained for worldwide application.

C.D. Ray
5758 George Washington Memorial Hwy, Yorktown, Virginia, USA

Correspondence to:
R. Vazquez
Raymedica, Inc.,
9401 James Avenue South, Suite 120, Bloomington, MN 55431 USA
(e-mail: r.vazquez@raymedica.com,
Tel.: +1-952-2773259,
Fax: +1-952-8850200)

Abstract The health of an intervertebral disc is based on a complicated interplay between physiology and biomechanics. The nucleus pulposus must remain well hydrated, and the surrounding anulus fibrosus must be competent in order for the disc to function properly. If either of these components fail, the disc will begin to degenerate, and clinically relevant symptoms may appear. Disc degeneration has traditionally been treated by either discectomy or immobilization of the affected vertebrae, and though these treatments can be effective, they also have their limitations. To help fill the therapy gap that exists for treating moderate degenerative disc disease, the PDN device has been developed. The device consists of a hydrogel core and a polyethylene jacket that are designed to assume the cushioning function of a healthy disc, while restoring/maintaining disc height and allowing normal range of motion. To receive the device, patients must have a preoperative disc height of at least 5 mm and the vertebral endplates must be free of significant defects such as Schmorl's nodules or fractures. Two approaches can be used for implanting PDN devices: a hemilaminotomy approach, where the disc is accessed through the back, or an Anterior-Lateral transPsoatic Approach (ALPA), where the disc is accessed from the side. In either case, the nucleus material is removed from the disc, and the devices are placed transversely within the nucleus cavity. The amount of research and development currently taking place in the field of disc arthroplasty gives hope that the treatment of degenerative disc disease will soon become multifaceted, with numerous choices being available to surgeons and their patients.

Keywords Intervertebral disc · Disc arthroplasty · PDN device · Degenerative disc disease · Nucleus pulposus

Introduction

On 26 January 1996, in Wiesbaden, Germany, a 40-year-old man with disabling degenerative disc disease at the L5-S1 level was given three choices for treatment: (1) to continue with his problem, perhaps with additional conservative management, (2) to undergo a spinal fusion at the affected level, or (3) to have a new experimental device implanted with the intended purpose of restoring disc function. He opted for the PDN prosthetic disc-nucleus device.

Six years later, over 550 patients have been implanted with this device [9], and the number of cases continues to increase as the advantages and efficacy of the device become more widely known and accepted. The PDN implant can be a valid choice – as opposed to fusion or pedicle screw fixation – due to the prospects of maintaining segmental flexibility, while requiring a less invasive surgical procedure. Based on these desirable goals, the device is currently in use by selected clinicians in several countries all over the world, including the Middle East, Europe, and Latin America. Additionally, clinical trials are proceeding in Canada and the United States [10, 11].

In order to clarify the structure and function of the PDN device, it is important to review the basic biomechanical and physiological principles involved. Nearly 18 years of research and development have gone into realizing the implant, its surgical method, and associated instruments. Several of these details are reviewed below.

Disc mechanics and physiology

The primary functions of an intervertebral disc are to provide cushioning and allow the axial skeleton to remain flexible. The structures of the disc are the ligamentous anulus fibrosus and the hygroscopic nucleus pulposus. The anulus is constructed of multiple (up to 20) circumferential laminations or plies. The inelastic type 1 collagen fibers of each lamination attach to each adjacent vertebral body in a diagonal orientation [2]. Each lamination is composed of right- and left-handed patches of these angulated fibers, which tighten with torsion of the disc space in either direction. This orientation is important to maintain bi-directional torsional stability. At the same time, the fibers and their laminations permit bulging under load, thereby creating the cushioning effect. Interestingly, the organization of the right- and left-handed patches in each lamination creates small imperfections. Between each lamination is a thin layer of glycosaminoglycan gel that permits limited motion between the plies [1]. Scanning electron microscopy of the anular surface subjected to high pressure shows that, if the anular imperfections happen to overlap, microherniations of the gel may pass through. In all probability, these may represent the starting point for macroherniations at some later date.

The content of fibers within the outer anulus is perhaps 90% of the entire mass. Progressively towards the center of the disc, the component of gel increases with each layer until, at the central nucleus, the gel content is about 90% with only 5 or 10% fiber. These internal fibers are shorter collagen fibers that do not directly attach to the vertebrae, but provide some substance to the nucleus mass. Under load, the semisolid nucleus pushes radially out from the center of the disc, causing the anulus to bulge [3, 7]. Effectively, the anulus dissipates the compressive forces via tensioning of its collagen fibers. In much the same way that a pneumatic tire absorbs shock, the intervertebral disc acts as a cushion between the vertebral bodies.

Even when at rest, discs are constantly under load. The pressure within the confines of the anulus is normally several atmospheres, and therefore many times greater than arterial pressure, preventing the normal disc from having a vascular bed. In fact, only the outermost layers of the anulus are fed by capillaries, which are naturally accompanied by 0.5–2 μm polymodal, pain-transmitting free nerve endings. With the high standing and loaded pressure within the nucleus, and in the absence of vascularity, the nucleus and inner anulus are anaerobic. Even the low-level nutritional exchange of intradiscal metabolites cannot pass through the anular layers, instead passing through the intact cartilaginous endplate and its macroscopic channels. These channels contain villus-like connections to a microvascular bed, where there are microscopic clusters of arteriolar cells comprising effective microglomeruli. These microglomeruli act as filters of fluids and small molecular constituents, effectively isolating the hygroscopic nucleus gel from potential attack by blood-borne enzymes and globulins [6]. Although the exchange of metabolites is related to osmotic differential pressures across the filter membranes, the process of ridding the nucleus of byproducts to conversely bring in fluids and nutrients is augmented by a diurnal pumping action [10]. That is, during the daytime hours, under increased skeletal load, the vertical forces cause the byproducts to exit through the endplate and into the capillary bed. This mechanism reverses at night when the axial load is minimal. With the fall in intradiscal pressure, the hydrophilic nucleus gel pulls fluid and nutrients into the disc through the endplates [4, 5]. This exchange of wastes and nutrients has been found to be essential for the disc health [12, 13].

The intervertebral disc continues to function correctly as long as both the anulus and the nucleus are intact. However, as a result of the normal aging process, the composition of the nucleus changes: by the third decade of life the nucleus is more fibrous and shows a loss of some water-absorbing and binding ability [13]. With this natural progression, by the fifth decade the nucleus is usually significantly dehydrated and has lost its mucoid consistency. This stiffening of the nucleus restricts its ability to push the anulus from within the disc, causing the anulus to bear more of the load by direct compression rather than centripetal tensioning of its fibers. Meakin and co-workers demonstrated that, in a fully functional nucleus, loading causes both the inner and outer margins of the anulus to bulge outward. However, when the nucleus no longer functions properly, under similar loading the inner anulus bulges or folds inward as the outer margin bulges outward [8]. As the gel layers between the laminations also dry out, this folding of the anulus permits tearing and delamination, weakening the disc. In addition to destabilizing the disc, tears in the anulus may permit internal disc metabolites to escape and reach the outer belt of free nerve endings, transmitters of pain impulses. The metabolites may further escape into the vertebral canal or outward to bathe the nearby root ganglion. A number of these anaerobic metabolites, such as lactic acid, stromelysin, metaloproteinases, and phospholipase-A2, normally concentrated in the disc, reach higher concentrations within the non-functioning, non-pumping degenerated nucleus. If and when they leak onto the free nerve endings or the root ganglion, they may precipitate acute or chronic back and/or leg pain. There may even be permanent changes in the ganglion under such chemical attack. This may be a common cause of severe, disabling discogenic back pain. Since only micromols of these metabolites can cause severe pain, a leakage sufficient to disable the patient can be provoked by very little motion of the segment. In the past, the most common method for removing the abnormal nucleus and stopping motion-induced discogenic back pain was to perform a fusion, discectomy alone often failing to stop the complex process.

Treating degenerative disc disease with a prosthetic nucleus

Fortunately, the clear majority of patients with natural disc degeneration never develop a clinically significant back problem, so no medical treatment is required. For others, however, the degeneration is accompanied by severe pain, and clinical intervention (conservative or surgical) may become necessary.

At present, the three standard options for treating degenerative disc disease are conservative treatment, discectomy, and immobilization. Conservative therapy largely consists of pain reduction by medication and various forms of applied therapy. The key indicators for surgical intervention are when the patient's lifestyle, work tolerance, emotional stability, or vocational activities are significantly altered due to debilitating pain. If the patient has psychiatric, legal, or social problems aggravating the condition, the indications become less clear and even confusing. Discectomy is primarily indicated in patients with direct nerve root compression, inflammation or vascular changes affecting the ganglion or root, but it is generally not indicated alone for the treatment of discogenic pain, due to the mechanical component of the problem that is inducing the back pain. Although the removal of most of the nucleus pulposus can relieve the nerve pressure and irritation, the segment is usually rendered less stable and less functional.

In many cases, the degeneration and pain may require some type of permanent immobilization of the segment. Numerous ways to stabilize degenerated vertebrae have been employed over the last 75 years, including bone grafting, plates, rods, pedicle screws, fusion cages, bone growth enhancing factors, or a combination of these. Although these methods usually succeed in relieving the motion-induced discogenic pain, they are highly invasive and permanently eliminate segmental function and mobility. Further, stiffening of a given segment may induce a more rapid degeneration of an adjacent segment.

The PDN disc-nucleus prosthesis has been developed to fill the therapy gap that exists between discectomy and fusion [10]. That is, the device offers a surgical solution to those patients whose discogenic back pain is sufficient to indicate the need for surgical intervention, but whose segment(s) are not so degenerated that immobilization of the affected vertebrae is the only reasonable alternative. The PDN device is designed to assume the cushioning function of a normal disc and simultaneously maintain disc height and flexibility.

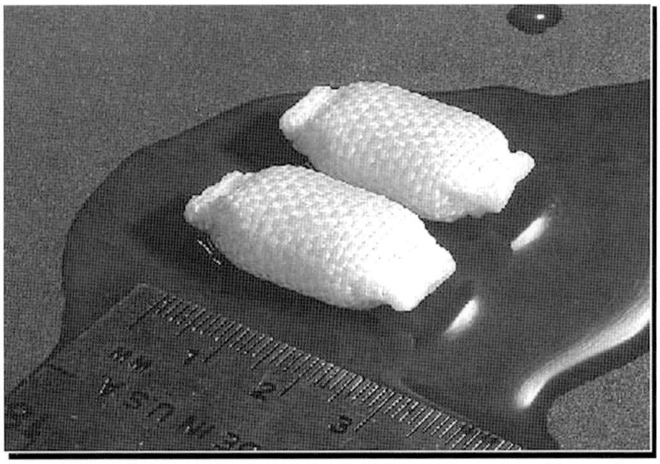

Fig. 1 The hydrophilic nature of the PDN hydrogel allows the devices to absorb fluid and swell

The PDN device is composed of a carefully formed hydrogel pellet that is encased in a polyethylene jacket (Fig. 1). The pellet is a copolymer of polyacrylonitrile (non-hydrophilic) and polyacrylamide (hydrophilic); the ratio of these two polymers determines the water absorbing and binding behavior of the finished hydrogel. The PDN pellets currently being used are designed to absorb 80% of their weight in water – this ability to absorb water and powerfully swell permits the device to restore or maintain disc height (Fig. 2). In order to limit the swelling, which unrestrained could potentially produce endplate fracturing, the pellet is surrounded by a very strong constraining jacket of high molecular weight and linear polyethylene fibers. The jacket also minimizes horizontal spreading, thus maintaining the implant shape so that it can retain the height of the disc even when subjected to heavy loading of the spine [11]. Each pellet (two are implanted in each enucleated disc space) has small platinum-iridium marker wires that are imbedded in the hydrogel in order to visualize the position and orientation of the implants by fluoroscopy during surgery and by ordinary X-ray imaging after surgery (Fig. 2).

It is very important to know that the PDN device and its component jacket have been subjected to mechanical and biological testing in order to ensure product safety and efficacy. Fatigue tests performed with loads of between 200 N and 800 N for 50 million cycles have shown that the device continues to function as designed, relative to load deflection, disc-height maintenance, and structural integrity. In addition, burst tests have been conducted using forces of up to 6000 N applied with no detrimental effects

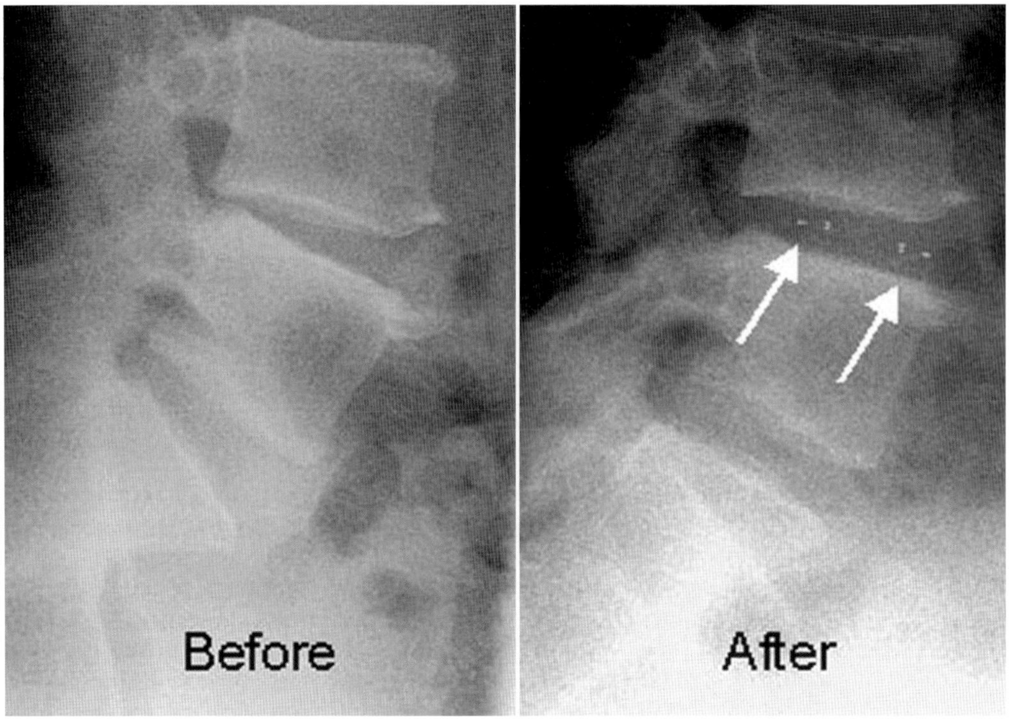

Fig. 2 Pre- and postoperative radiographs of L4-L5 disc space. Disc height has noticeably increased following implantation of PDN devices. Wire markers within the hydrogel allow for better X-ray and magnetic resonance imaging visualization

on the hydrogel or the jacket. Biocompatibility tests for systemic toxicity, genotoxicity, and carcinogenicity have all been negative. Studies have also been done to test for polyethylene wear debris, a problem that has resulted in osteolysis with other total joint-replacement devices. However, the polyethylene used to manufacture the PDN jacket is of a higher molecular weight than that ordinarily used in artificial joints (hip and knee), and mechanical testing has consistently shown no wear debris production for the PDN device [11].

Appropriate patient selection

With any medical device, proper patient selection is crucial, and the PDN implant is no exception. Five years of research and over 550 cases have allowed us to correctly determine the patients who should receive devices. Important anatomical selection criteria include the lack of advanced disc degeneration, namely the height of the central disc cavity must be 5 mm or greater and the vertebral endplates must be free of significant defects such as Schmorl's nodules or fractures. Moreover, the patient's body mass index (BMI = weight in kg / height in m^2) must be less than 30, and total body weight must be less than 90 kg if the implant is to be inserted at the L5–S1 level, to reduce the potential for angular slippage.

Additionally, the anterior-posterior (AP) dimension of the affected disc (as indicated on magnetic resonance imaging films) must be large enough to accommodate the pair of PDN devices. Data suggest that an AP diameter of at least 37 mm is necessary for two devices to fit properly – our studies have shown that when smaller disc spaces are implanted with the two devices, there is a greater rate of migration or dislodgment. When the disc diameter is less than 37 mm, a single implant may be used, or the case may be abandoned.

Implantation techniques

Two techniques are commonly used to implant PDN devices: a posterior hemilaminotimy approach or an Anterior-Lateral transPsoatic Approach (ALPA). In the posterior approach, the patient is placed in the usual prone-sitting position, with knees and hips flexed. The disc is approached as in a standard discectomy, with minimal removal of bone and ligament. The dura and nerve root are retracted, and a stab incision is made in the posterior anulus, after which an anulus dilator is used to provide wider access to the nucleus. The disc is enucleated thoroughly using straight and angled pituitary rongeurs. The goal is to completely evacuate the nucleus before the PDN devices are implanted. After the nucleus has been prepared, the jacket is grasped with an Allis clamp, and a smooth curving steel band is inserted into the disc cavity to act as a guide. Small impactors are then used to drive the PDN devices through the dilated anulus opening and properly align them transversely across the prepared disc space (Fig. 3).

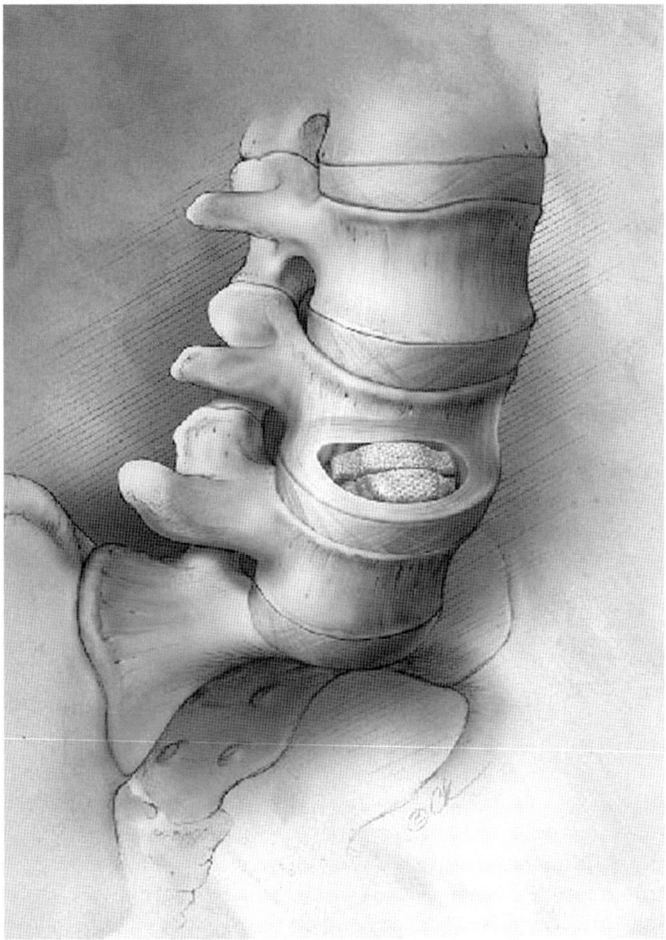

Fig. 3 Anterior and posterior PDN devices implanted at the L4-L5 disc space. The devices are situated transversely within the vacated nucleus cavity

The ALPA technique, developed by Rudolf Bertagnoli, differs from the posterior approach in that the disc is accessed laterally. The patient is placed in a lateral-decubitus position on an adjustable surgical table, and the table is flexed slightly to arch the upper flank, which will increase the distance between the iliac crest and the rib cage. The dissection passes through the external oblique, internal oblique, and transversus muscles. The retroperitoneal area is accessed and followed medially to the lumbar spine, where blunt dissection through the psoas muscle in a strict lateral direction is used to access the disc. A hinged flap is cut into the anulus and sufficient nucleus material is removed to accommodate the PDN devices. This approach is minimally traumatic, and the PDN devices are implanted directly into the disc space without having to be rotated 90° inside the nucleus cavity, as is the case in the posterior approach. As such, the implantation is faster and requires less surgical manipulation.

The future of the PDN device

The future of the PDN device and of artificial disc technology in general appears promising. The large number of patients requiring surgical relief from debilitating back pain, and the desire for more physiological methods of restabilizing the disc, are constant reminders of the need to find better solutions to this worldwide health condition. Presently there appear to be ten or more different types of prosthetic disc devices under development, with some currently in clinical trial. Those involving replacements of the nucleus, pioneered by the author, now include the Aquarelle, SINUX, and the PDN device. The total disc replacements include the Link SB Charité Artificial Disc, the ProDisc, and the Acroflex. Continued innovation and data from clinical outcomes will certainly advance disc arthroplasty technology over the next decade, greatly enhancing reasonable treatments for degenerative disc disease. It is also anticipated that cervical prostheses will arrive shortly. In this way, patients and surgeons will have additional, valid choices for care of various stages of symptomatic disc degeneration.

References

1. Bushell GR, Ghosh P, Taylor TF, Akeson WH (1977) Proteoglycan chemistry of the intervertebral disks. Clin Orthop 129:115–123
2. Cassidy JJ, Hiltner A, Baer E (1989) Hierarchical structure of the intervertebral disc. Connect Tissue Res 23:75–88
3. Fennell AJ, Jones AP, Hukins DW (1996) Migration of the nucleus pulposus within the intervertebral disc during flexion and extension of the spine. Spine 21:2753–2757
4. Ghosh P (1988) The biology of the intervertebral disc, vols I, II. CRC Press, Boca Raton
5. Holm S, Maroudas A, Urban JPG, Selstam G, Nachemson A (1981) Nutrition of the intervertebral disc: solute transport and metabolism. Connect Tissue Res 8:101–119
6. Hukins DW (1992) A simple model for the function of proteoglycan and collagen in the response to compression of the intervertebral disc. Proc R Soc Lond B Biol Sci 249:281–285
7. Klein JA, Hickey DS, Hukins DW (1983) Radial bulging of the anulus fibrosus during compression of the intervertebral disc. J Biomech 16:211–217
8. Meakin JR, Redpath TW, Hukins DW (2001) The effect of partial removal of the nucleus pulposus from the intervertebral disc on the response of the human anulus fibrosus to compression. Clin Biomech 16:121–128
9. Ray CD (1991) Lumbar interbody threaded prostheses. In: Brock M, Mayer HM, Weigel K (eds) The artificial disc. Springer, Berlin Heidelberg New York, pp 53–67

10. Ray CD (1992) The artificial disc: introduction, history, and socioeconomics. In: Weinstein JN (ed) Clinical efficacy and outcome in the diagnosis and treatment of low back pain. Raven Press, New York, pp 205–225
11. Ray CD, Sachs BL, Norton BK, Mikkelsen ES, Clausen NA (2002) Prosthetic disc nucleus implants: an update. In: Gunzburg R, Szpalski M (eds) Lumbar disc herniation. Lippincott Williams & Wilkins, Philadelphia
12. Urban MR, Fairbank JCT, Etherington PJ, Loh L, Winlove CP, Urban JPG (2001) Electrochemical measurement of transport into scoliotic intervertebral discs in vivo using nitrous oxide as a tracer. Spine 26:984–990
13. Yu S, Haughton VM, Ho PS, et al (1988) Progressive and regressive changes in the nucleus pulposus. II. The adult. Radiology 169:93–97

R. Bertagnoli
R. Schönmayr

Surgical and clinical results with the PDN® prosthetic disc-nucleus device

Abstract The PDN prosthetic disc-nucleus device has been in use for 6 years, both in clinical trials and through commercial sale. Surgical and clinical data for the device have been collected and analyzed to help determine the strengths and limitations of the implant. The shape of the device has been found to be an important element in predicting surgical success, with wedge and rectangular devices being the most stable. The patient's disc dimensions are also critically important. Data indicate that patients with a disc height of less than 5 mm should be excluded from surgery. Moreover, the anterior-posterior (AP) diameter of the disc endplates must be 37 mm or more in order to properly situate two devices within the disc – patients with a smaller AP diameter should receive only a single device. Body mass and overall patient weight are also good predictors of surgical success. If the patient's body mass index is 30 or greater, then the patient should not receive the implants. Complications related to the PDN implant have included migration of the device and endplate remodeling in some patients. This endplate remodeling has usually been mild, and has occurred in response to the change in load distribution. In a few cases there has been more pronounced remodeling with a loss of disc height. To minimize endplate remodeling, the PDN hydrogel has been reformulated to be softer, absorbing 80% of its weight in water. Subsequent to implementing changes in device design and patient selection, and with the introduction of the ALPA (Anterior-Lateral transPsoatic Approach) technique for implanting the devices, there has been an increase in surgical success with a concomitant reduction in the number of revision surgeries. The current surgical success rate for patients implanted from 1999 through 2001 is 88%. Clinical results are also very encouraging, with marked decreases in Oswestry and visual analog scale pain levels, and disc height also shows improvement and stabilization.

Keywords Degenerative disc disease · Disc arthroplasty · PDN device · Intervertebral disc · on-fusion treatment

R. Bertagnoli
St. Elisabeth Klinikum, Straubing, Germany

R. Schönmayr
Dr.-Horst-Schmidt-Kliniken GmbH, Wiesbaden, Germany

Correspondence to:
R. J. Vazquez
Raymedica, Inc., 9401 James Ave South, Bloomington, MN 55431, USA
(r.vazquez@raymedica.com, Tel.: +1-952-2773259).

Introduction

The PDN prosthetic disc nucleus has been developed for treating moderate forms of degenerative disc disease [7]. The goal of the device is to relieve low-back pain while maintaining disc height and allowing normal flexibility in the affected vertebral segments. The PDN device tries to fill the therapy gap that exists between discectomy and immobilization [6]. Unlike discectomy, the PDN implant restores disc height by increasing anular tension, which is essential for adequate segmental function [5, 8]. In contrast to fusion, the PDN device does not affect mobility at the implanted or adjacent vertebral segments [1, 4]. This approach has played a major role in shifting orthopedic research for the treatment of disc degeneration away from immobilization, and focusing it more on maintaining or restoring segmental flexibility. Indeed, the development of many nucleus replacement products such as Newcleus, DPD (Dampening Posterior Device), SINUX, Aquacryl, and Aquarelle can be attributed to the guiding concept of the PDN device.

The PDN device has been in use for the past 6 years, both in clinical trials and through commercial sale. As such, there is a growing pool of data and follow-up information that can be used to gauge the effectiveness of the device. In this paper we examine past and current surgical success rates for the PDN prosthesis, as well as clinical outcomes for low-back pain and disc height. By analyzing our results and reviewing what has been learned over the years, we can continue improving the device and helping our patients regain quality of life.

Surgical results for the PDN device

Clinical trials for the PDN device began on 26 January 1996. Twelve patients were implanted that year, 11 in Germany and one in South Africa. In this initial group, the first three cases were implanted with the devices oriented parallel to the sagittal plane. Thereafter, the surgical technique was modified, and in the remaining patients the devices were placed transversely within the disc. All patients were implanted through an open posterior approach (hemilaminotomy), as is standard in spine decompression surgery. The outcome from this initial group was very encouraging, with marked improvements in Oswestry scores and disc height measurements. Surgical success rates were also good, with only one patient requiring revision surgery in the 1st year of implantation – a laudable result for a new device.

These initial clinical trials were followed by additional implants in Germany, Saudi Arabia, South Africa, Sweden, and the United States between 1997 and 1998. These implant surgeries were performed using the same posterior hemilaminotomy technique as before. This latter patient cohort, however, did not show the same surgical success as the initial group (Fig. 1). Though Oswestry and disc height measurements were satisfactory for those patients with successful implants, overall there was a high rate of device migration (26%), with a concomitant need for revision surgeries.

A multivariate statistical analysis was made of all factors that might be responsible for the high revision rate. This analysis included such variables as device size and shape, aspects of the surgical procedure, and elements of the postoperative patient protocol. The results of the study identified a number of important changes that needed to be implemented to reduce the number of postoperative complications.

The statistical analysis revealed that certain device configurations were less likely to undergo migration. The rectangular and wedge-shaped devices were found to be most stable, as their shapes and sizes could be combined in different ways to best match the angle and shape of the vertebral endplates.

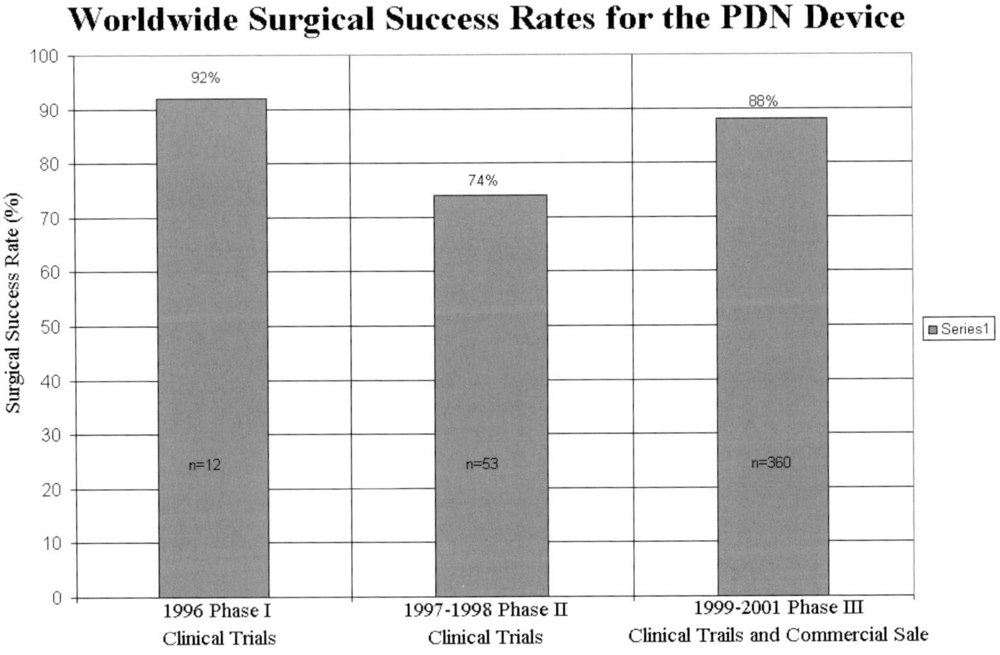

Fig. 1 Worldwide surgical success rates for the PDN device shown in three phases

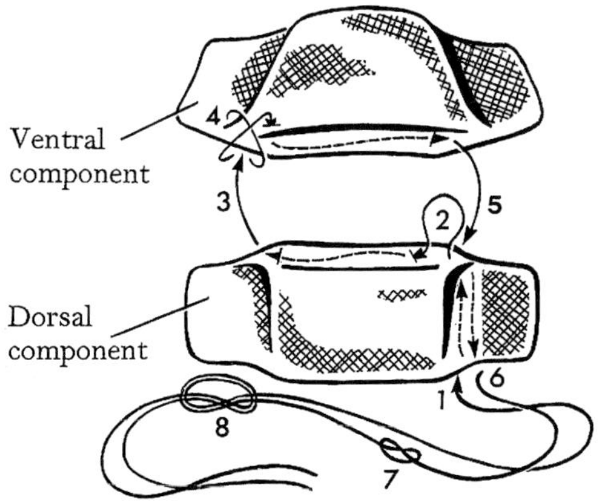

Fig. 2 Anterior (ventral) and posterior (dorsal) PDN devices are tethered together using a #2 polyester suture. Each device is implanted separately into the disc space, but they are pulled together after implantation so that the two devices act as a single system

In order to further stabilize the devices within the disc, a tethering system was developed using a #2 polyester suture. The anterior and posterior PDN devices are now threaded together in such a way that they can be implanted separately, but once within the disc space, they can be secured together (Fig. 2). The resulting implant, though composed of two separate devices, functions as a single system, which is less likely to undergo significant displacement.

Indications/contraindications and patient selection were identified as crucial variables in predicting surgical success. Available data suggested that those patients with disc heights less than 5 mm had a high risk of experiencing device migration. Also important was the patient's anterior-posterior (AP) disc-endplate diameter. When patients with AP disc dimensions of less than 37 mm were implanted with two PDN devices, not only was it difficult to fit both devices into the disc space, but also there was a higher rate of device migration. As such, it is currently recommended that only those patients with AP disc dimensions of 37 mm or greater be implanted with two PDN devices, while patients with smaller discs should be implanted with a single device.

Apart from intervertebral disc size, patient body mass and weight have also been found to be important variables. Those patients with a body mass index of 30 or greater were shown to have significantly higher rates of surgical complications (BMI = weight in kg / height in m^2). For these reasons, careful attention is now given to a patient's body mass before deciding to proceed with PDN implant surgery.

Another significant step towards reducing the number of revision surgeries has been the implementation of the Anterior-Lateral transPsoatic Approach (ALPA), which was introduced in the late 1990s as an alternative method for implanting the PDN device [2, 3]. In contrast to the posterior hemilaminotomy approach, where the disc is accessed from the back, in the ALPA technique the disc is accessed laterally through a minimal invasive approach in a strict lateral plane. After blunt dissection through the lateral abdominal muscles, the retroperitoneal region is accessed and followed laterally to the psoas muscle, where blunt dissection is again used to reach the disc. This approach offers access to the largest possible anatomical area of the disc circumference without impairing important anatomical structures. Once the nucleus material has been removed, the devices are implanted directly into the disc without needing to be turned, as is the case with the posterior surgical approach. Another advantage of ALPA is that the anterior longitudinal ligament and posterior longitudinal ligament (as well as all posterior structures) are kept intact and the anular incision is made on the biomechanically less important lateral aspect. These factors could explain why migration rates are significantly lower with ALPA compared to the posterior approach.

The need for changes to the postoperative patient protocol was also indicated by the analysis. The use of orthosis was found to be beneficial during the first 6 weeks after surgery to keep patients from putting too much strain on their lumbar spine while the PDN devices are conforming to the shape of the endplates.

The aforementioned changes began to be implemented in 1999, and subsequently the number of revision surgeries for the PDN device has decreased significantly. From 1999 through 2001, there have been 462 patients implanted, and of these, 12% have required some type of revision surgery to either reposition or explant the devices – yielding a cumulative rate of 88% successful implantations. This is a remarkable improvement compared to the earlier 1997–1998 implants, where the explant rate had been 26%. It is also important to note that the PDN does not prevent future treatment for those patients who do require some type of surgical revision. Because the devices do not promote fusion of the vertebrae, they can be replaced with other implants such as total disc replacements, or cages and bone grafts (alone or in combination with dorsal instrumentation).

Clinical results for the PDN device

The primary reason for using the PDN device in cases of moderate degenerative disc disease is the great improvement in the low-back pain of our patients. Worldwide clinical results for Oswestry score and pain on a visual analog scale (VAS) have shown marked improvement in pain levels. For 243 patients, the mean preoperative Oswestry score was 52.7. At the 6-month follow-up the average score dropped to 17.4, and at the 24-month follow-up, the mean score had declined further, to 9 (Fig. 3). VAS scores are equally compelling: for 213 patents, the preoperative mean was 7.1. At the 12-month follow-up visit, this pain level had decreased to 2.49, and at the

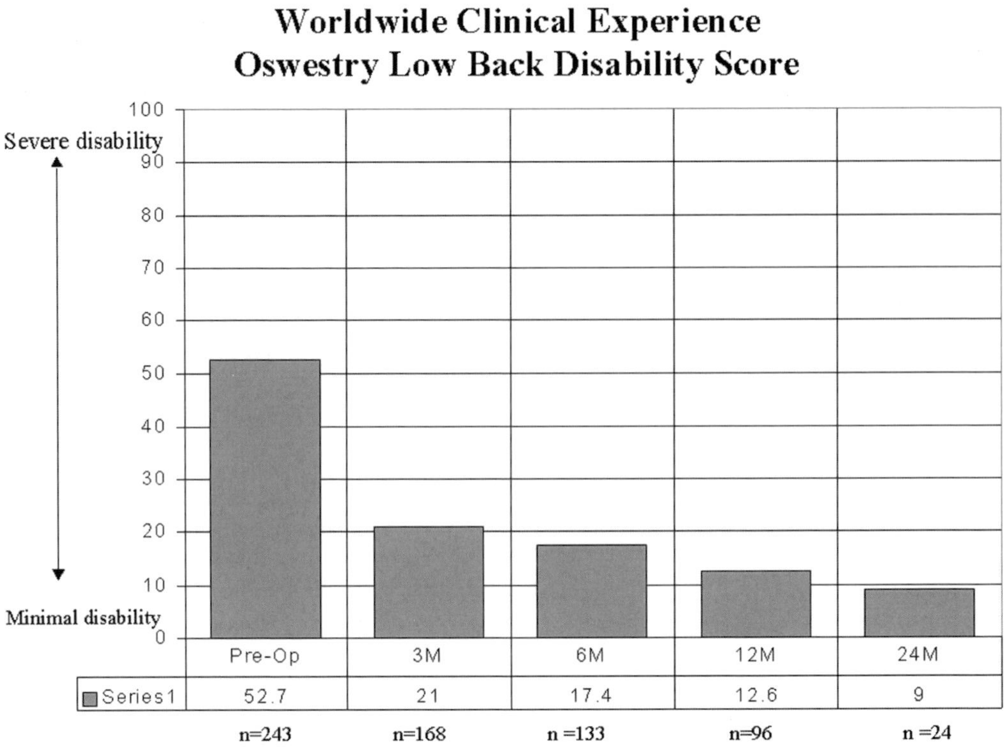

Fig. 3 Oswestry disability scores for the PDN device. Pain levels drop significantly after PDN device implantation

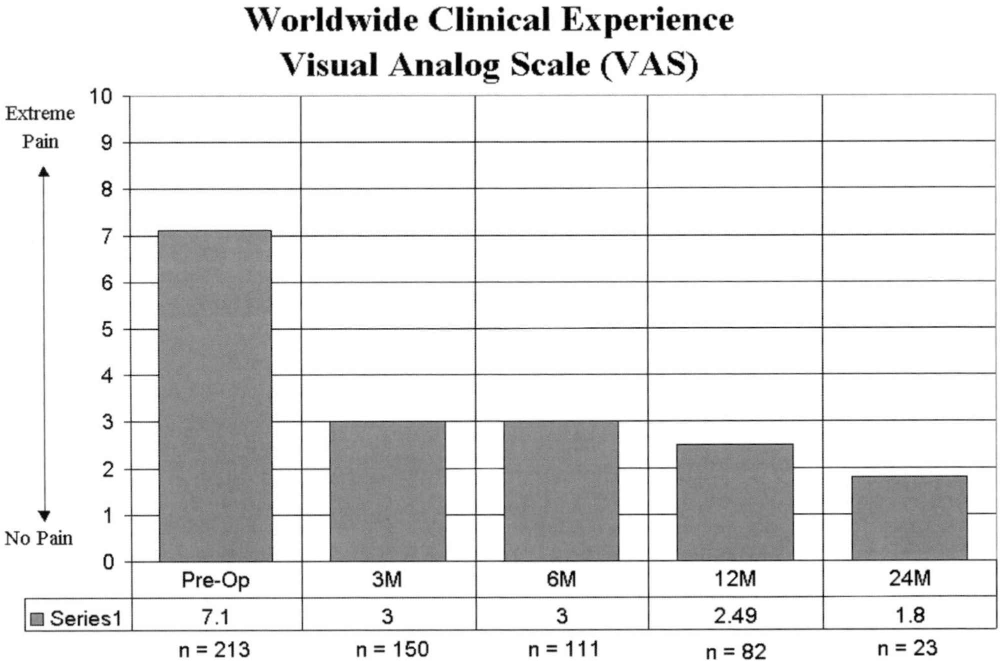

Fig. 4 Visual analog scale (VAS) for patients implanted with PDN devices. Pain levels drop significantly after PDN device implantation

24-month follow-up the level of pain had declined further to 1.8 (Fig. 4). As the number of patients with follow-up information at 24 months is still relatively low, these figures still are of a preliminary character.

This postoperative reduction in low-back pain is accompanied by an increase in disc height, which is a prerequisite for segmental stability to minimize nonphysiologic movements that may cause additional tearing of the anulus. For 218 patients, preoperative disc height averaged 8.1 mm. This measurement increased postoperatively to 9.7 mm at the 12-month follow-up, and 10.2 mm in the cohort measured after 24 months (Fig. 5, Fig. 6).

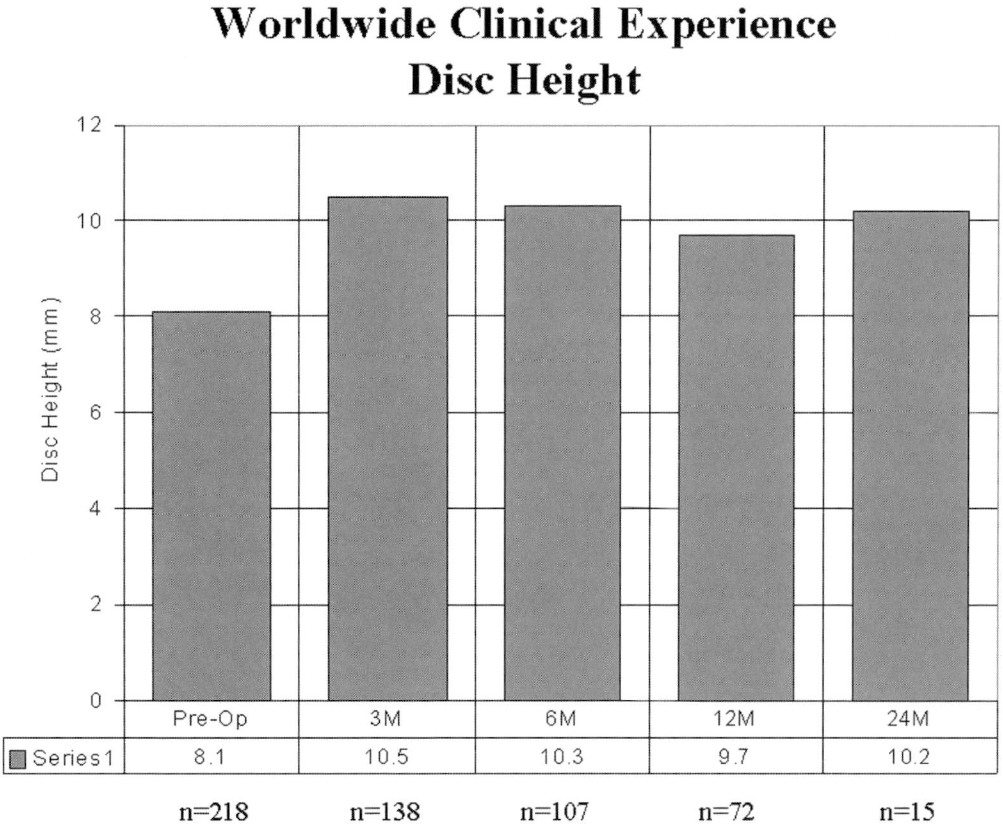

Fig. 5 Disc height measurements before and after PDN device implantation. The device restores/maintains disc height postoperatively

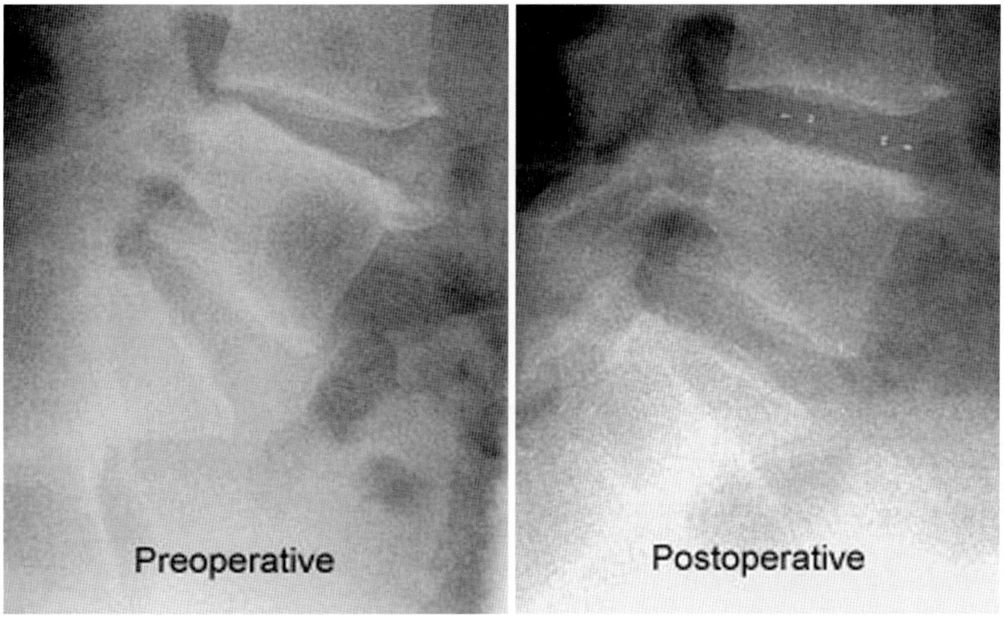

Fig. 6 A 42-year-old man with vertical instability at L4–L5, severe low-back pain, and unsuccessful conservative treatment. PDN devices were implanted via the ALPA (Anterior-Lateral transPsoatic) approach, with subsequent improvements in clinical symptoms and disc height

Discussion

The primary source of complications with the posterior surgical approach for PDN device implantation has been migration. Though not all device migrations have produced clinically relevant symptoms, some have caused discomfort requiring surgical revision or explantation. It is interesting that many patients, having the choice of replacing the PDN implants versus converting to an interbody fusion, have decided in favor of replacing the implants, as the concept of preserving segmental function remained attractive.

In some patients implanted with PDN devices, there has been a temporary postoperative increase in low-back pain. Such pain has usually been minor, lasting a relatively short period of time, and probably represents a reaction to segmental distraction caused by the hydrating implants.

Moderate to severe endplate changes have also been noted on some patients implanted with PDN devices. Mild endplate remodeling is probably due to changes in load distribution – the endplates appear to adapt to the contours of the implants. From a biomechanical perspective, endplate remodeling is not unexpected, and when it does occur it tends to be minor and stabilizes fairly quickly, typically within 6 weeks after surgery. It is important, however, to monitor all patients for 12 months to ensure that endplate remodeling has indeed stabilized and that there has not been a significant loss of disc height. Only a few cases of severe remodeling have been reported, strongly suggesting that in these cases there was a mismatch between the strength of the endplates and the stiffness of the implants. To avoid this problem, patients with osteoporosis or osteopathies should be excluded from PDN device surgery.

In response to the possibility of endplate remodeling, the material properties of the PDN hydrogel have been reformulated to be less stiff. The original hydrogel formulation 68, which was used in the first group of patients, has been changed to a formulation 80 – capable of absorbing 80% of its weight in water, with less possibility of having a negative lasting impact on the endplates.

Conclusion

The success of any medical device is measured by its clinical results. No matter how well conceived and engineered the device may be, or how elegant a surgical technique has been developed for implanting the device, the ultimate determination of efficacy is made by patients: Have their lives improved significantly enough to warrant the treatment?

The successful implantations and clinical results of the PDN over the last 2 years certainly seem to indicate that the benefits of implanting a PDN device outweigh the risks. A surgical success rate of 88%, coupled with a marked reduction in back pain and an increase in disc height, suggests that the PDN device is an effective treatment mode for cases of moderate degenerative disc disease that are associated with chronic low-back pain.

As with any new device, there are questions that still remain unanswered and deserve ongoing observation. The long-term reaction of the vertebral endplates to the new load distributions is a focus of our current interest. Radiological findings in a few patients suggest that some adaptation of the endplates to the surface contours of the PDN device is to be expected. Patients should be monitored to guard against significant disc height reductions. In addition, more long-term clinical data are necessary to gauge the efficacy of the PDN device in preventing or retarding progressive segmental degeneration.

It seems that the nucleus replacement concept of the PDN device bears great potential. Six years after the first implantation, we have learned much concerning the surgical technique and indications for the PDN device, and we have learned about the device limitations as well as its benefits. We have also learned that proper indication and patient selection are crucial factors for successful results. There is no doubt that improvements in device design and surgical technique will continue to be made, but already today the clinical results justify the efforts and support the soundness and effectiveness of this concept.

References

1. Aota Y, Kumano K, Hirabayashi S (1995) Postfusion instability at the adjacent segments after rigid pedicle screw fixation for degenerated lumbar spinal disorders. J Spinal Disord 8:464–473
2. Bertagnoli R (2000) Anterior mini-open approach for nucleus prosthesis – a new application technique for PDN. Thirteenth Annual Meeting of the IITS, St. Williamsburg, Virginia, 8–10 June 2000
3. Bertagnoli R, Sachs BL, Ray CD, Pimenta L (2001) Modified surgical technique for implantation of prosthetic disc nucleus devices. Presented at the International Meeting of Advanced Spine Techniques, Paradise Island, Bahamas, July 2001
4. Lee CK (1988) Accelerated degeneration of the segment adjacent to a lumbar fusion. Spine 13:375–377
5. Meakin JR, Redpath TW, Hukins DW (2001) The effect of partial removal of the nucleus pulposus from the intervertebral disc on the response of the human anulus fibrosus to compression. Clin Biomech 16:121–128
6. Ray CD (1992) The artificial disc: introduction, history, and socioeconomics. In: Weinstein JN (ed) Clinical efficacy and outcome in the diagnosis and treatment of low back pain. Raven Press, pp 205–225
7. Yu S, Haughton VM, Ho PS, et al (1988) Progressive and regressive changes in the nucleus pulposus. II. The adult. Radiology 169:93–97
8. Zollner J, Heine J, Eysel P (2000) Effect of enucleation on the biomechanical behavior of the lumbar motion segment. Zentralbl Neurochir 61:138–142

A. Korge
Th. Nydegger
J. L. Polard
H. M. Mayer
J. L. Husson

A spiral implant as nucleus prosthesis in the lumbar spine

A. Korge (✉) · H.M. Mayer
Spine Center,
Orthopedic Clinic Munich-Harlaching,
Harlachinger Strasse 51,
81547 Munich, Germany
e-mail: AKorge@schoen-kliniken.de,
Tel.: +49-89-62112011,
Fax: +49-89-62112012

Th. Nydegger
Biomechanical Research,
Sulzer Orthopedics,
Winterthur, Switzerland

J.L. Polard · J.L. Husson
Service Orthopédie-Traumatologie A,
CHU Hôtel Dieu, Rennes, France

Abstract Microdiscectomy represents the gold standard in disc surgery on the lumbar spine. The remaining defect in the intervertebral disc space can be filled with a newly developed nucleus prosthesis presented in this paper. This prosthesis consists of polycarbonate urethane (Sulene™ PCU), and takes the form of a memory coiling spiral. It can be easily implanted using the standard microdiscectomy approach with no further tissue damage. Biomechanical tests have shown that anatomical distances can be restored by the spiral for both the facet joints and the endplates. Endplate deformations are not statistically different when compared to intact conditions. Inclusion and exclusion criteria of an in vivo pilot study are presented. The paper describes the insertion setup for the spiral and the technique of implantation. Five patients have been supplied with the implant to date. The first results on postoperative magnetic resonance images are presented.

Keywords Nucleus prosthesis · Artificial disc · Non-fusion treatment · Spine arthroplasty · Discogenic pain

Introduction

In many cases, low-back pain arises from pathological discogenic changes of the lumbar motion segment. Autopsy studies have shown that by the age of 21, in nearly every second person, at least one lumbar disc is already damaged. Moreover, even in healthy symptom-free adults, disc protrusions and disc herniations are found frequently [1].

With conservative treatment being routinely the initial treatment in discogenic low-back pain, clinical symptoms such as an increasing sensomotoric deficit or a more or less complete cauda equina syndrome as well as therapy-resistant radicular pain may require surgical intervention. So far, microsurgical discectomy, whether performed through an open endoscopic or microscope-assisted procedure, represents the gold standard procedure for herniated discs.

Depending in part on the amount of disc material being removed, more or less dramatic changes may threaten the lumbar motion segment [2, 3, 8, 13]. With progressive loss of the pressure-absorbing function of the disc, the height of the affected segment will be reduced, resulting in a further degeneration of annulus and remaining nucleus. Finally, the segment will collapse, increasing the load on both facet joints, leading to accelerated spondylarthrosis and reduced mobility.

For many decades, several attempts were made to create an efficient implant to replace the herniated or degenerated nucleus, including the concepts of a waterbladder [7], a hydrophilic elastomer [4] and a silicone polyethylene implant [5]. More or less ineffective, these implants never went into clinical studies or into routine use. Recently, the PDN device (Prosthetic Disc Nucleus; RayMedica, Inc., USA), developed by Charles Ray, has been gaining influence [11]. Briefly summarizing, it consists of a hydrogel core with a polyethylene coating serv-

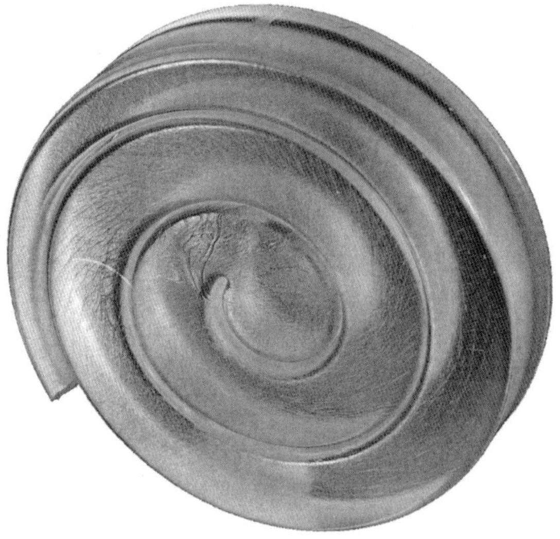

Fig. 1 New spiral implant

ing for nucleus augmentation. However, difficulties in the implantation technique as well as reports on dislocation are important drawbacks that still prevent the routine use of this device.

A different approach was taken in 1997 by J. L. Husson in cooperation with SulzerMedica [9, 10]. They developed an intervertebral spacer for nucleus replacement in the form of a memory coiling spiral (Fig. 1). The memory effect is based on a specifically validated manufacturing process, with modulation of the molecular chains of the basic component – polycarbonate urethane – into a spiral form. Being in rectilinear position before application, the implant will roll automatically into a spiral shape and will cover in situ the intervertebral disc cavity with no fixed mechanical axis.

Material

The basic implant material – polycarbonate urethane (Sulene™ PCU) – is a well-established material in medicine (used, for instance, in other spinal implants and cardiovascular surgery), and has been extensively and successfully tested for biocompatibility and biostability. When comparing polycarbonate urethane with polyurethane (PUR) in a fatigue test model, electron microscopic studies after five million cycles have shown microcracks in PUR, but not in Sulene™ PCU.

When comparing an intact lumbar motion segment with a nucleotomized segment without and with the spiral, biomechanical cadaver tests have revealed that the spiral is able to restore both the cranio-caudal distance of a lumbar facet joint, and the cranio-caudal distance between the adjacent endplates [12]. In additional biomechanical tests comparing intact, nucleotomized and nucleoplastically supported functional spinal units, the effects of axial compression and eccentric loading in different directions were measured, with special emphasis on the endplate deformation [6]. The coiling spiral increased central endplate deformation when compared to nucleotomy. Furthermore, the endplate deformations were not statistically different when compared to the intact condition, with the exception of posterior shear loading. In all biomechanical tests, no implant migration was seen.

Patient selection

At the moment, two main indications exist for nucleus replacement by an implanted spiral (Table 1):

1. Single-level radiculalgia without back pain due to disc herniation
2. Single-level radiculalgia with predominant leg pain and some back pain, due to disc herniation and degenerative disc disease

Both indications must be confirmed by patient history, physical examination and radiographic findings. In both indication groups, conservative treatment, if indicated, must have failed. In addition, in the present pilot study, other inclusion criteria are: a posterior disc height of more than 5 mm (due to the implant height currently available); a symptomatic pathology restricted to one level between L2 and S1; an age limit between 18 and 65 years and, finally, the absence of any associated severe vertebral pathology. Some exclusion criteria are currently in place during the pilot study, which are detailed in Table 2. They

Table 1 Inclusion criteria

Pure disc herniation with leg pain only *or* disc herniation + degenerative disc disease with predominant leg pain
Candidate for one-level discectomy from L2 to S1
Posterior disc height at affected level ≥5 mm
Patient age between 18 and 65 years

Table 2 Main exclusion criteria

Previous spine surgery
Spinal problem at more than one level
Globular disc
Central disc herniation
Pronounced Schmorl's nodules at the involved level
Endplate lesions
Significant spinal, foraminal or lateral recess stenosis
Symptomatic degenerated facet joints
Degenerative spondylolisthesis greater than grade I
Lytic spondylolisthesis
Severe osteoporosis
Bone tumors or congenital bony abnormalities
Active infection
Presence of malignant tumors

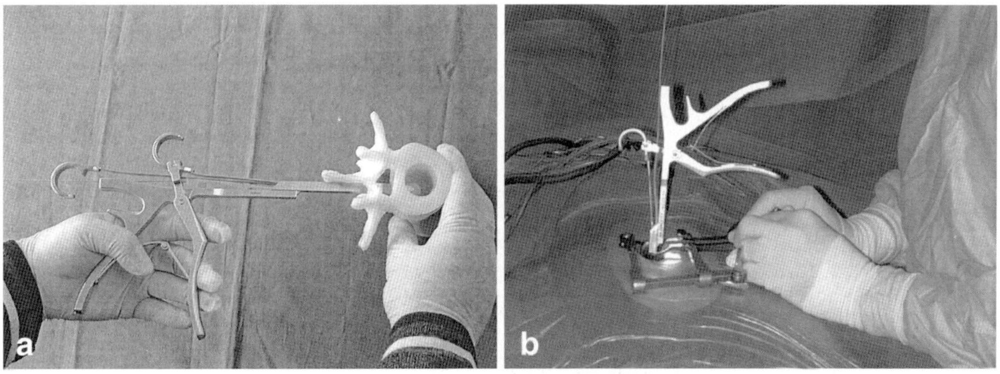

Fig. 2 Insertion instrument filled with spiral, guard and pusher: **A** in vitro, using a saw bone model, **B** in situ (due to technical and approach-related improvements, the instrument now is turned around with the handle towards the midline and its open mouth laterally, thus enabling a permanent microscopic visual control of instrument, dura and nerve root while inserting the spiral)

will probably be slowly modified as the implant comes into routine use.

Surgical technique

The complete insertion setup for the spiral consists of five parts: an insertion instrument (subsequently filled with the spiral) with a guard and spiral pusher, a cutting blade and a measuring gauge (Fig. 2). In combination with lumbar disc surgery, an established microsurgical microscope-assisted approach can be used for the application of the insertion instrument. No additional substantial defect of soft tissue or bony structures has to be performed to place the filled insertion instrument. Microdiscectomy should include clearance of the intervertebral disc space, with removal of as much nucleus material as possible, in order to create a cavity with enough space for a large spiral volume. Then, under microscopic control of the neural structures, the loaded insertion instrument is placed into the intervertebral disc space, extending at least half of the diameter of the disc space. The final position of the insertion instrument should be controlled and documented fluoroscopically (Fig. 3). If the insertion instrument is not inserted deep enough, the spiral might not fill sufficiently the anterior part of the cleared intervertebral disc space. Then, by slowly pushing forward the handle of the insertion instrument, the spiral is inserted into the disc space. As soon as the spiral has reached the anterior border of the created cavity, the surgeon feels the insertion instrument moving slowly backwards out of the middle of the disc space with every push. As soon as the insertion instrument does not carry any further spiral material forward, due to the resistance of the completely filled cavity, the insertion process is finished. Using a guard and replacing the spiral pusher by a cutting blade, with a final strong forward movement of the handle of the insertion instrument, the spiral is then cut in the disc space and beneath the level of the posterior wall of the vertebral body. The insertion instrument with the remainder of the spiral is then removed. In both situations – with the insertion instrument still in situ without the cut spiral as well as with the insertion instrument having already been removed with the remainder of the spiral – the amount and diameter of covered disc area can be measured. A microscopical control of the end of the spiral should be performed. The end of the spiral should be rotated forward to the anterior part of the disc space in order to avoid any theoretically imaginable dislocation of this end into the spinal canal. Finally, wound closure follows traditional principles, with drainage being not necessary routinely. Mobilisation starts at the latest the day after surgery, without any bracing support. In accordance with valid study guidelines, the position of the spiral is controlled on the second day after surgery by magnetic resonance imaging in axial, frontal and sagittal planes (Fig. 4).

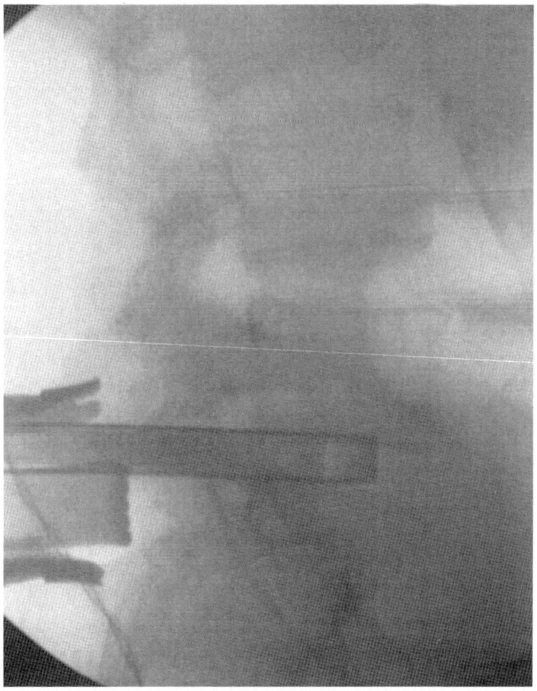

Fig. 3 Loaded insertion instrument in situ in the intervertebral disc space under lateral fluoroscopic control

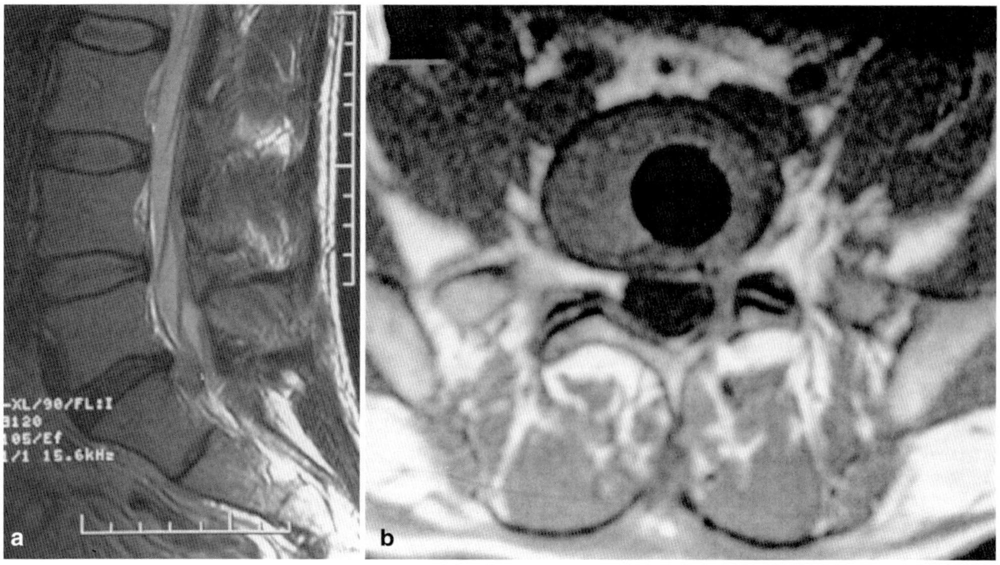

Fig. 4 **A** Preoperative sagittal magnetic resonance (MR) image showing a disc herniation L5/S1 left-side, in a 52-year-old man with typical radicular leg pain. **B** Postoperative axial MR image at postoperative day 4 of the same patient, with the spiral in place

Preliminary experiences

To date, five patients (two female, three male; age range: 24–52 years) have been supplied with a spiral implant. In all cases, a disc herniation with radicular symptoms presented the indication for surgery. Affected levels were L4/5 or L5/S1. In all of these patients, disc surgery and insertion of the spiral were performed without complications. Postoperative rotational CT scans performed in the first patient at 2 years follow-up demonstrated the completely maintained function of the facet joints. All patients were satisfied with the result of the operation, and scored better values in the postoperative VAS and Oswestry score. However, due to both the small number of patients and short follow-up, no statistical analysis has been carried out so far.

Conclusion

In summary, the major advantage of this new implant for nucleus replacement is its easy application due to both the standardized approach and the memory coiling mechanism of the spiral. Due to the spiral shape of the implant, the filling and covering of the intradiscal space is enlarged, resulting in a reduced risk of migration. The larger surface of the device in situ improves the pressure distribution on both endplates, thereby minimizing the risk of the implant sinking into the endplates. Biomechanical tests have shown a restoration of the kinematics of a lumbar motion segment by the spiral after disc removal when compared to unsupported segments. Both the disc height and the position of the facet joints were restored and/or maintained by the spiral implant. As verified in biomechanical tests, no implant migration occurred. The implant itself sufficiently supports the anterior column of a functional spinal unit under compression conditions. Cadaver studies as well as in vivo surgery showed that the spiral is usable in the established minimal invasive microscope-assisted techniques for both anterior and posterior approaches.

In the clinical pathway for low-back pain, this new spiral implant promotes the philosophy of non-fusion technologies in spine arthroplasty and fills a gap between the semi-invasive non-open procedures, such as intraspinal injections or the IDET technique, and the next step of complete disc replacement by disc prostheses and finally fusion surgery. An international multicenter study is currently underway, focussing on outcome parameters such as subjective improvement of quality of life, objective clinical results and radiological findings, to establish the long-term effectiveness of this new spiral implant.

References

1. Boden SC, Davis DO, Dina TS, Patronas NJ, Wiesel SW (1990) Abnormal magnetic-resonance scans of the lumbar spine in asymptomatic subjects. J Bone Joint Surg Am 72:403–408
2. Brinckmann P, Grootenboer H (1991) Change of disc height, radial disc bulge, and intradiscal pressure from discectomy. An in vitro investigation on human lumbar discs. Spine 16: 641–646
3. Dunlop RB, Adams MA, Hutton WC (1984) Disc space narrowing and the lumbar facet joints. J Bone Joint Surg Br 66:706–710

4. Edeland HG (1981) Suggestions for a total elasto-dynamic intervertebral disc prosthesis. Biomater Med Dev Artif Organs 9:65–72
5. Edeland HG (1989) Some additional suggestions for an intervertebral disc prosthesis. J Biomed Mater Resources Appl Biomater 23:189
6. Frei HP, Rathonyi G, Orr TE, Nolte LP, Oxland T (1999) Effect of a nucleus prosthetic device on the biomechanical behavior of the functional spinal unit. Eur Spine J 8:S36–S37
7. Froning EC (1975) Intervertebral disc prosthesis and instruments for locating same. US Patent Office, Patent No. 3,875,595, April 8
8. Gotfried Y, Bradford DS, Oegema TR (1986) Facet joint changes after chemonucleolysis-induced disc space narrowing. Spine 11:944–950
9. Husson JL, Baumgartner W, Le Nihouannen JC (1996) Nucléoplastie inter-somatique par voie postérieure per-discectomie: concept et étude espérimentale. In: Husson JL, Le Huec JC (eds) Restabilisation inter-somatique du rachis lombaire. Sauramps, Montpellier, pp 311–320
10. Husson JL, Schärer N, Le Nihouannen JC, Freudiger S, Baumgartner W, Polard JL (1997) Nucleoplasty during discectomy: concept and experimental study. Rachis 9:145–152
11. Ray CD, Schönmayr R, Kavanagh SA, Assell R (1999) Prosthetic disc nucleus implants. Riv Neuroradiol 12 [Suppl 1]: 157–162
12. Schärer N, Husson JL, Froehlich M (1999) Translation of the endplate during flexion and extension on intact human spines: an in-vitro study. Annual Meeting of the Spine Society of Europe, Munich/Germany (poster)
13. Steffen R, Wittenberg RH, Nolte LP, Hedtmann A, Kolditz D, Herchenbach T (1991) Experimentelle Untersuchungen zur Drehpunktveränderung des Bewegungssegmentes nach Bandscheibenausräumung. Z Orthop Ihre Grenzgeb 129:248–254

Armin Studer

Nucleus prosthesis: a new concept

Abstract In a large number of low-back pain patients, the pain is related to disc herniation or prolapse of the nucleus pulposus. Although the pathogenesis is still the topic of debate, the nucleus seems to play an important role not only in the progression of low-back pain, but also in its treatment. Numerous surgical treatment solutions have been patented or described in the literature; however, only a few seem promising and are in use today. After the development of numerous ideas, for instance metallic implants, the concept of a compressible material encased by a strong, inelastic outer layer emerged as the logical conclusion. Specific requirements during operation and during the entire life of the implant have to be taken into consideration in developing new solutions. In this paper, the development of the nucleus prosthesis will be discussed and a new concept presented.

Keywords Low-back pain · Disc replacement · Nucleus prosthesis · Nucleus prolapse

A. Studer
Mathys Medical Ltd,
Güterstrasse 5, P.O. Box,
2544 Bettlach, Switzerland
e-mail: armin.studer@mathysmedical.com,
Tel.: +41-32-6441751,
Fax: +41-32-6441173

Introduction

Back pain is a major reason for consultations. Almost 15 million visits to a doctor were counted in the US for this diagnosis, making low-back pain the fifth leading diagnosis cluster [10]. Behind the diagnosis "non-specific backache", accounting for 57% of low-back pain diagnoses, the most specific categories were 12.5% "probable degenerative changes" and 11.1% "herniated discs". These figures emphasize the size of the problem related to mechanical low-back pain. Although the pathogenesis of mechanical low-back pain related to degenerative disc disease is still the topic of debate, the nucleus seems to play an important role. It is not only the centre of spinal motion segments, but also the origin of the degenerative cascade, and therefore the target of old and new treatment options.

The nucleus: origin and target

Origin of pain development

The nucleus pulposus is the central soft and gelatinous region of each intervertebral disc, surrounded by multilayered fibres of the annulus fibrosus. It is situated closer to the posterior border of the annulus fibrosus than to the anterior one [15]. The main organic structural components are collagens and proteoglycans. While collagens account for less than 20% of the dry weight of the central nucleus, proteoglycans represent as much as 50% in a child. The proteoglycans provide the tissue with its stiffness and resistance against compression by their interactions with water [6]. The presence of these hydrophilic proteins is the reason for the water-binding capacity of the nucleus (swelling pressure). The equilibrium of water content also depends on the external disc load. Increased loads squeeze water into the adjacent vertebral endplates. Unloading leads to return of water. This pumping mechanism provides the metabolism to the vessel-free nucleus [3]. Consequently, the fluid content of the nucleus shows diurnal variations. In the morning after rest, the turgor, and with it the thickness, is higher; by the evening the nucleus has lost some turgor.

The water content of the nucleus is highest in youth, at about 80%, and decreases gradually with age [12]. It starts reducing in the fourth decade due to a gradual change in the type of proteoglycans [2]. Loss of height is the consequence. In an experimental study by Brinckmann and Grootenboer [5], for instance, about 1 g of tissue loss in the nucleus pulposus led to a loss of height of approximately 0.8 mm. This influences the load sharing between nucleus pulposus, annulus fibrosus and facet joints. The decrease in interdiscal pressure reduces the engagement of the nucleus in the load flow, thus increasing the portions of the load carried by the annulus fibrosus and facet joints. Finally, it may result in damage to the joint cartilage, reactive hypertrophy and inflammation, and the neuroforaminal space of the exiting nerve roots may be impaired as well. The increasing load and the tissue alterations of the annulus fibrosus are the base for radial tears, cracks and fissures. The nucleus will finally prolapse if the mechanisms for self-healing are insufficient. The deformation of a nerve root clinically imposes radicular pain. In contrast, the irritation and inflammation of the facet joints lead to so-called pseudoradicular pain.

Since, in many cases, the nucleus pulposus seems to be the starting point of the degenerative cascade, it should also be the treatment target. But in the past, surgical interventions consisted either in a decompression of the nerve roots alone, in a fusion of motion segments or in a combination of both. All methods lead to an improvement in the clinical symptoms for a certain time. However, these methods do not solve the real problem. The problems are shifted to the adjacent motion segments because of the fusion or the contrasting instability of the segment [21].

Treatment target

The idea of restoring the biomechanical function of the disc by replacing only the nucleus as the cause of degeneration and pain seems very elegant, but has several limitations. The nucleus replacement is based on the assumption that the annulus and the endplates are still functioning properly [3]. This boundary condition has an important impact on patient selection and the indications for surgery. Potential patients are young and without many accompanying degenerative changes in the spine. Implanting an artificial substance into the spine of a young patient, however, raises questions about the longevity of the implant [13]. Wear problems, known from total hip replacements [20], and possible degradation processes within the nucleus material may lead to a need for re-intervention after 15–20 years. Furthermore, the risk of herniation of the new, artificial nucleus has to be minimised. The likelihood of this event should be lower than that of a normal prolapse [19]. The latter requirement has a direct impact on the surgical technique. While inserting the nucleus, the intraoperative damage to the annulus fibrosus must be kept to a minimum.

Numerous solutions have been patented or described in the literature, but only a few seem promising and are in use today. Initially attempts were made by injecting an acrylic mass [7, 9], and this was later followed by silicone [19]. Roy-Camille et al. used a latex bag to reduce the probability of material herniation and to decrease fatigue behaviour [18]. Nucleus replacement by means of metallic implants was attempted, but was abandoned because of migration and subsidence problems [8].

The concept of a compressible material, encased by a strong, inelastic outer layer, emerged as the logical consequence of the first ideas, and was first tested in vivo by Hou et al. [11], and brought to clinical use by Ray and Corbin [17]. However, clinical studies that prove the long-term efficiency of the device have yet to be done. More recent work is directed towards the development of materials (e.g. hydrogel) that better mimic the physiological behaviour of the nucleus [13, 16] and towards reducing invasiveness during insertion of the nucleus. This latter aim should be achieved by using devices with a memory effect. They are guided into the central disc cavity in a straight shape, but return to their pre-formed (in most cases spiral) structure [4, 14] once they are within the cavity. This solution offers two interesting features: the opening for the insertion of the implant is minimal, while the risk of a re-prolapse is reduced because of the overall size of the nucleus prosthesis after implantation. However, this exciting idea requires an excellent interaction between the materials used and the structure. The shear strength of the spiral's elastic contents, which is not an issue in homogeneous devices such as the PDN, becomes a major issue. Furthermore, delaminating between core and cover of the spiral has to be prevented. When using a hydrogel for the core, the cover sheath has to be guaranteed to remain intact.

New treatment concept

All above-mentioned requirements for a nucleus replacement were taken into consideration during the development of a new nucleus prosthesis design. Mathys Medical Ltd has realised a concept using a "snail" design for the final implant. A complex manufacturing process has been developed to specify the memory effect of the device, and to ensure that it has the required biomechanical properties such as shear strength, etc. The opening required by this specific design is minimal. Insertion into the disc is possible through a cross-stitched incision of the annulus. A tube is used to guide the straight-shaped prosthesis into the cleaned cavity of the disc. The insertion is possible through a percutaneous or minimal open posterior as well as a retroperitoneal approach. Once inside the empty cavity of the former nucleus, the device can return to its snail shape. Different lengths and diameters allow for compensation in disc height or diameter [1]. No intraoperative shortening of the device is necessary. The hydrogel of the nucleus prosthesis will start to swell after insertion. The prosthesis thus mimics diurnal changes and creep behaviour under mechanical load. As a consequence, the annulus fibrosus should be protected from overload. The core material possesses elastic and reversible plastic behaviour. Unlike other core materials such as polyurethane, nutrients can be transported via the nucleus to the annulus fibrosus. The materials used for both device components are biologically inert, to minimise adverse reactions.

The next steps towards a device for clinical use will include extensive biomechanical testing with respect to complex three-dimensional and fatigue behaviour. Next year, the biocompatibility will be tested before the first clinical studies. A clinical multicentre study will follow.

Conclusions

The newly developed nucleus prosthesis by Mathys Medical Ltd has biomechanical and biological properties that come very close to those of the original nucleus. The intraoperative damage to the surrounding tissue, especially the annulus fibrosus, is minimal, thus reducing the risk of herniation of the nucleus prosthesis. However, the indication for this device has to be established very carefully with respect to accompanying damage of the disc.

The proposed concept may find its place as a first – even prophylactic – treatment option for disc herniation. Especially in young patients, it can offer a long-term solution without limiting further treatment options. If the degeneration of the affected disc continues, replacement of the whole disc or even a fusion is still possible at a later time.

References

1. Aharinejad S, Bertagnoli R, Wicke K, Firbas W, Schneider B (1990) Morphometric analysis of vertebrae and intervertebral discs as a basis of disc replacement. Am J Anat 189:69–76
2. Akeson WH, Woo SL, Taylor TK, Ghosh P, Bushell GR (1977) Biomechanics and biochemistry of the intervertebral discs: the need for correlation studies. Clin Orthop 129:133–140
3. Bao QB, McCullen GM, Higham PA, Dumbleton JH, Yuan HA (1996) The artificial disc: theory, design and materials. Biomaterials 17:1157–1167
4. Baumgartner W (1992) Intervertebral prosthesis. US patent 5,171,280
5. Brinckmann P, Grootenboer H (1991) Change of disc height, radial disc bulge, and intradiscal pressure from discectomy. An in vitro investigation on human lumbar discs. Spine 16:641–646
6. Buckwalter JA (1995) Aging and degeneration of the human intervertebral disc. Spine 20:1307–1314
7. Cleveland DA (1955) The use of methylacrylates for spinal stabilization after disc operations. Marquette Med Rev 20:62–64
8. Fernstrom U (1966) Arthroplasty with intercorporal endoprosthesis in herniated disc and in painful disc. Acta Chir Scand Suppl 357:154–159
9. Hamby WB, Glaser HT (1959) Replacement of spinal intervertebral discs with locally polymerizing methyl methacrylate. J Neurosurg 16:311–313
10. Hart LG, Deyo RA, Cherkin DC (1995) Physician office visits for low back pain. Frequency, clinical evaluation, and treatment patterns from a U.S. national survey. Spine 20:11–19
11. Hou TS, Tu KY, Xu YK, Li ZB, Cai AH, Wang HC (1991) Lumbar intervertebral disc prosthesis. An experimental study. Chin Med J (Engl) 104: 381–386
12. Humzah MD, Soames, RW (1988) Human intervertebral disc: structure and function. Anat Rec 220:337–356
13. Kadoya K, Kotani Y, Abumi K, Takada T, Shimamoto N, Shikinami Y, Kadosawa T, Kaneda K (2001) Biomechanical and morphologic evaluation of a three-dimensional fabric sheep artificial intervertebral disc: in vitro and in vivo analysis. Spine 26:1562–1569
14. Lin C-I (1998) Artificial intervertebral disk and method for implanting the same. US patent 5,716,416
15. Markolf KL, Morris JM (1974) The structural components of the intervertebral disc. A study of their contributions to the ability of the disc to withstand compressive forces. J Bone Joint Surg Am 56:675–687
16. Meakin JR, Reid JE, Hukins DW (2001) Replacing the nucleus pulposus of the intervertebral disc. Clin Biomech 16:560–565
17. Ray CD (1988) Percutaneous discectomy. A new day-surgical method for herniated lumbar discs. Minn Med 71: 485–488
18. Roy-Camille R, Saillant G, Lavaste F (1978) Experimental study of lumbar disc replacement. Rev Chir Orthop Reparatrice Appar Mot 64 [Suppl 2]: 106–107
19. Schneider PG, Oyen R (1974) Plastische Bandscheibenchirurgie. I. Mitteilung: Bandscheibenersatz im lumbalen Bereich mit Silikonkautschuk. Theoretische und experimentelle Untersuchungen. Z Orthop Ihre Grenzgeb 112:1078–1086
20. Urban RM, Jacobs JJ, Tomlinson MJ, Gavrilovic J, Black J, Peoch M (2000) Dissemination of wear particles to the liver, spleen, and abdominal lymph nodes of patients with hip or knee replacement. J Bone Joint Surg Am 82: 457–476
21. Weber H (1983) Lumbar disc herniation. A controlled, prospective study with ten years of observation. Spine 8:131–140

Alan Gardner
Ketan C. Pande

Graf ligamentoplasty: a 7-year follow-up

Abstract Graf ligamentoplasty is seen as a means of stabilising and reducing the mobility of one or more severely symptomatic motion segments associated with degenerative disc disease. It is a less invasive procedure than fusion and appears to have a similar or slightly better success rate. Some studies have reported mixed results at early follow up; generally, they have suffered from poorly defined indications for the procedure, which are now much clearer. Reports on the first 50 patients undergoing Graf stabilisation in 1990/1991 were published in the *European Spine Journal* in 1995, with a 2-year follow-up. In the present study, the results of which were independently reviewed by the second author (K.C.P.), a spinal research fellow from an unrelated centre, we were able to establish postal contact with 40 of those patients, of whom 31 still had Graf instrumentation in situ. Examination of the clinical records of the ten non-responders when last seen indicated no particular bias of the results. The average age at surgery and average follow-up were 41.8 years (range 17.2–60 years) and 7.4 years (range 5.6–8.5 years) respectively. Excellent and good subjective results were reported in 62% of patients; 61% reported significant or total relief of low-back pain and 77% never or occasionally used analgesics. Patients were evaluated using the Oswestry Disability Score and the MSPQ (Modified Somatic Perception Questionnaire) and Zung Depression Index with the DRAM (Disability and Risk Assessment Method). Additional information was obtained from the clinical notes and radiographs at last review. The mean Oswestry Disability Score was 59± 10% pre-operatively and 37.7±14% after 7 years. There was a statistically significant correlation between the Oswestry scores and the subjective outcome (P=0.009). The results of this study suggest that the beneficial effects of Graf ligamentoplasty are sustained in the longer term in spite of the presence of an established degenerative process.

Keywords Graf ligamentoplasty · Flexible stabilisation · Low-back pain · Disc degeneration

A. Gardner (✉)
The Essex Spine Centre, BUPA
Hartswood Hospital, Brentwood,
Essex CM13 3LE, UK
e-mail: gardner@adhg.demon.co.uk,
Tel.: +44-1245-223456,
Fax: +44-1245-222130

K.C. Pande
Orthopaedic Department,
Queen's Medical Centre,
University of Nottingham,
Nottingham, UK

Introduction

The mechanical model of the pathogenesis of discogenic back pain predicts that if the motion segment is immobilised then there will be no further stimulation of nociceptive receptors. All of us with any extensive experience of the surgical treatment of low-back pain will know that things are not that simple. Firstly, fully rigid fixation is probably not achieved by posterior or intertransverse fusion alone – 360° fusion is necessary.

Secondly, the causes of pain in degenerative disc disease are not well understood and are difficult to investigate. Laboratory testing, with demonstration of various

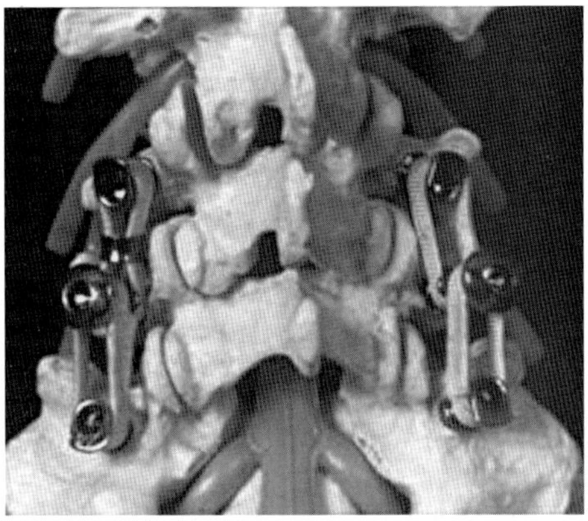

Fig. 1 Graf pedicle screws and polyester bands. The optional diabolo on the left protects the band from chafing against the facet joint

modes of mechanical instability, is suggestive and provides circumstantial evidence; however, the main complaint of pain, being a symptom, is not amenable to verification in the laboratory or in an animal model.

We are all aware that over the past 20 years the bio-psycho-social model of back pain and its associated disability has gained much greater appreciation and is better understood [13]. A great array of psychometric tools has been described, along with a variety of educational, physical and therapeutic management programmes designed to reorientate the individual's attitude to their pain and to lessen their disability.

We strongly believe, however, that a proper understanding of back pain and its consequences must include both the mechanical and bio-psycho-social models. Neither has a monopoly of wisdom, as some would have us believe. We have no doubt that either surgery or rehabilitation programmes or both, when applied to well-selected patients without undue delay, will provide the key for the great majority of back sufferers and enable them to live a reasonably fulfilling life. However, there are those who slip through the net and receive either delayed or inappropriate treatment, and also those who are psychologically vulnerable, who make their own lives a misery and challenge the resources of those who try to help them.

This article describes the Graf technique which, like all stabilising back pain surgery, is applicable only to a small percentage of back sufferers who are psychologically robust and have a demonstrable pain source verified, so far as is possible, by clinical assessment, plain radiography, magnetic resonance imaging (MRI) and discography, where necessary.

Graf ligamentoplasty (Fig. 1) may be described as a stabilising and splinting procedure, designed to substantially immobilise a symptomatic and presumably damaged motion segment made vulnerable by the degenerative process or injury.

The prime clinical indication for Graf ligamentoplasty may be described as "the lumbar instability syndrome."

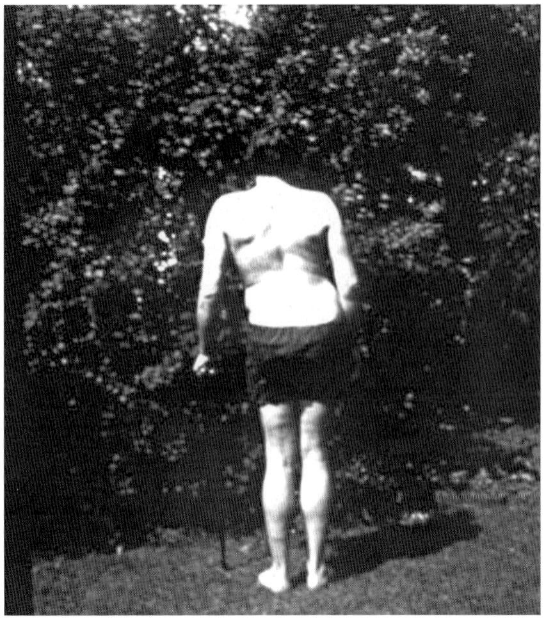

Fig. 2 Characteristic spasm of lumbar instability syndrome. The lumbar spine is immobilised in extension, the position of maximum stability, as in the Graf operation. This man had no leg pain and his symptoms resolved with time with no surgery being necessary

The important word here is "syndrome," meaning a collection of symptoms. Frequently patients are highly symptomatic, with pain sources that are difficult to demonstrate objectively. The surgeon has to decide on the relative importance of the mechanical model and the bio-psycho-social model. Surgeons and physicians have to become expert at resolving this conflict and assessing the correct balance, so that they can recommend the treatment mode most likely to help that individual.

The lumbar instability syndrome (Fig. 2) is often characterised by recurrent or chronic low-back pain with disabling episodes of acute muscle spasm. The longer the history and the more intense the back pain, the more likely it is to be referred down one or both legs, sometimes to the feet.

The pain is often described as a vague, dead, heavy ache with tingling into the feet and toes in a non-dermatomal distribution. Objective neurological signs are absent unless there is associated lumbar nerve root involvement.

Needless to say, patients do not become candidates for surgery unless they have been through a thorough course of non-operative treatment. A pre-operative functional restoration or self-management programme is often helpful anyway, because of its educational content and instruction in physical therapy.

Indications

The indications for Graf ligamentoplasty may be summarised as follows:

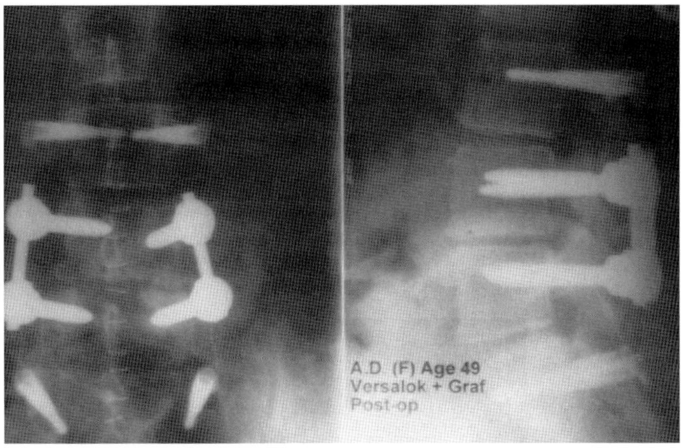

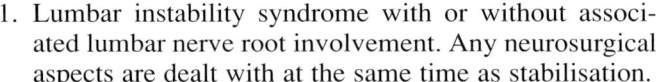

Fig. 3 Hybrid stabilisation. L4/5 fusion with L3/4 and L5/S1 Graf. This school-teacher, who was about to retire because of her back, was able to return to full duties 4 months after surgery and rehabilitation

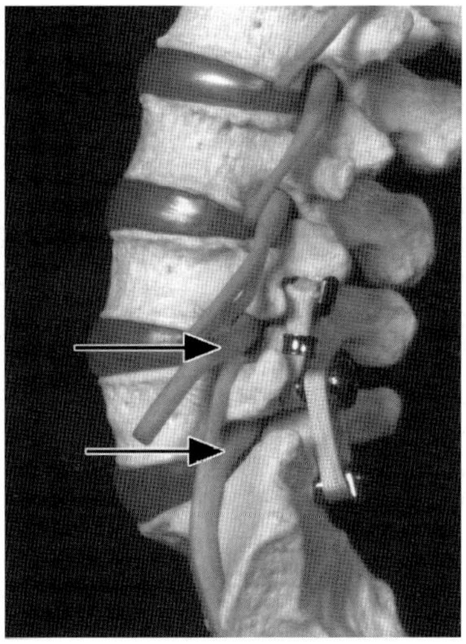

Fig. 4 The arrows indicate where nerve root compression can occur

1. Lumbar instability syndrome with or without associated lumbar nerve root involvement. Any neurosurgical aspects are dealt with at the same time as stabilisation.
2. Stabilisation of degenerate and symptomatic discs above or below an existing fusion. Fusing yet another level with its invasiveness and biomechanical consequences is often undesirable and unnecessary.
3. Stabilisation of a symptomatic adjacent disc to a spondylolysis which is repaired at the same time, as an alternative to fusion.
4. Stabilisation of three-level disc degeneration as a more successful alternative to three-level fusion. We have found that ligamentoplasty up to three levels is as successful as one-level stabilisation, provided the correct levels are stabilised. Four-level stabilisations have been disappointing.
5. "Hybrid" stabilisation (Fig. 3). Graf stabilisation in combination with fusion of an adjacent severely degenerate disc or spondylolisthesis not suitable for Graf stabilisation. In these cases the Graf bands are placed deep to the pedicle screw-rod junction. A slightly longer screw (5 mm) may be necessary to allow for the thickness of the band. Allowance should also be made for the difference in band length, because of any difference in screw diameter from that of the Graf screw (6.5 or 7.5 mm).

Contra-indications

The contra-indications for Graf ligamentoplasty are as follows:

1. Isthmic or degenerative spondylolisthesis greater than grade 1. Such cases are better treated by fusion if necessary.
2. Severe degenerative disc disease. It seems illogical to preserve movement of a severely degenerate disc, and fusion is probably preferable. However, good results have been reported in some such cases. When marked disc narrowing is present, the risk of lateral recess and foraminal compression is much greater, as the motion segment is immobilised in lordosis with Graf bands. It is often not possible to carry out an adequate decompression without excessive partial facetectomy in these cases.
3. Tumours, infection or trauma, where rigid stabilisation is required.
4. Patients with prolonged and severe disability for more than 1 year and those with unsatisfactory psycho-social profiles. In this group, stabilising surgery may produce some benefits, but a good or excellent result is not to be expected.

As a general consideration, it is necessary to appreciate that application of appropriate Graf bands immobilises the motion segment in lordosis with the facet joints in a position of full extension, in which position they are very stable. As a consequence, the lateral recess and the exit foramen will be narrowed to some extent.

If significant disc narrowing is present or there is a constitutional tendency to stenosis, then nerve root compression may result if ligamentum flavum removal or partial facetectomy is not carried out as a precaution (Fig. 4).

The clinical history and the MRI scan will give some guidance as to the need for decompression, but the exit foramen should always be probed to ensure there is adequate space if there is any doubt. In the experience of the first author, around 60% of operated levels need bilateral decompression, but some surgeons will decompress all levels.

In our report [5] of the first 50 Graf stabilisation patients, new post-operative lumbar nerve root compression symptoms were the commonest complication and, although the majority resolved with time, epidural injections etc., a small number did not. Lessons were learnt.

All these matters are reviewed in greater detail in other publications [2, 3, 4].

Materials and methods

The first 50 patients operated upon by the first author (A.G.) were independently reviewed and reported in the *European Spine Journal* in 1995 [6]. For the purposes of the present study, as many as possible of these patients, who had undergone surgery between August 1990 and December 1991, were subject to a further independent review conducted by the second author (K.C.P.), an orthopaedic surgeon from another, unrelated, centre.

The objective was to assess the long-term outcome of patients with the Graf implant in situ. Patients were evaluated using a postal questionnaire, which included the Oswestry Disability Score [1], the MSPQ (Modified Somatic Perception Questionnaire) [9] and the Zung Depression Index [14]. This enabled calculation of the DRAM (Disability and Risk Assessment Method) score [10]. Additional information was obtained from the clinical notes and radiographs at last review.

Results

Data were available on 40 patients (ten non-responders). For the final analysis, 31 patients with the Graf implant in situ were considered after excluding patients who had undergone subsequent fusion or removal of the Graf implant. Four had undergone fusion, with indifferent results. They probably represented errors of case selection. Three patients had had screws removed for late loosening, with symptomatic relief. One patient had had the implant removed because of persistent pain with no relief, and one patient, a 35-year-old policeman, had developed an acute infection 8 weeks after surgery; the implant was removed, with an excellent long-term outcome and return to full duties. The combination of surgical stabilisation and infection seemed to cure his "instability".

The clinical records of the ten non-responders were reviewed and the spread of results showed no particular bias compared with the responders.

The average age at the time of surgery was 41.8 years (range 17.2–60 years). No significant difference in the subjective result was seen between patients below and those above the age of 40 years.

The average follow up was 7.4 years (range 5.6–8.6 years).

Twenty-two patients had undergone single-level instrumentation and nine had had more than one level instrumented. Patients instrumented at more than one level appeared to have better results, although this difference did not reach statistical significance (P=0.06).

Additional information was obtained from the clinical notes and radiographs at last review.

The results of the questionnaire are given in Fig. 5. Sixty-one percent of patients were still rated as good or excellent 7.4 years after surgery, but 10% were rated worse than their preoperative condition.

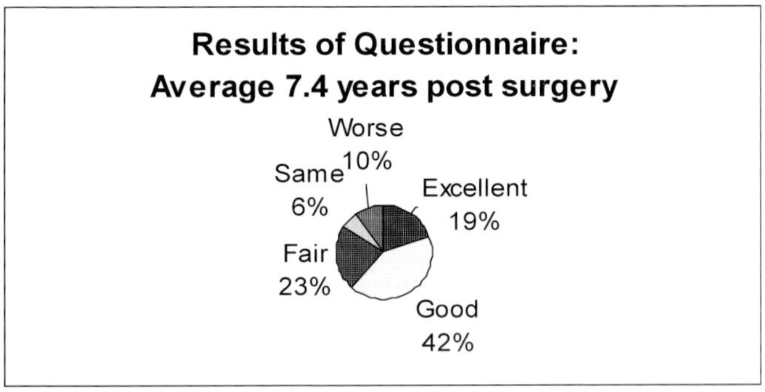

Fig. 5 Results of questionnaire assessing the outcome of surgery at an average of 7.4 years after the operation

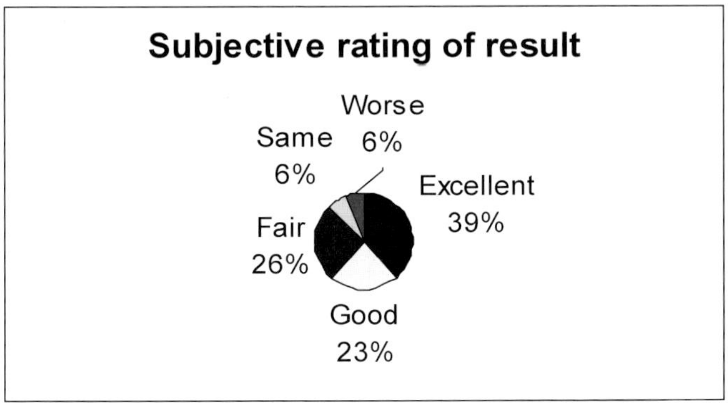

Fig. 6 Subjective rating of the results

This is always a cause for concern, but there was no particular pattern to this group of patients. It has been a noticeable, but anecdotal, feature that patients who are worse after Graf stabilisation do not seem to be severely worse; they have simply gone on deteriorating, in contrast to those who are worse after fusion, who seem to be a great deal worse and complain bitterly. The first author's telephone has been very much quieter since Graf stabilisation replaced the majority of fusions for degenerative disc disease.

The subjective ratings of the result by the patients when asked to place themselves in one of five categories was, as usual, somewhat optimistic (Fig. 6). The percentage of good and excellent results, at 62%, remained much the same as the doctor's grading in Fig. 5, but within this group, the percentage who considered themselves excellent was doubled.

In the questionnaire, patients were asked whether, if they had the choice again, they would be willing to undergo the same surgery (Fig. 7). Sixty-eight percent responded in the positive, with none responding that they would not have made that decision. This was understandable, as nobody likes to be proved wrong. It was encouraging that nobody admitted to being misled or misinformed.

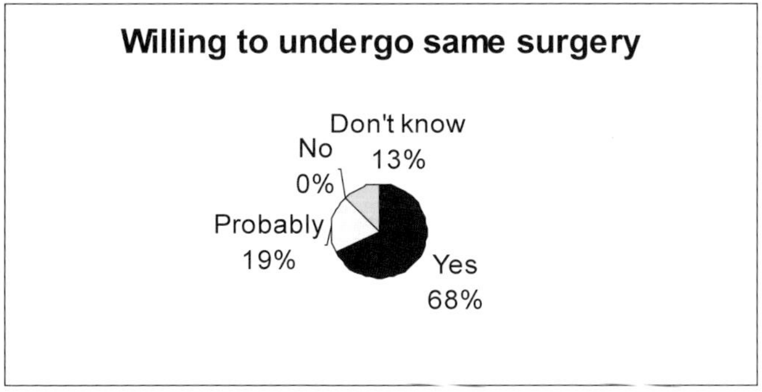

Fig. 7 Responses to item on whether patient would be willing to undergo the same surgery

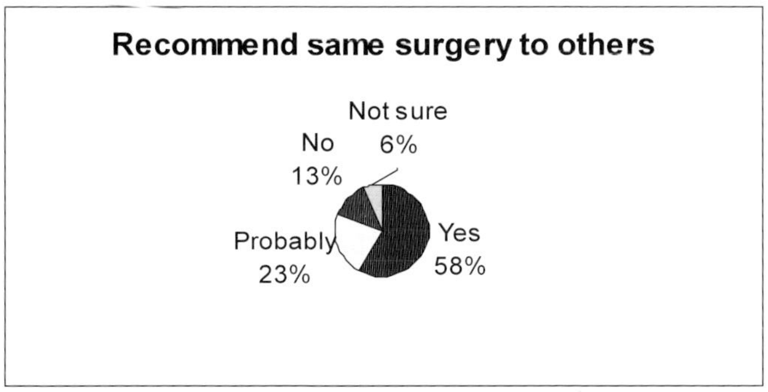

Fig. 8 Responses to item on whether the patient would recommend the same surgery to others

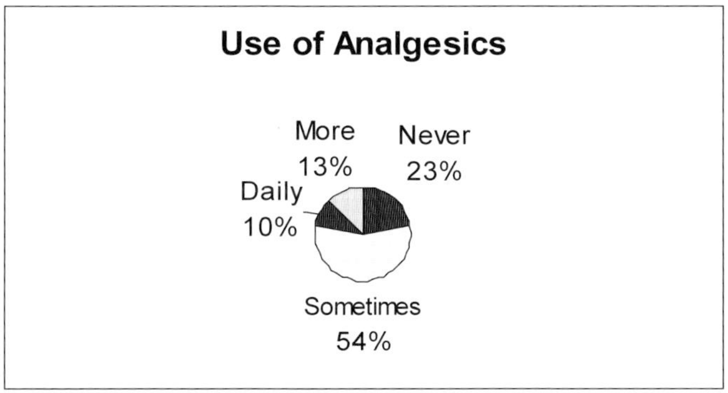

Fig. 9 Use of analgesics

The question as to whether patients would recommend the same surgery to others (Fig. 8) was less encouraging, with only 58% being sure and 13% (four patients) responding in the negative.

Patients were also asked about their analgesic consumption (Fig. 9). One-quarter said they never used analgesics, and 54% said they sometimes used them, with 13% using them more than daily. Given that the average Oswestry score prior to surgery was 59%, it was considered reasonably satisfactory that 77% of patients (24 out of 31) used analgesics sometimes or never.

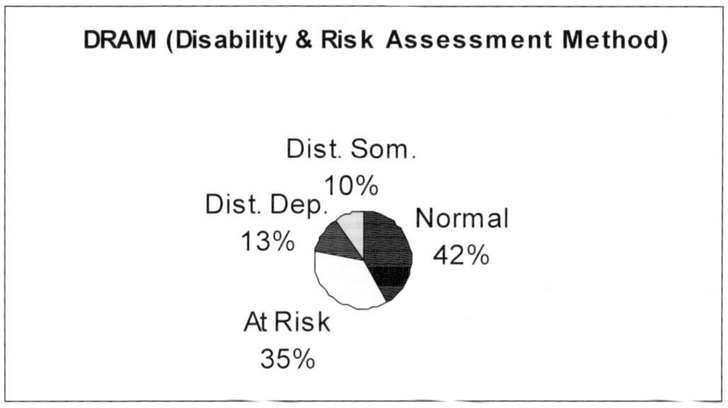

Fig. 10 Results of the Disability and Risk Assessment Method (DRAM)

Finally, the DRAM category (Fig. 10) of each patient was calculated using the MSPQ and Zung scores to establish the psychological profile. Seventy-seven percent of patients were considered to be normal or at risk, with 23 being rated as distressed. This series was too small to obtain any statistical correlation between psychological category and outcome. However, it is worth making the point that while the first author has operated on distressed depressive patients with good or excellent results, the outcomes for distressed somatic patients have been generally disappointing.

Discussion

A previous series of 268 patients, independently reviewed (K.C.P.), produced results sufficiently encouraging to maintain that Graf stabilisation for patients experiencing intolerable symptoms from degenerative disc disease is a useful procedure [4]. The results were considered to be as good as, if not better than, those obtained by spinal fusion for this condition.

The above assertion will no doubt be challenged by many with an equal lack of objective information. There is an undoubted need for more carefully structured clinical trials to answer the following questions, to which we have partial answers only:

1. What precisely is the place for surgical stabilisation, either fusion or ligamentoplasty, in degenerative disc disease? Some maintain that there is no place, and they are probably wrong, as is usual with a dogmatic point of view. On the other hand, many surgeons, including the first author, have probably over-operated in the past, before the bio-psycho-social model of back pain and its associated treatment options became appreciated. The mechanical model of back pain remains important in many patients.
2. Flexible or soft stabilisation appears to be a more physiological and less mechanically disruptive procedure than fusion, particularly for three-level instrumentations. It is also a less invasive procedure. The

Graf and Dynesys methods appear to be the most popular. Is one method more effective than the other in both the short and the long terms?

3. Which patients and which spinal levels should undergo fusion and which flexible stabilisation? Severe degeneration and bone problems should be fused and soft tissue problems need soft tissue surgery, i.e. Graf.
4. Do patients undergoing flexible stabilisation benefit from reduced symptomatic disc degeneration at adjacent levels compared with those undergoing fusion? This remains to be established, but it is probably the case.
5. Should MRI dehydrated discs, which are thought to be asymptomatic and are adjacent to a symptomatic disc, be stabilised? The first author, prior to the advent of MRI around 15 years ago, generally fused the lower two lumbar discs if either was symptomatic, whether or not they were both degenerate. Since MRI, it has been easier to discriminate. The first author has generally advised extending Graf stabilisation to cover degenerate discs that are thought to be asymptomatic and are adjacent to symptomatic degenerate discs up to a maximum of three levels. Failure to do this has resulted in secondary surgery in some patients. It has to be admitted that this information is anecdotal, but at present there is little other information.
6. Finally, we come to the largely philosophical question as to whether we should advise major surgery for which the main indication is pain – a symptom that is difficult to measure and whose sources we do not fully understand. Perhaps the best that can be said on this is that spinal surgeons with experience in this field can probably produce a majority of patients who are grateful for their surgery, although there are some who are undoubtedly worse as a result.

Increasingly, we in the UK, and also surgeons in many other countries, are being advised and often instructed by administrators that we should use only evidence-based medical and surgical techniques. However, unfortunately, in many cases they fail to supply the resources and infrastructure to enable clinicians to collect that evidence. Meanwhile, is it not unethical to deny substantially disabled patients a probable route back to a more satisfactory and productive life? Clinical experience should not be ignored. It was many years before clinical trials established the efficacy of antibiotics and decades before their mode of action was understood.

Conclusions

The first author now has experience of over a thousand Graf stabilisations carried out between 1990 and 2000. Independent reviews have been conducted by Michael Grevitt reporting on a 2-year follow-up of the first 50 cases in 1995 [6], and the second author (K.C.P), who conducted the subsequent follow-up reported in this article. In addition, he also reviewed results of a further 268 patients reported elsewhere [3, 4]. Grevitt and Pande were Spinal Fellows from the University of Nottingham, with no medical or administrative connection to the Essex Spine Centre. It is considered reasonable to draw the following conclusions.

1. Graf ligamentoplasty has proved successful in the majority of patients undergoing stabilisation of up to three motion segments for highly symptomatic degenerative disc disease not responding to non-operative management. It is of course essential to establish which discs are symptomatic by clinical examination, plain radiology, MRI scanning and discography, where necessary. (Discography is particularly valuable in younger patients under the age of 25, who may have normal MRI scans but highly symptomatic discs.)
2. Graf ligamentoplasty is quicker, less invasive and, in experienced hands, less prone to complications than spinal fusion, being a simpler procedure with less to go wrong. Pseudarthrosis and donor site pain, in particular, are avoided. Since it is a less invasive procedure than a posterior or posterolateral fusion, and since there is no bone graft to worry about, recovery and rehabilitation can proceed more quickly and the majority of patients are back to light work within 6–8 weeks.
3. It has been suggested that Graf stabilisation either has inferior results to fusion [7] or that the results are not sustained. Neither criticism has been substantiated on independent review of the above series, and it is clear that some studies have had major structural defects [5] and others errors of case selection. Other studies [8, 11, 12] have had satisfactory results, similar to those reported in the present series.

The concept of flexible stabilisation is a soft tissue solution to what is essentially a soft tissue problem. Significant spondylolisthesis and severe degenerative disc disease with secondary bone changes are bone problems requiring a bone solution such as spinal fusion. The overkill of spinal fusion for most symptomatic degenerate discs is unnecessary and over-elaborate. Flexible stabilisation merits serious consideration in psychologically stable individuals when the symptomatic disc or discs can be identified with reasonable certainty and the response to non-operative treatment has been poor.

References

1. Fairbank JCT, Couper J, Davies JB, et al (1980) The Oswestry Low Back Pain Disability Questionnaire. Physiotherapy 66:271–273
2. Gardner ADH (1996) An alternative concept in the surgical management of lumbar degenerative disc disease: flexible stabilisation. In: Margulies JY, Flomaon Y, Farcy J-P, Neuwirth M (eds) Lumbosacral and spinopelvic fixation. Lippincott-Raven, Philadelphia, pp 889–905
3. Gardner ADH (1997) Flexible lumbar stabilisation: the Graf technique. Spine State Art Rev 11:479–507
4. Gardner ADH, Pande KC, Hassaan AM, Declerck G (1999) Graf stabilisation of intractable lumbar instability syndrome. In: Szpalski M, Gunzburg R, Pope M (eds) Lumbar segmental instability. Lippincott Williams & Wilkins, Philadelphia, pp 175–190
5. Gardner ADH, Declerck GM, Hardcastle P, Markwalder TM, Moon MS, Salanova C, Shim YS, Fraser RD (2000) Letter and reply concerning the article by Hadlow, Fraser, et al. in *Spine* 1998. Spine 25:2
6. Grevitt MP, Gardner ADH, Spilsbury J, et al (1995) The Graf stabilisation system: early results in 50 patients. Eur Spine J 4:169–175
7. Hadlow SW, Fagan AB, Hillier TM, Fraser RD (1998) The Graf ligamentoplasty procedure – comparison with postero-lateral fusion in the management of low back pain. Spine 23: 1172–1179
8. Leeks N, Skinner I, Hardcastle P (1999) Soft stabilisation of the lumbar spine using the Graf system for spinal instability syndromes and pseudarthrosis – 5 years results. J Musculo-skeletal Med 3:143–155
9. Main CJ (1983) The Modified Somatic Perception Questionnaire (MSPQ). J Psychosom Res 27:503–514
10. Main CJ, Wood PLR, Hollis S, et al (1992) Distress and Risk Assessment Method. A simple patient classification to identify distress and evaluate the risk of poor outcome. Spine 17:42–52
11. Markwalder TM, Dubach R, Brann M (1995) Soft stabilisation of the lumbar spine as an alternative surgical modality to lumbar arthrodesis in the facet syndrome. Acta Neurochir (Wien) 134:1–4
12. Salanova C, Moreno P, Benlot J (1998) Middle term results of flexible Graf stabilisation. Reson Eur Rachis 6:842–843
13. Waddell G (1998) The back pain revolution. Churchill Livingstone, Edinburgh
14. Zung WWK (1965) A self-related depression scale. Arch Gen Psychiatry 32:63–70

J. Sénégas

Mechanical supplementation by non-rigid fixation in degenerative intervertebral lumbar segments: the Wallis system

J. Sénégas
Clinique Saint Martin, Allée des Tulipes, 33608 Pessac Cedex, France
e-mail: js@cad-fr.com,
Tel.: +33-5-57020000,
Fax: +33-5-57020202

Abstract A first-generation implant for non-rigid stabilization of lumbar segments was developed in 1986. It included a titanium interspinous blocker and an artificial ligament made of dacron. Following an initial observational study in 1988 and a prospective controlled study from 1988 to 1993, more than 300 patients have been treated for degenerative lesions with this type of implant with clinical and mechanical follow-up. After careful analysis of the points that could be improved, a second-generation implant called the "Wallis" implant, was developed. This interspinous blocker, which was made of metal in the preliminary version, is made of PEEK (polyetheretherketone) in the new model. The overall implant constitutes a "floating" system, with no permanent fixation in the vertebral bone, to avoid the risk of loosening. It achieves an increase in the rigidity of destabilized segments beyond normal values. The clinical trials of the first-generation implant provided evidence that the interspinous system of non-rigid stabilization is efficacious against low-back pain due to degenerative instability and free of serious complications. The first-generation devices achieved marked, significant resolution of residual low-back pain. These results warrant confirmation. A randomized clinical trial and an observational study of the new implant are currently underway. Non-rigid fixation clearly appears to be a useful technique in the management of initial forms of degenerative intervertebral lumbar disc disease. This method should rapidly assume a specific role along with total disc prostheses in the new step-wise surgical strategy to obviate definitive fusion of degenerative intervertebral segments. At present, the Wallis system is recommended for lumbar disc disease in the following indications: (i) discectomy for massive herniated disc leading to substantial loss of disc material, (ii) a second discectomy for recurrence of herniated disc, (iii) discectomy for herniation of a transitional disc with sacralization of L5, (iv) degenerative disc disease at a level adjacent to a previous fusion, and (v) isolated Modic I lesion leading to chronic low-back pain.

Keywords Non-rigid fixation · Degenerative lumbar disc · Low-back pain

Introduction

We began studying and developing non-rigid stabilization of lumbar segments in 1984, because at that time it was already clear that the progress achieved in these techniques in other joints of the locomotor system would sooner or later be applicable to the joints of the vertebral column. The current continued use of intervertebral fusion procedures, which totally eliminate mobility, cannot be attributed solely to insufficient mastery of spinal prosthesis techniques or ligament reconstruction. Spinal surgeons also continue to use fusion because of the unique organization of the intervertebral articulations forming a kinetic chain. This multi-articular system provides the capacity to compensate relatively well for damage to a single segment, regardless of whether such lesions result from a degenerative process or surgical fusion.

From 1984 to 1986, we carried out biomechanical cadaver studies, mechanically testing various non-rigid systems of stabilization of lumbar intervertebral segments. Ultimately, we opted for a "floating" system with no bony fixation, because it is illusory to hope for durable functioning of a system that includes, for example, pedicle screw fixation. The system that we developed and first implanted in 1986 included a titanium interspinous blocker and an artificial ligament made of dacron. The results of an initial observational study were published in 1988 and 1991 [6, 7]. This was followed by a prospective controlled study from 1988 to 1993 [8]. Since then, more than 300 patients have been treated for degenerative lesions with this type of implant, with clinical and mechanical follow-up.

Despite satisfactory findings and the absence of serious complications, the initial device was never commercially developed while waiting for assessment of long-term results. Finally, after careful analysis of the points that could be improved, we have developed a second-generation implant called the "Wallis" implant, which is awaiting use with a maximum of precautions. A randomized clinical trial and an observational study of the new implant are currently underway.

Basic concepts

As in any dynamic system, a mobile intervertebral segment undergoes acceleration inversely proportional to the moment of inertia when it is submitted to a force. The rigidity of the system limits the displacement. This braking action preserves a margin of security and helps protect against tissue lesions involving the disc or the intervertebral ligaments. "Rigidity" is a mechanical parameter defined in terms of load for a given displacement. It corresponds to the slope of the load/deformity curve.

The stretching of the elements of articular union leads to a force resisting the displacement. The dissipation of kinetic energy in the form of heat is mediated by the viscoelastic properties of the connective tissue (passive damping). This damping phenomenon would, in fact, be quite insufficient to protect the disc if it were not constantly supplemented by a much more effective active damping provided by the reflex contraction of the powerful paravertebral muscles. Although the dynamic equilibrium of the intervertebral articular system is dependent on a combination of muscle activity and tension of the passive elements of union, the active system constantly protects the passive elements, which consequently are never submitted to the limits of their elasticity under normal conditions.

Under these specific mechanical conditions, the intervertebral disc cells that produce the extracellular matrix exhibit normal activity. These cells are, in fact, mechanodependent, as demonstrated by Lotz and Chin [2]. They function normally only under a precise range of mechanical loading. Outside of this range, they initiate apoptosis. When loading is excessive or the active system of damping is deficient, the passive system represented by the disc and intervertebral ligaments can be overloaded and rupture. If these lesions are not excessively severe, or if the lesional process takes place over time analogously to stress fractures, cell activity can repair the damage, as is the case in any connective tissue. However, when the constraints persist, the reparative process can be overwhelmed, and irreversible degenerative lesions develop if the loss of rigidity persists. Laxity or a diminution in the rigidity of an intervertebral segment is constant in the degenerative process, as demonstrated by Ebara et al. [1] and Mimura et al. [3]. This is true regardless of the stage of degeneration. At the beginning of the degenerative process, before alteration of the disc height, an increase in the range of motion is observed on bending studies because of the greater laxity. When the disc lesions are more severe, intervertebral mobility is reduced because of the narrowing of the disc space. However, mechanical testing shows that the system is still less rigid than normally, the decrease being reflected by an increase in the neutral zone.

Basically, nonetheless, the disc tissue, notably the annulus, has healing capacity, as do all connective tissues. In fact, an indisputable healing process can be observed in the intervertebral disc, with a fibroelastic reaction and neovascularization, at least at the beginning of degenerative lesions. However, the persistence of excessive mechanical loading leads to the failure of this healing process, similar to that observed in pseudarthrosis of long bones or in meniscal lesions.

The principle of mechanical supplementation by nonrigid fixation consists in both increasing the rigidity of the intervertebral system and limiting the amplitude of mobility to stop the irreversible course of the degenerative lesions, and possibly, in some cases, to foster the healing of the least severe lesions.

The Wallis implant

We believe that it is not possible to rigidify all joint elements of the intervertebral segment with a simple system. In designing the implant (Fig. 1, Fig. 2), we decided to supplement only damping of the motions of flexion and rotation. We chose to limit extension with an interspinous blocker, which is intended to act as a posterior shock absorber. This interspinous blocker, which was made of metal in the preliminary version, is now made of PEEK

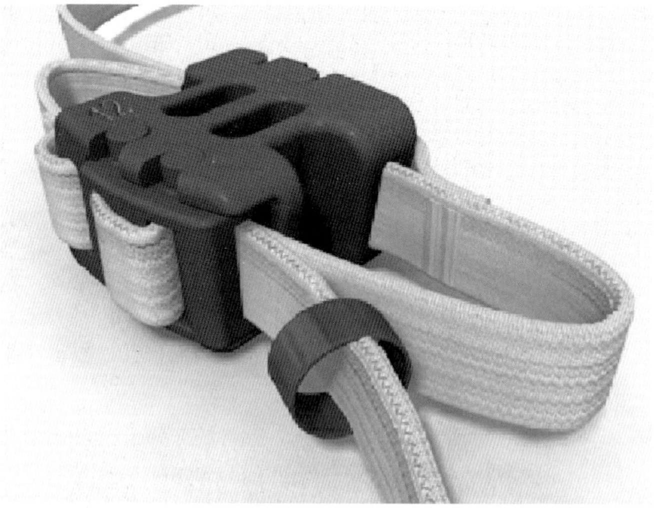

Fig. 1 The non-rigid fixation "Wallis" implant

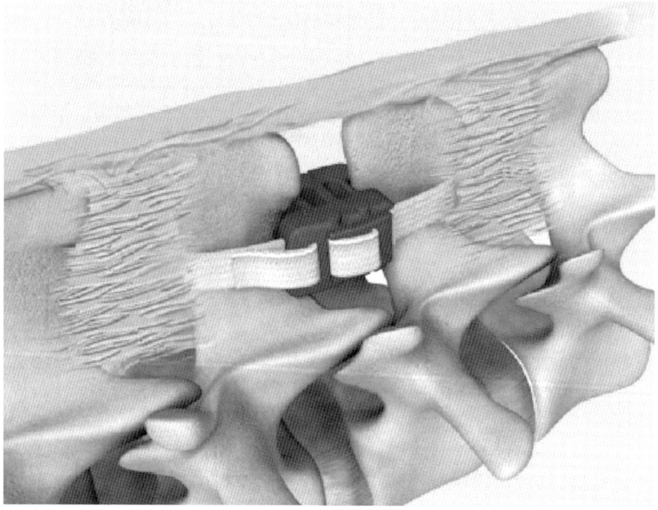

Fig. 2 Schematic view of the Wallis implant in place

(polyetheretherketone) in the "Wallis" model. Thanks to its shape and the properties of PEEK, the new blocker has much greater elasticity (the PEEK blockers are 30 times less rigid than the former, titanium, model). Moreover, the use of an interspinous blocker confers substantial mechanical advantages, as shown by Minns et al. [4]. When the spinal column is submitted to loading, the interspinous blocker displaces the mechanical constraints dorsally and reduces the load upon the disc and the facet joint system (by as much as 50% for a blocker 12 mm in thickness).

In addition, the implant includes two ligaments made of woven dacron that are wrapped around the spinous processes and fixed under tension to the blocker. This is facilitated by the design of the implant and dedicated instrumentation. The ligaments resist traction of 200 daN and stretch approximately 20% before failure by overloading.

The overall implant constitutes a "floating" system with no permanent fixation in the vertebral bone, which might otherwise expose it to the risk of loosening. As yet unpublished mechanical human cadaver studies conducted on the implant have shown that it permits a reduction in the mobility of intervertebral segments previously destabilized by discectomy and that it achieves an increase in the rigidity of the destabilized segment beyond normal values.

Furthermore, animal studies have shown that it was possible to obtain fibrous healing of a disc space after total discectomy by use of non-rigid fixation, whereas in the absence of fixation, only complete destruction of the intervertebral tissue is observed.

Clinical results

From 1988 to 1993, we carried out a non-randomized prospective controlled study comparing two homogeneous groups of patients, both of which underwent surgery for recurrence of herniated disc after an initial L4-L5 discectomy [8]. One group was treated by a second discectomy alone (group A), whereas the other group underwent discectomy and implantation of the first-generation device. Before the second intervention, all patients underwent neurologic examination, assessment of pain on a visual analog scale, and a functional evaluation using the Oswestry score. The preoperative radiologic work-up included conventional X-rays and dynamic bending films in all patients, as well as myelography followed by computed tomography, or, in most of the patients, magnetic resonance imaging (MRI). There were 40 patients in each group. At follow-up, the same clinical assessments that were obtained preoperatively were performed again, and MRI was obtained systematically. The mean follow-up after the intervention was 3 years and 4 months (range 1 year to 4 years and 8 months).

Group A (discectomy alone) included 26 men and 14 women, the average age of whom was 41 years (range 22–58 years). Twenty-eight of these patients (70%) had no motor deficits. Among the remaining 12 patients (30%), seven (17%) had a motor deficit evaluated at 3 or 4 on the ASIA scale, three (7.5%) had a deficit of 2, and two (5%) had a deficit of 0 to 1. In every case, patent recurrence of herniated disc was observed during the operation. The following complications were observed in group A: two superficial infections, four cases of intraoperative dural tear, and, subsequent to one of the latter, one infectious meningitis, which healed without sequelae.

Two patients in group A were reoperated because of chronic low-back pain. They underwent lumbar fusion. A neurostimulation device was implanted in one patient who had constant pain.

Group B (discectomy and implant) included 29 men and 11 women, the average age of whom was 42 years

Fig. 3 Recurrence of herniated disc

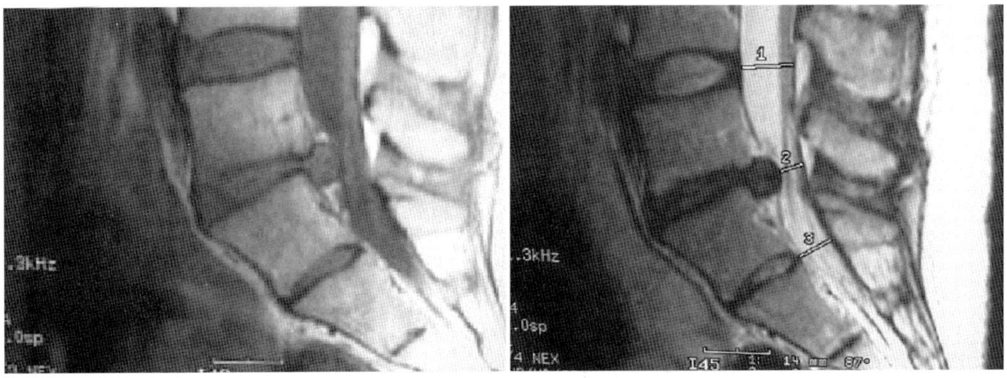

Fig. 4 Magnetic resonance imaging aspect 11 years after non-rigid fixation

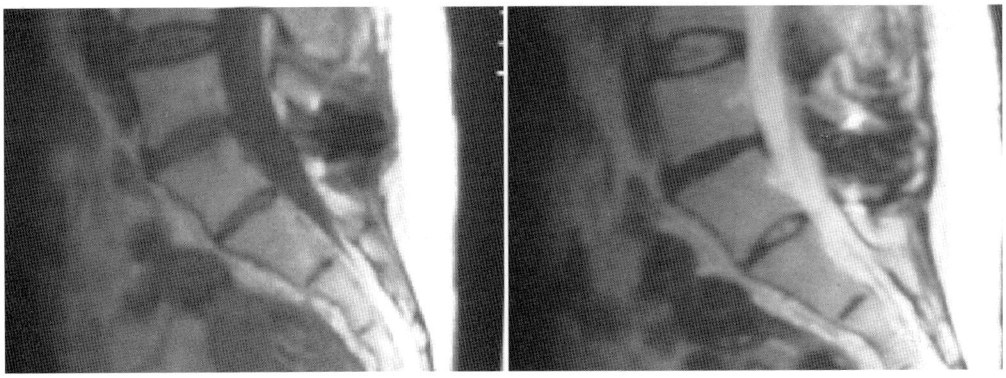

(range 25–62 years). In 20 patients (50%), there was no detectable motor deficit before the second intervention. Among the remaining patients, 14 (35%) had a motor deficit evaluated at 3 or 4 on the ASIA scale, five (12.5%) had a deficit of 2, and one (2.5%) had a deficit of 0 to 1. In 38 patients, we found a patent recurrence of disc herniation, and in two cases, the nerve-root compression was caused by migration of biocompatible osteoconductive (hydroxyapatite) polymer that had been inserted in the disc space during the initial intervention.

The complications in group B were essentially limited to dural violation (seven cases) with no resulting adverse consequences. No case of infection or worsening of neurologic deficit occurred. None of the spinous processes was fractured and none of the dacron ligaments failed.

Three patients in group B underwent revision surgery, one for persisting low-back pain 3 months after the procedure. The revision operation showed that the ligament was loose due to failure of the system of fixation to the metallic blocker. Arthrodesis was performed after removal of the implant. In two patients, a second revision operation was necessary after a new recurrence of disc herniation in the same segment. In one, the implant was easily removed after discectomy and arthrodesis was performed. In the other patient, after decompression, the implant was left in place with a satisfactory result. In all three of these revision procedures, the excellent tolerance of the implant was confirmed. The non-rigid fixation device was found embedded in a homogeneous fibrous mass with no sign of inflammatory reaction.

Analysis of clinical results

The percentage of improvement in low-back pain over the preoperative VAS score was 52% at follow-up in group A (discectomy alone) and 74% in group B (discectomy and implant). Nerve root pain was improved by 87% in group A and by 92% in group B.

At follow-up, 20% of the patients in group A were no longer taking analgesic medication, as opposed to 42.5% in group B. The Oswestry functional score in group A changed from 54.7 (SD ±16) preoperatively to 22 (SD ±11) at follow-up. In group B, the mean preoperative score was 58.2 (SD ±22) and 16.4 (SD ±10) at follow-up.

In the patients who received the implant, we studied the course of the instability of the segment involved using dynamic bending films. The preoperative disc space height varied from 2 to 10 mm. In eight patients, a postoperative diminution in disc height was observed (mean 2 mm) and in three patients, an approximately 3-mm ventral displacement of the cephalad adjacent vertebral body was noted with no correlation to the clinical outcome of these patients.

The angle of flexion-extension mobility varied from 0° to 12° (mean 5°). In four patients, the angle of mobility was greater than 10°.

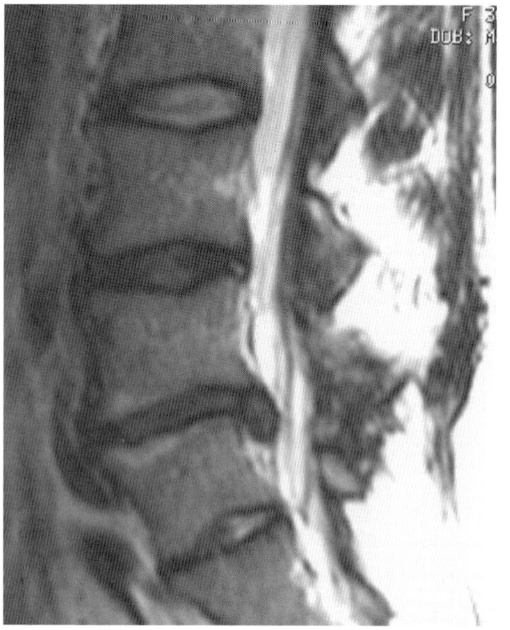

Fig. 5 Recurrence of herniated transitional disc at L4-L5 (due to sacralization of L5)

Postoperative analysis of the MR images (Fig. 3, Fig. 4) showed marked improvement in the bony lesions on both sides of the operated disc. In six cases, exacerbation of adjacent disc lesions was visible.

Discussion

The clinical trial results of the first-generation implant provide evidence that the interspinous system of non-rigid stabilization is efficacious against low-back pain due to degenerative instability, while remaining technically straightforward to implement and free of serious complications. Moreover, in case of failure, removal of the implant poses no technical problem, and revision by arthrodesis, if necessary, has proven to be simple.

The first-generation devices achieved marked, significant resolution of residual low-back pain. The functional improvement assessed using the Oswestry score was less marked, because it fails to distinguish between nerve-root pain and purely low-back pain.

We believe that these results warrant confirmation and that they can be improved by use of the second-generation implant, concerning which two clinical trials are currently underway.

Non-rigid fixation clearly appears to be a useful technique in the management of initial forms of degenerative intervertebral lumbar disc disease. This method should rapidly assume a specific role along with total disc prostheses in the new step-wise surgical strategy to obviate definitive fusion of degenerative intervertebral segments.

At present, we consider that the Wallis system can be used for lesions of grade II, III, and IV in the MRI classification proposed by Pfirrmann et al. [5] in the following indications:

- Discectomy for voluminous herniated disc leading to substantial loss of disc material
- A second discectomy for recurrence of herniated disc
- Discectomy for herniation of a transitional disc with sacralization of L5 (Fig. 5, Fig. 6)
- Degenerative disc disease at a level adjacent to a previous fusion
- Isolated Modic I lesion leading to chronic low-back pain

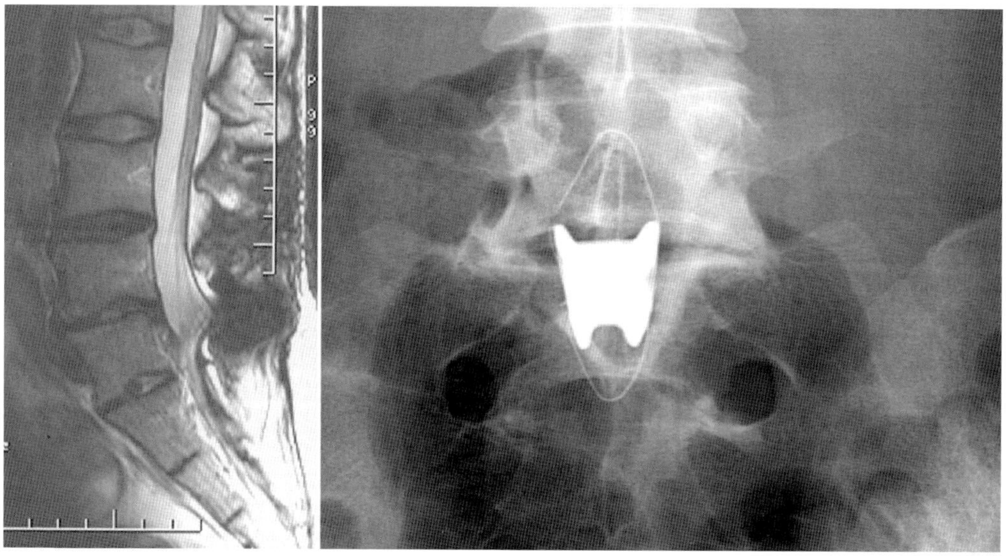

Fig. 6 Same patient as in Fig. 5, 8 years after discectomy and non-rigid stabilization (first-generation implant with titanium blocker)

References

1. Ebara S, Harada T, Hosono N, et al (1992) Intraoperative measurement of lumbar spinal instability. Spine 17 [3 Suppl]:44–50
2. Lotz JC, Chin JR (2000) Intervertebral disc cell death is dependent on the magnitude and duration of spinal loading. Spine 25:1477–1483
3. Mimura M, Panjabi M, Oxland TR, et al (1994) Disc degeneration affects the multidirectional flexibility of the lumbar spine. Spine 19:1371–1380
4. Minns RJ, Walsh WK (1997) Preliminary design and experimental studies of a novel soft implant for correcting sagittal plane instability in the lumbar spine. Spine 22:1819–1825; discussion 1826–1827
5. Pfirrmann CWA, Metzdorf A, Zanetti M, Hodler J, Boos N (2001) Magnetic resonance classification of lumbar intervertebral disc degeneration. Spine 26: 4873–4878
6. Sénégas J (1991) La ligamentoplastie intervertébrale, alternative à l'arthrodèse dans le traitement des instabilitiés dégénćratives. Acta Orthop Belg 57 [Suppl 1]:221–226
7. Sénégas J, Etchevers JP, Baulny D, Grenier F (1988) Widening of the lumbar vertebral canal as an alternative to laminectomy, in the treatment of lumbar stenosis. Fr J Orthop Surg 2:93–99
8. Sénégas J, Vital JM, Guérin J, Bernard P, M'Barek M, Loreiro M, Bouvet R (1995) Stabilisation lombaire souple. In: GIEDA – Instabilités vertébrales lombaires. Expansion Scientifique Française, Paris, pp 122–132

Thomas M. Stoll
Gilles Dubois
Othmar Schwarzenbach

The dynamic neutralization system for the spine: a multi-center study of a novel non-fusion system

Abstract Various forms of lumbar instability require a surgical stabilization. As an alternative to fusion, a mobile, dynamic stabilization restricting segmental motion would be advantageous in various indications, allowing greater physiological function and reducing the inherent disadvantages of rigid instrumentation and fusion. The dynamic neutralization system for the spine (Dynesys) is a pedicle screw system for mobile stabilization, consisting of titanium alloy screws connected by an elastic synthetic compound, controlling motion in any plane (non-fusion system). This prospective, multi-center study evaluated the safety and efficacy of Dynesys in the treatment of lumbar instability conditions, evaluating pre- and post-operative pain, function, and radiological data on a consecutive series of 83 patients. Indications consisted of unstable segmental conditions, mainly combined with spinal stenosis (60.2%) and with degenerative discopathy (24.1%), in some cases with disc herniation (8.4%), and with revision surgery (6.0%). Thirty-nine patients additionally had degenerative spondylolisthesis, and 30 patients had undergone previous lumbar surgery. In 56 patients instrumentation was combined with direct decompression. The mean age at operation was 58.2 (range 26.8–85.3) years; the mean follow-up time was 38.1 months (range 11.2–79.1 months). There were nine complications unrelated to the implant, and one due to a screw malplacement. Four of them required an early surgical reintervention. Additional lumbar surgery in the follow-up period included: implant removal and conversion into spinal fusion with rigid instrumentation for persisting pain in three cases, laminectomy of an index segment in one case and screw removal due to loosening in one case. In seven cases, radiological signs of screw loosening were observed. In seven cases, adjacent segment degeneration necessitated further surgery. Mean pain and function scores improved significantly from baseline to follow-up, as follows: back pain scale from 7.4 to 3.1, leg pain scale from 6.9 to 2.4, and Oswestry Disability Index from 55.4% to 22.9%. These study results compare well with those obtained by conventional procedures; in addition to which, mobile stabilization is less invasive than fusion. Long-term screw fixation is dependent on correct screw dimension and proper screw positioning. The natural course of polysegmental disease in some cases necessitates further surgery as the disease progresses. Dynamic neutralization proved to be a safe and effective alternative in the treatment of unstable lumbar conditions.

Keywords Lumbar spine · Surgical treatment · Non-fusion · Instrumentation · Instability

T.M. Stoll (✉)
Department of Spinal Surgery,
Bethesda Spital,
Gellertstrasse 144,
4020 Basel, Switzerland
e-mail: thomas.stoll@bethesda.ch,
Tel.: +41-61-3152333,
Fax: +41-61-3152338

G. Dubois
Nouvelle Clinique de l'Union,
St. Jean, France

O. Schwarzenbach
Spital Thun-Simmental, Thun, Switzerland

Introduction

Spinal instrumentation has always pursued one main aim: to stabilize the motion segment. Stabilization is aimed at stopping noxious motion, holding position, and preventing deformity. It has always addressed the two main sequelae of spinal pathology: pain and dysfunction by neurocompression as well as pain by loading and moving pain-generating tissues such as the disc, facet joints, ligaments, muscles or fracture fragments [30]. In the individual life cycle, degenerative spondylosis frequently leads to instability, as Kirkaldy-Willis and Farfan [22] depicted well with their concept of three phases of degenerative spondylosis: (1) dysfunction, (2) unstable phase, (3) restabilization. This concept is supported by Husson et al. [19]. Thus, spinal instrumentation has always aimed at dealing with some form of instability.

The dynamic neutralization system for the spine (Dynesys) is a non-fusion pedicle screw system for the stabilization of the lumbar spine [8, 11]. It is designed for uni- or multisegmental use. It aims at pathological conditions with some form of segmental instability and various forms of sequelae. Dynesys was developed based upon all the current knowledge of and experience with conventional rigid pedicle systems. It establishes a mobile load transfer and controls motion of the segment in all planes, whilst inducing stability. Thus, the bilateral implant system controls motion in all planes. Stability with controlled segmental motion is established, achieving a more physiological condition as compared with the sole decompression of an unstable segment or as compared with fusion of such a segment. In connection with decompressive procedures, the system re-establishes stability and avoids iatrogenic instability. Some disadvantages of fusion could be expected to be overcome, for instance the "transition syndrome" caused by overloading adjacent segments or increased invasiveness. The first implantation of this novel system was performed in 1994 by one of the authors of the present paper, G. D., who is the author of the system.

The study presented here was performed with the primary objective of proving the safety and efficacy of this novel posterior instrumentation system. It is a multi-center study reflecting the first clinical experience with this implant based upon a prospective protocol and including frequent indications for surgery, for which conventional procedures would otherwise have been applied.

The results should be compared to series of patients with similar pathologies, but surgically treated differently, be it by direct decompression or some fusion procedure.

Materials and methods

Patients

The study covers 83 consecutive patients who underwent surgery with Dynesys instrumentation performed by the three authors. At two centers (T.S., O.S.) it included the first consecutive series.

Table 1 Indications

	N	%
Primary diagnosis		
Spinal stenosis	50	60.2
Degenerative discopathy (DDD)	20	24.1
Disc herniation	7	8.4
Revision surgery	5	6.0
Other	1	1.2
Total	83	100
Secondary diagnosis		
Degenerative spondylolisthesis	39	47.0
Previous therapeutic lumbar interventions	30	36.1

Patient selection: inclusion criteria

The selection criteria for the procedure included patients with neurogenic, radicular pain and/or chronic low-back pain resistant to any conservative treatment, presenting with some form of instability, where stabilization was judged to be beneficial. Most of these patients would have undergone fusion if Dynesys had not been available. Some would have undergone only a direct decompression. The range of indications was determined upon the theoretical concept and on an understanding of the mechanical qualities of the implant, gained from existing clinical and biomechanical knowledge and from biomechanical tests [8, 11].

The primary indications (Table 1) were: spinal stenosis in 50 patients, degenerative discopathy in 20 patients, disc herniation in 7 patients and revision surgery in 5 patients. Spinal stenosis was often combined with other secondary pathologies: with degenerative olisthesis in 29 patients, with degenerative olisthesis and degenerative scoliosis in 3 patients and with a degenerative scoliosis in another 3 patients.

The average age at operation was 58.2 (range 26.8–85.3) years. The gender distribution was 49 women, 34 men. Figure 1, Fig. 2, Fig. 3 and Fig. 4 show cases demonstrating typical pathologies for which Dynesys was applied.

Preoperative assessment

The preoperative assessment included patient history, physical assessment, neurological assessment and the assessment of imaging. Imaging included antero-posterior, lateral and dynamic lateral X-rays as well as at least one form of additional imaging (myelography, MRI, CT-scan, discography). The Prolo score [32] was assessed. The patient answered the Oswestry Questionnaire (Oswestry Disability Index) and two pain score questionnaires, one for axial low back pain and one for leg pain.

Assessment at follow-up

The assessment at follow-up was performed by independent examiners. It included the same protocol as the preoperative assessment, with the exception of the additional imaging studies.

Surgical technique

Surgery was performed by a mid-line approach and instrumentation by the surgical technique for Dynesys, with the pedicle screw positioned at the conventional (Magerl) site. Decompression, where indicated, was performed directly by undercutting laminae

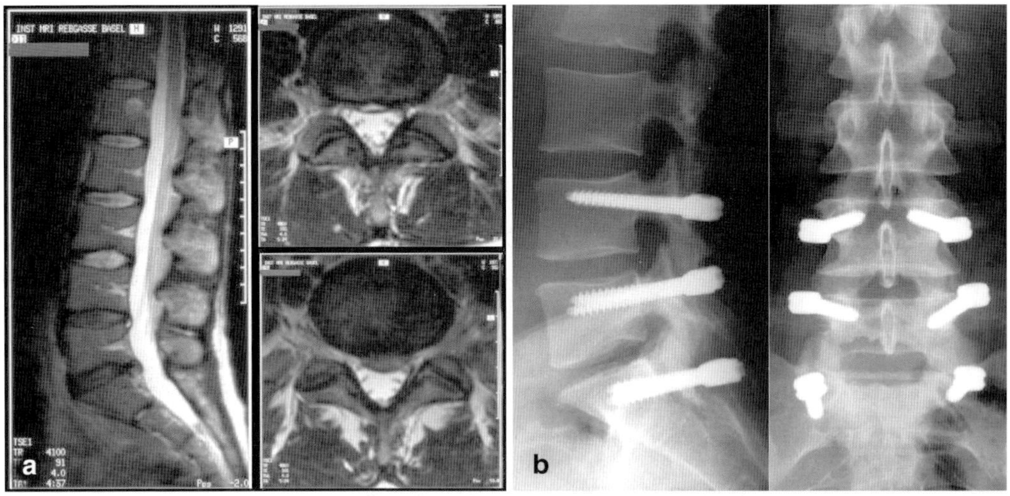

Fig. 1 **A** Magnetic resonance (MR) image of a 39-year-old woman presenting with low-back pain and S1 root pain, which demonstrates disc disease at L4/5, and L5/S1; L4/5 with annular tear, L5/S1 with medial herniation. Both discs produced positive provocative pain sign on discography. **B** Radiographs of the same patient as in **A**, following L5/S1 nucleotomy and instrumentation with Dynesys at L4–S1

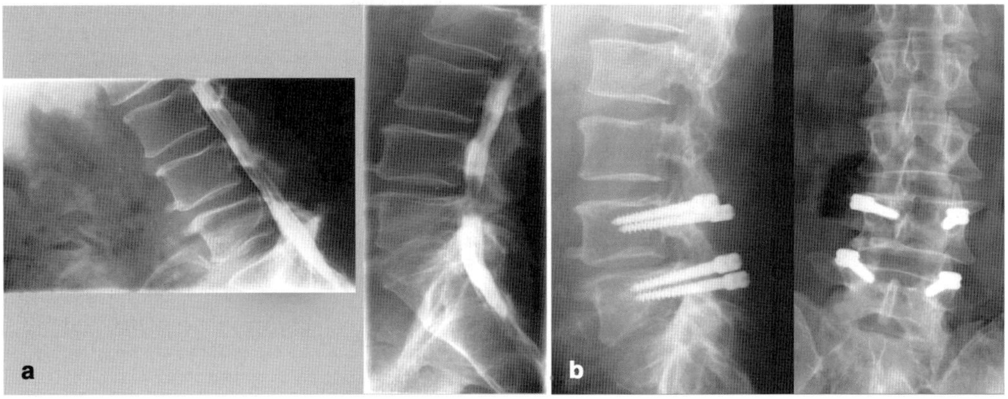

Fig. 2 **A** Preoperative myelographs of a 65-year-old man, demonstrating L4/5 dynamic stenosis with instability. **B** Same patient as in **A**, following direct decompression and L4/5 instrumentation with Dynesys

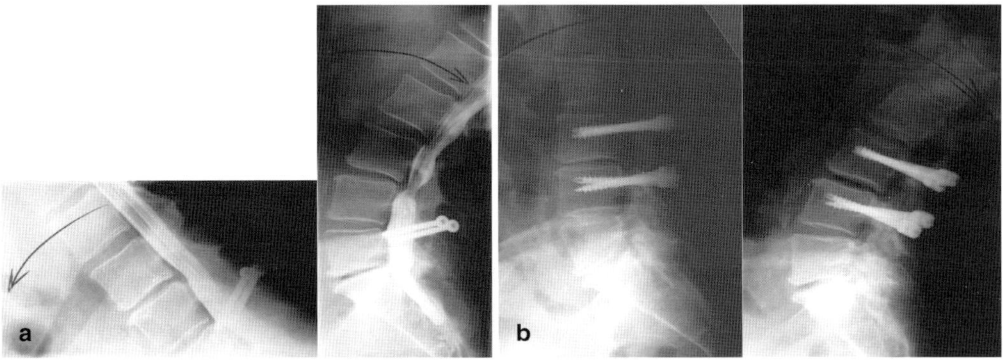

Fig. 3 A 56-year-old woman with previous postero-lateral fusion at L4/5 and L5/S1, instrumented with translaminar screws at L4/5. Myelography demonstrates dynamic stenosis at the adjacent L3/4 segment. **B** Same patient as in **A**, 12 months after L4/5 screw removal, direct decompression and L3/4 Dynesys instrumentation. L3/4 angular motion is apparent

and facet joints. Postoperative bracing was applied only in exceptional cases.

Implants

The Dynesys system is composed of titanium alloy (Protasul 100) pedicle screws, polyester (Sulene-PET) cords, and polycarbonat-urethane (Sulene-PCU) spacers (Fig. 5). The surface of the screw is sandblasted. The screws anchor the Dynesys system in the pedicle and in the vertebral body. The modular spacer fits between the pedicle screw heads. The stabilizing cord connects the pedicle screw heads via the hollow core of the spacer and holds the spacer in place. Its preload provides a uniform system rigidity. The stabilizing cord carries tensile forces and the spacers resist compressive forces. The inherent stability of the whole construct also resists bending and shear forces.

Biomechanical testing

All components underwent various biomechanical and biological tests. This included fatigue testing of the whole construct for distraction and compression over 10 million cycles. The non-metallic parts were additionally tested in terms of biocompatibility.

In the majority of cases (66.3%), a monosegmental instrumentation was performed (Table 2). The most frequently instrumented segment was L4/5. Frequently, direct decompression was also per-

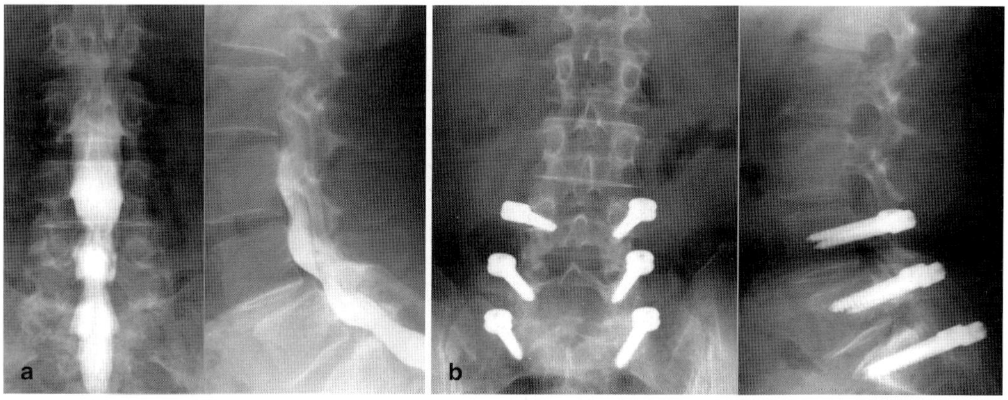

Fig. 4 Antero-posterior and lateral myelographs of L4/5 and L5/S1 stenosis in a 67-year-old woman. **B** Same patient as in **A**: antero-posterior and lateral standing radiographs following direct decompression and L4–S1 stabilisation with Dynesys

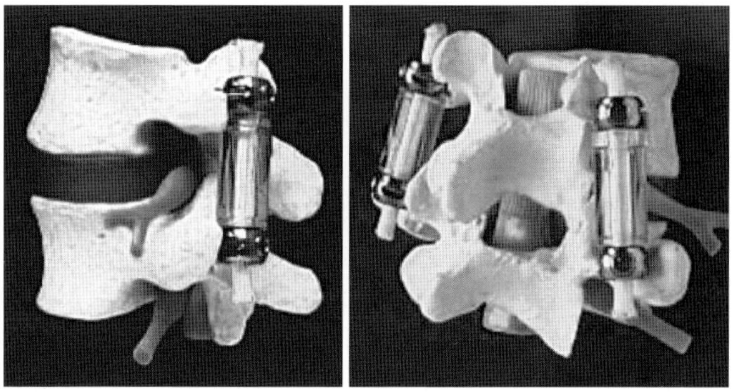

Fig. 5 Photographs of monosegmental Dynesys on a spine model

Table 2 Instrumented segments

	N	%
No. of levels treated		
One	55	66.3
Two	17	20.5
Three	8	9.6
Four	3	3.6
Distribution of levels treated[a]		
L1/2	2	2.4
L2/3	8	9.6
L3/4	23	27.7
L4/5	44	53.0
L5/S1	6	7.2

[a] Highest level treated for multi-level patients

Table 3 Additional procedures

Additional procedure	*N*	%
Direct decompression	56	67.5
Nucleotomy	3	3.6
Other	8	9.6
Decompression + Other	1	1.2
None	15	18.1

formed, not only at the instrumented levels, but also at adjacent levels that were judged not to be unstable (additional procedures are shown in Table 3).

The mean duration of surgery was 163 min (±58 min) and the mean blood loss was 407 cc (range 50–2500 cc).

Statistics

Statistics were calculated using the Statistica for Windows, by StatSoft, Inc. (2000).

Results

A total of 73 patients were available for follow-up. Two patients had died of non-related causes and eight patients had undergone implant removal for various reasons that are discussed later. The mean follow-up time was 38.1 months (range 11.2–79.1 months).

Complications

Complications were divided up into two groups. The nine complications unrelated to the implant were of usual quality and quantity (Table 4). One dural lesion necessitated a reoperation. In one case a paresis led to a revision (extension of instrumentation) 1 month postoperatively. Eventually, the cause of this progressive multilevel paresis was found to be a systemic non-Hodgkin lymphoma, and the patient died 4 months postoperatively of this disease. In one case a seroma had to be drained, and in another case a scar neuroma was excised.

Complications related to the implant included two screw misplacements; one patient had to be reoperated 2 weeks postoperatively because of root compression

Table 4 Complications unrelated to implant

Dural lesion	2 (1[a])
Infection	1
Paresis	1[a]
Hypesthesia (resolving)	1
Seroma	1[a]
Scar neuroma	1[a]
Cardiovascular	1
Thromboembolism	1

[a] Reoperated

Table 5 Complications related to implant

Pedicle fracture (intraop.)	1
Screw loosening	1[a]
Signs of screw loosening on radiograph	7
Screw malplacement	2 (1[a])

[a] Reoperated

signs (Table 5). The symptoms resolved soon after the reoperation.

In seven cases a screw loosening was suspected, based upon the radiological appearance of a screw halo or migration. In one case, a radiologically suspected screw loosening in combination with clinical symptoms necessitated a further intervention 14.5 months postoperatively. The loosening of two bilateral screws was confirmed and the screws were removed without re-stabilization.

Later, additional surgery

Apart from the above-mentioned reoperations due to complications, 11 patients needed additional lumbar surgery in the follow-up period (Table 6). In three cases with unresolved persisting pain the implant was removed, at 17.6, 18.8 and 39.7 months postoperatively, and in two of them a fusion was added. In one patient the index segment needed an additional laminectomy 22 months postoperatively.

Table 6 Later, additional surgery

Complete implant removal	8
Dynesys extension (adjacent stenosis)	2
Decompression of adjacent segment (1 patient, later fused)	2
Laminectomy of index segment	1

In seven patients, adjacent segment degeneration necessitated further surgery. One of these patients underwent direct decompression procedures of the adjacent level at 11.3 and 24.7 months postoperatively, followed by implant removal and extended fusion 29.6 months postoperatively; four patients underwent implant removals and extended fusions at 5.8, 9.1, 15 and 17.6 months postoperatively, and two received extensions of the Dynesys instrumentation to an adjacent segment at 14.5 and 20.8 months postoperatively.

Radiological evaluation

The radiological evaluation revealed ten loose screws (in seven patients, including two removed screws) out of a total number of 280 screws (3.6%). Loose screws were defined as screws with a radiologically visible lytic zone (halo) and/or with migration. In all cases, the most cranial or/and most caudal screws were involved. Most loose screws appeared in early postoperative radiographs (less than 6 months postoperatively), and none appeared later than 1 year postoperatively.

Functional and economic status

The patients improved significantly in functional (Table 7) and economic (Table 8) status. However, the interpretation of these data is much restricted as a significant proportion of the patients were retired at the time of surgery.

Pain

The pain scale (visual analog scale 1–10) for low-back pain improved from a mean preoperative value of 7.4

Table 7 Prolo functional status [32]

Functional score	Preoperative		Follow-up	
	N	%	*N*	%
Total incapacity	35	47.9	2	2.7
Back pain mild to moderate, able to perform all daily tasks of living	19	26.0	13	17.8
Low level of pain, able to perform all activities except sports	19	26.0	23	31.5
No pain, but patient has had one or more occurrences of back pain	–	–	25	34.2
No recurrent episodes of back pain, all previous sports/social activities	–	–	10	13.7

Table 8 Prolo economic status

Economic score	Preoperative		Follow-up	
	N	%	*N*	%
Complete invalid	7	9.6	–	–
No gainful occupation (capable of indep. locomotion & self-care, unable to hold job, perform housework etc.)	39	53.4	13	17.8
Able to work	21	28.8	27	37.0
Working on part-time or limited status	4	5.5	15	20.5
Working with no restrictions of any kind	2	2.7	18	24.7

(±2.6) to a postoperative mean value of 3.1 (±2.3). For leg pain, the preoperative value was 6.9 (±3.0), which improved to 2.4 (±2.1) at follow-up. The VAS for low-back pain and leg pain improved with a statistical significance ($P<0.01$, Wilcoxon's matched-pair test).

Disability Index

The Oswestry Disability Index (ODI) is scored on a scale of 0–100%, where 0–20% means minimal disability, 20–40% means moderate disability, 40–60% means severe disability, 60–80% means crippled, and 80–100% means either bed-bound or exaggerating symptoms.

The preoperative mean Oswestry score was 55.4% (±19.5%, range 10–92%), which expresses a severe disability of the average patient. At follow-up it was 22.9% (±19.3%, range 0–71%), which expresses just a moderate disability of the average patient. This improvement was also statistically significant ($P<0.01$). In patients with more than 2 years follow-up, the Oswestry score stayed at the same low level.

Discussion

Degenerative spondylosis can create spinal instability of various forms and characters. Instability can produce axial local low-back pain and pseudoradicular pain, as well as radicular pain and neurological deficit. Decompressive procedures may induce or increase instability [1, 5, 12, 20, 21]. In order to treat the various conditions degenerative spondylosis can create, surgical stabilization is frequently needed. Currently this is performed by some form of fusion (uninstrumented, instrumented, pedicular, PLIF, TLIF, ALIF). All these procedures have their specific disadvantages. They all generate a considerable amount of morbidity and high rates of complications [9, 27, 29, 31, 40, 41, 42, 43]. Moreover, fusion eliminates motion of the functional spinal segment and may overload the adjacent segments, thereby generating the "transition syndrome" and a high frequency of re-interventions [4, 23, 24, 33, 36, 37, 38].

These disadvantages lead to alternative procedures and techniques for stabilization without fusion – non-fusion systems.

Mobile stabilization systems have to neutralize noxious forces and restore normal function of the spinal segments on the one hand, and protect the adjacent segments on the other. Implants for a mobile connection have been proposed for intervertebral (disc arthroplasty), for transpedicular and for interspinous application. Sénégas [39] introduced an interspinous system for stabilization following decompression procedures in spinal stenosis, with the main aim being the prevention of long, polysegmental fusions. Graf [15] introduced a transpedicular ligament replacement system for the treatment of painful degenerative disc disease, arousing many expectations [6, 26] that eventually probably can not be met [13, 17, 34]. The suggested action of this pedicle screw system was based upon the interlocking of the facet joints in maximal extension.

Dynesys is a pedicle system providing mobile stabilization controlling motion in any plane. It is designed for the treatment of degenerative conditions of the lumbar spine that present with unstable motion segments [11]. It aims at the restoration of stability in unstable conditions of degenerative origin, as presented by some forms of degenerative disc disease as well as unstable forms of lumbar stenosis, be this dynamic or permanent. Thus, indications are conditions of instability with local lumbar pain as well as radicular pain and/or deficit. Dynesys is also designed to stop further progression of minor deformity, which is frequently combined with spinal stenosis as, for instance, in degenerative spondylolisthesis, early degenerative scoliosis, and the combination of the two.

The posterior approach of the Dynesys is highly compatible with direct decompression procedures, and in the treatment of axial segmental pain it can be applied with less morbidity than a formal posterolateral fusion with pedicle instrumentation. It can also be applied through a Wiltse [44] approach, for less muscle damage, though in this series this approach was not used, as most cases needed additional direct decompression.

Interpretation of the results of the presented study must take into account some possible sources of bias; namely, it included the first series of patients operated with this technique, and therefore involved a learning curve, the average age of the patients was high, and 36.1% had undergone prior lumbar surgery.

This study on the efficacy and safety of this novel instrumentation includes a variety of diagnostic entities, among which the common denominator was a state of degenerative spondylosis. The main group, comprising patients with stenosis combined with some form of instability, is large enough ($n=50$, 60.2%) to offer a statistically valid database. While this is less true for the smaller subgroup of degenerative discopathy ($n=20$, 24.1%) and the other subgroups, some aspects of the study can nonetheless be used for comparison for these diagnostic subgroups as well.

The problem of all non-controlled clinical studies is the difficulty of comparing them with other similar series because important parameters are different. Nevertheless, it is still appropriate to compare some aspects of other studies with our own results. There are few studies published covering similar pathologies with fusion or pure decompression procedures. Many studies on pedicle fixation in non-traumatic pathologies include lytic spondylolisthesis, which we regard as a specific pathological entity with specific biomechanics. In 1999 the Chochrane Review of Surgery was still lamenting the absence of a randomized controlled study dealing with the surgical decompression of degenerative lumbar spondylosis or spinal stenosis [14], although the following year Amundsen [3] reported on the beneficial effects of decompressive surgery based on a randomized controlled study. Other randomized studies compared different surgical procedures for spinal stenosis [7, 10, 16, 18], which provide convincing evidence that, for spinal stenosis with instability and spondylolisthesis, fusion is beneficial, and this is clearly supported by the meta-analysis of Mardjetko et al. [25]. Hence, although there is excellent evidence that surgical decompression and added fusion for stenosis with degenerative spondylolisthesis is beneficial, it is debatable (evidence is sparse) whether added instrumentation is beneficial for this condition. And for this pathology, Dynesys may combine advantages, for instance by providing more stability than decompression alone, with being less invasive than instrumented fusion.

Invasiveness is reflected by morbidity. Morbidity generated by a procedure is expressed by the overall complication rate. With respect to morbidity, the mid-term results of this study compare favourably with fusion procedures. The overall complication rate in this study was 20 events in 83 patients (24%), but this includes seven cases with radiological signs of screw loosening at follow-up, of which probably only three are symptomatic, one case was reoperated prior to follow-up. The total complication rate also includes one complication that arose completely independent of the surgical procedure (rapidly developing systemic lymphoma). In a series of 107 patients with non-traumatic disorders treated with lumbar and lumbosacral fixation, Pihlajamäki et al. [31] reported 76 complications with 65 reoperations in an average follow-up period of 40 months. This high percentage may be partially explained by the inclusion of 40 cases of spondylolysis with olisthesis. In a selected survey of ABS (American Board of Surgeons) members, looking at complications in 617 cases of pedicle screw fixation, Esses et al. [9] reported a total of 169 (27.4%) complications. In a series of 148 cases (79 with degenerative olisthesis) treated with PLIF and pedicle fixation, Okuyama et al. [29] actually reported 91 complications in 75 cases.

Of the nine non-implant related complications in our series, some are of minor importance and none of them are severe. They compare favorably with other studies on similar pathologies and are rather few in number, bearing in mind the elevated age of the patients – a fact that supports Dynesys as a less invasive procedure than fusion.

The low rate of infections (there was only one and it was superficial), and the lack of serious cardiovascular complications in our series may be explained by the fact that Dynesys is less invasive as compared with most posterior fusion procedures. There are three main reasons for this. First, there is no need for graft site preparation with posterolateral enlargement of the soft tissue damage and no harvest site morbidity. Second, it is more rapidly performed. Third, it allows the treatment of degenerative lumbar disease in a segment by segment manner. This means that with multisegmental degeneration, the stabilizing procedure can be restricted to one segment above or below a degenerative but stable segment – a decision that would not be considered with fusion, resulting in the extremely invasive, and probably unnecessary, extensions of fusions frequently observed.

The rate of implant-related complications was also moderate in this series [42]: two screw malpositionings, one intraoperative pedicle fracture, seven cases of radiographic screw loosening and one case of confirmed screw loosening, which had to be reoperated. The rate of pedicle screw misplacement in this series is low [2, 9, 43], but this is independent of the specific qualities of Dynesys and probably reflects the experience of the three surgeons, as no procedure was performed with the help of a computed navigation system.

In this series, no screw breakage was observed. This compares favorably with rates recorded for rigid pedicle systems [28, 29, 31, 40]. Reason for this may be the elasticity of the spacer/cord compound, which may cause cyclic peak loads on the implant to be lower than in rigid constructs.

Screw loosening was defined as the radiological appearance of halo formation and/or screw migration. This was observed in seven patients (including one patient in whom screws at a different site had previously been removed bilaterally). Only one of these patients had to be reoperated, and six of them had no accompanying symptoms and a low level of pain.

This screw-loosening rate seems to be similar or even low compared with studies on rigid pedicle instrumentations. In the above-mentioned study of Pihlajamäki et al. [31], of 102 cases 18 showed screw loosening, one screw bending and 20 screw breakage. Ohlin et al. [28] reported implant failure in 64 of 163 procedures (153 patients). Soini et al. [40] reported screw breakage in eight and screw loosening in 14 of 51 patients with olisthetic and degenerative conditions of the spine. Adding an anterior, intervertebral support to the pedicle instrumentation certainly lowers the rate of screw loosening and breakage, as the above-mentioned study of Okuyama et al. [29] reports, but it increases the rate of other complications and morbidity.

As Dynesys is a prosthetic device that theoretically ought to act as such for the remaining life-time, screw loosening deserves special analysis. Implant loads in a segmental lumbar setting are of high complexity [35]. It is hypothesized that, due to its lower stiffness, Dynesys and therefore also the screw-bone interface may see less load than conventional internal fixator systems. But load transfer is substantially different, since the screws are not rigidly linked by a rod. Screws radiologically presenting with a halo may be surrounded by fibrous tissue withstanding the cyclic load and preventing any further progression of the loosening. However, the appropriate amount of interface loading for optimal initiation of bone formation around the screw is not known and needs to be subjected to further research. Some loosening in this series is probably due to technical faults in the preparation of the screw hole and positioning of the screw (depth of placement, manipulation while inserting cord), and some may be due to incorrect choice of screw dimensions, as until December 1998 only two screw widths were available. This judgement is based on two observations: First, screw loosening seems to develop very early, as the authors made the observation that the halo appeared in early postoperative radiographs (less than 6 months postoperatively), and with one exception it never appeared later in the course. Second, the rate of loosening seems to have decreased with the growth of the series, which expresses aspects of the learning curve and the availability of a wider choice of screw dimensions.

Reoperations and later, additional surgery

Reoperations for complications were necessary in six cases. They were either unrelated (n=4) or related (n=2) to the implant. This has been discussed above. Later additional surgery was performed in a total of 11 patients. In three patients, Dynesys was removed and a fusion procedure was performed because of persisting low-back pain. One patient had undergone two decompression procedures before the removal. The most frequent cause for later additional surgery (nine in 13 events or seven in 11 patients) in this series was adjacent segment degeneration. Some of these segments had been decompressed at the initial operation, and some had not. The main question remains, however: in which cases was the development of adjacent stenosis due to the natural progression of the disease (degenerative lumbar stenosis) and in which was it due to transferred overload? Studies on fusions provide much evidence of the overload sequelae [4, 23, 33, 36, 37, 38], but are not comparable because of different study parameters. A reduction of acceleration of adjacent segment degeneration with Dynesys can theoretically be stated on the basis of the protective effect of persisting segmental motion. Based upon the number and the follow-up time of this series, a reduction of acceleration of adjacent segment degeneration cannot be proven. However, with respect to adjacent degeneration, it has to be emphasized that it is under any circumstances very difficult to differentiate the degeneration rate due the natural course of the disease from the one that is due to acceleration of this process by the elevated load transfer or other factors related to the procedure and the instrumentation. The iatrogenic contribution to this process could perhaps be defined statistically only in large comparative, randomized series, which are not available to date. This is especially true in the age group and the specific selection of indications of this study. The progressive natural history of plurisegmental degenerative lumbar disease challenges the result of any kind of surgical treatment.

Conclusions

This study proves Dynesys to be a safe and efficient procedure for stabilization of unstable conditions of the lumbar spine presenting with neurocompression. The mid-term results are highly comparable to fusion procedures, with the difference that Dynesys is less invasive and theoretically produces less degeneration of adjacent segments in the long term.

Dynesys allows the treatment of degenerative lumbar disease in a segment by segment manner. In early stages, as well as in more advanced stages of degeneration of the motion segment, Dynesys re-establishes stability.

Acknowledgements The authors are grateful to Ms Elke Rometsch, Sulzer Medica, for the excellent preparation of the data base and the extensive statistical analysis. They thank Mark Myers MD, Minneapolis, for the radiological evaluation at follow-up.

References

1. Abumi K, Panjabi MM, Kramer KM, Duranceau J, Oxland T, Crisco JJ (1990) Biomechanical evaluation of lumbar spine stability after graded facetectomies. Spine 15:1142–1147
2. Amiot LP, Lang K, Putzier M, Zippel H, Labelle H (2000) Comparative results between conventional and computer-assisted pedicle screw installation in the thoracic, lumbar, and sacral spine. Spine 25:606–614
3. Amundsen T, Weber H, Nordal HJ, Magnaes B, Abdelnoor M, Lilleas F (2000) Lumbar spinal stenosis: conservative or surgical management? Spine 25:1424–1436
4. Aota Y, Kumano K, Hirabayashi S (1995) Postfusion instability at the adjacent segments after rigid pedicle screw fixation for degenerative lumbar spinal disorders. J Spinal Disord 8: 464–473
5. Boden SD, Martin C, Rudolph R, Kirkpatrick JS, Moeini SMR, Hutton WC (1994) Increase of motion between lumbar vertebrae after excision of the capsule and cartilage of the facets. J Bone Joint Surg Am 76:1847–1853
6. Brechbühler D, Markwalder TM, Braun M (1998) Surgical results after soft system stabilization of the lumbar spine in degenerative disc disease – long term results. Acta Neurochir 140: 521–525
7. Bridwell KH, Sedgewick TA, O'Brien MF, Lenke LG, Baldus C (1993) The role of fusion and instrumentation in the treatment of degenerative spondylolisthesis with spinal stenosis. J Spinal Disord 6:461–472

8. Dubois G, de Germay B, Schaerer NS, Fennema P (1999) Dynamic neutralization: a new concept for restabilization of the spine. In: Szpalski M, Gunzburg R, Pope MH (eds) Lumbar segmental instability. Lippincott Williams & Wilkins, Philadelphia, pp 233–240
9. Esses SI, Sachs BL, Dreyzin V (1993) Complications associated with the technique of pedicle screw fixation. Spine 18:2231–2239
10. Fischgrund JS, Mackay M, Herkowitz HN, Brower R, Montgomery DM, Kurz LT (1997) Volvo Award Winner in Clinical Studies. Degenerative lumbar spondylolisthesis with spinal stenosis: a prospective, randomized study comparing decompressive laminectomy and arthrodesis with and without spinal instrumentation. Spine 22:2807–2812
11. Freudiger S, Dubois G, Lorrain M (1999) Dynamic neutralisation of the lumbar spine confirmed on a new lumbar spine simulator in vitro. Arch Orthop Trauma Surg 119:127–132
12. Frymoyer JW, Selby DK (1985) Segmental instability. Rationale for treatment. Spine 10:280–286
13. Gardner AD, Pande KC, Hassaan AM, Declerck G (1999) Graf stabilization of intractable lumbar instability syndrome. In: Szpalski M, Gunzburg R, Pope MH (eds) Lumbar segmental instability. Lippincott Williams & Wilkins, Philadelphia, pp 175–190
14. Gibson JNA, Grant IC, Waddell G (1999) The Cochrane rewiew of surgery for lumbar disc prolapse and degenerative lumbar spondylosis. Spine 24:1820
15. Graf H (1992) Lumbar instability: surgical treatment without fusion. Rachis 412:123–137
16. Grob D, Humke T, Dvorak J (1995) Degenerative lumbar spinal stenosis. J Bone Joint Surg Am 77:1036–1041
17. Hadlow SV, Fagan AB, Hillier TM, Fraser RD (1998) The Graf ligamentoplasty procedure – comparison with posterolateral fusion in the management of low back pain. Spine 23: 1172–1179
18. Herkowitz HM, Kurz LT (1991) Degenerative lumbar spondylolisthesis with spinal stenosis: a prospective study comparing decompression and intertransverse arthrodesis. J Bone Joint Surg Am 73:802–808
19. Husson JL, Poncer R, Polard JL (1996) Dérangement intervertebral acquis (DIVA). In: Husson JL, Le Huec JC (eds) Restabilisation intersomatique du rachis lombaire. Sauramps Medical, Montpellier, pp 13–21
20. Johnsson KE, Willner S, Johnsson K (1986) Postoperative instability after decompression for lumbar spinal stenosis. Spine 11:107–110
21. Jönsson B, Akesson M, Jonsson K, Strömqvist B (1992) Low risk for vertebral slipping after decompression with facet joint preserving technique for lumbar spinal stenosis. Eur Spine J 1:100–104
22. Kirkaldy-Willis WH, Farfan HF (1982) Instability of the lumbar spine. Clin Orthop 165:110–123
23. Kumar MN, Jacquot F, Hall H (2001) Long-term follow-up of functional outcomes and radiographic changes at adjacent levels following lumbar spine fusion for degenerative disc disease. Eur Spine J 10:309–313
24. Lehmann TR, Spratt KF, Tozzi JE, Weinstein JN, Reinarz SJ, El-Khoury GY, Colby H (1987) Long-term follow-up of lower lumbar fusion patients. Spine 12:97–104
25. Mardjetko SM, Connolly PJ, Shott S (1994) Degenerative lumbar spondylolisthesis. Spine 19:S2256–S2265
26. Markwalder TM, Dubach R, Braun M (1995) Soft system stabilization of the lumbar spine as an alternative surgical modality to lumbar arthrodesis in facet syndrome. Preliminary results. Acta Neurochir 134:1–4
27. Matsuzaki H, Tokuhashi Y, Matsumoto F, Hoshino M, Kiuchi T, Toriyama S (1990) Problems and solutions of pedicle screw plate fixation of lumbar spine. Spine 15:1159–1165
28. Ohlin A, Karlsson M, Düppe H, Hasserius R, Redlund-Johnell I (1994) Complications after transpedicular stabilization of the spine. Spine 19:2774–2779
29. Okuyama K, Abe E, Suzuki T, Tamura Y, Chiba M, Sato K (1999) Posterior lumbar interbody fusion. Acta Orthop Scand 70:329–334
30. Panjabi MM (1992) The stabilizing system of the spine. 2. Neutral zone and instability hypothesis. J Spinal Disord 5: 390–397
31. Pihlajamäki H, Myllynen P, Böstman O (1997) Complications of transpedicular lumbosacral fixation for non-traumatic disorders. J Bone Joint Surg Br 79:183–189
32. Prolo DJ, Oklund SA, Butcher M (1986) Toward uniformity in evaluating results of lumbar spine operations. A paradigm applied to posterior lumbar interbody fusions. Spine 11:601–606
33. Rahm MD, Hall BB (1996) Adjacent-segment degeneration after lumbar fusion with instrumentation: a retrospective study. J Spinal Disord 9:392–400
34. Rigby MC, Selmon GPF, Foy MA, Fogg AJB (2001) Graf ligament stabilisation: mid- to long-term follow-up. Eur Spine J 10:234–236
35. Rohlmann A, Graichen F, Weber U, Bergmann G (2000) 2000 Volvo Award winner in biomechanical studies. Monitoring in vivo implant loads with a telemeterized internal spinal fixation device. Spine 25:2981–2986
36. Schären S, Dick W (1998) Erfolge und Probleme langstreckiger Fusionen der degenerativen Lendenwirbelsäule. Osteosynthese Int 6:173–179
37. Schlegel JD, Smith JA, Schleusener RL (1996) Lumbar motion segment pathology adjacent to thoracolumbar, lumbar and lumbosacral fusions. Spine 21:970–981
38. Schulitz KP, Wiesner L, Wittenberg RH, Hille E (1996) Das Bewegungssegment oberhalb der Fusion. Z Orthop 134:171–176
39. Senegas J, Etchevers JP, Vital JM, Baulny D, Grenier F (1988) Widening of the lumbar vertebral canal as an alternative to laminectomy in the treatment of lumbar stenosis. Fr J Orthop Surg 2:93–99
40. Soini J, Laine T, Pohjolainen T, Hurri H, Alaranta H (1993) Spondylodesis augmented by transpedicular fixation in the treatment of olisthetic and degenerative conditions of the lumbar spine. Clin Orthop 297:111–116
41. Turner JA, Ersek M, Herron L, Haselkorn J Kent D, Ciol M, Deyo R (1992) Patient outcomes after lumbar spinal fusions. JAMA 268:907–911
42. Turner JA, Herron L, Deyo RA (1993) Meta-analysis of the results of lumbar spine fusion. Acta Orthop Scand [Suppl 251] 64:120–122
43. West JL, Ogilvie JW, Bradford DS (1991) Complications of the variable screw plate pedicle screw fixation. Spine 16:576–579
44. Wiltse LL, Spencer CW (1988) New uses and refinements of the paraspinal approach to the lumbar spine. Spine 13:1008–1012

Donal S. McNally

The objectives for the mechanical evaluation of spinal instrumentation have changed

D.S. McNally
Institute of Biomechanics,
School of Mechanical, Materials,
Manufacturing Engineering
and Management,
University of Nottingham, University
Park, Nottingham NG7 2RD, UK
e-mail: donal.mcnally@nottingham.ac.uk,
Tel.: +44-115-8466375,
Fax: +44-115-9513800

Abstract The objectives for the mechanical evaluation of spinal implants have changed because many modern devices are designed to modify the mechanics of the disc rather than to simply fix the segment. This means that a biomechanical objective must be decided, a priori, for a particular device. It is then relatively straightforward to design a biomechanical evaluation protocol that can either test whether this objective is fulfilled, or optimise the device in the context of the objective. Because 'soft stabilisation' systems are soft, their performance is affected by the magnitude of the loading sustained by the bridged segment. This means that is vital to reproduce a realistic loading regime for the biomechanical evaluation, if its results are to be relevant to a clinical problem. Similarly, the condition of the segment in terms of disc degeneration, facet joint condition, etc. affect the mechanical performance of the segment and must be relevant to the performance objectives set for the device. Loading protocols for testing short and long segments are discussed. Since the aim of many spinal devices is to modify the loading of the intervertebral disc, it is important to quantify their effect in terms of how both the internal loads and deformations are changed. A number of different technologies for quantifying both loads and deformations in intact discs are described and discussed.

Keywords Biomechanics · Motion segment · Intervertebral disc · Instrumentation · Evaluation

Introduction

Historically, the major application of spinal instrumentation has been to provide motional stability in arthrodesis and deformity correction. As such, the principal mechanical objective of the instrumentation has been to control movement of the bridged segment. Consequently, a series of mechanical evaluation protocols have been proposed and developed [1, 33, 35, 49], which are based on the standardised analysis of segment movements resulting from the application of pure rotational moments. This form of biomechanical evaluation is now the gold standard for the characterisation of spinal instrumentation. However, with the increasing introduction of new implants such as soft stabilisation devices, such evaluation protocols need to be revised.

The primary driver for the development of new assessment protocols is the change in mechanical objective of the devices themselves. They are no longer designed simply to control rotational motion of the bridged segment, but also to change particular features of the internal mechanical environment of the disc itself, for example to offload the whole disc or modify the loading of the posterior annulus. Assessment protocols must be designed to test that such mechanical objectives are being met, and this requires both a range of experimental techniques that characterise the internal mechanics of intact intervertebral discs and a loading protocol that simulates realistic functional loading.

A secondary driver for the development of new protocols arises from the fact that many of the new fixation devices are not in themselves rigid. With rigid fixation devices, compressive loading in addition to the applied bending moments has little effect on the rotation of the segment [43]. This means that parameters such as ligament tension are largely unaffected, and hence the measurements of rotational motion are largely unaffected. However, compressive load has been found to influence the relative loading of the segment and the fixation device [50]. Implants such as the Graf ligament or the Dynesys device will deform under compressive loading of the segment, and hence their mechanical performance will be changed (as has been demonstrated in intact segments [21]). Consequently, it becomes much more important to test the devices under more realistic loading conditions, where muscle forces are simulated. Similarly, the mechanical condition of the bridged segment in terms of disc degeneration, facet joint condition, etc. can have a significant effect both on the behaviour of the segment and on how a fixation device modifies it. Thought must therefore be given to the condition of the specimens used in biomechanical investigations.

The purpose of this paper is to identify a range of novel assessment technologies and to suggest how they might be incorporated into a protocol to evaluate the mechanical performance of spinal instrumentation. Since the mechanical objectives of current spinal instrumentation systems are highly varied, the protocols used to assess their performance must necessarily be diverse. However, the underlying principles of the mechanical evaluation remain consistent and are addressed here.

Defining objectives for biomechanical evaluation

The primary roles of biomechanical evaluation are to confirm that a particular fixation device achieves its functional objectives and to compare the performance of a range of devices in meeting such objectives. It is therefore of vital importance to decide, a priori, exactly what functional behaviour is required from the fixation device.

In the case of soft stabilisation systems, determining such an objective is not as easy as it may first appear. For example, a major application of such devices is the relief of discogenic pain through modification of the mechanics of the affected disc. However, at the moment it is not completely clear what features of disc mechanics are responsible for the generation of pain. Clinical measurement of the internal loading of painful discs have shown that there are loading features in the posterior annulus that probably correspond to inward bulging and severe fracturing [24], and disc degeneration has been found to correspond to reduced nucleus loads [44], whilst studies of motion combined with electromyography have indicated that pain is related to increased compression and lateral shear [20]. However, these features of internal load distribution may be a consequence of the process that causes pain rather than the cause itself. This having been said, such soft fixation devices are designed on the basis of a hypothesis of mechanical modification of a painful process, and therefore it is possible to construct a mechanical objective for the device.

There are two further roles of mechanical evaluation. The first of these is to ensure that the device affects the internal and external mechanical behaviour of the bridged segment in ways that are clinically acceptable; ensuring, for example, that they do not cause undue loading of other structures. The second role is to ensure patient safety by confirming that the device will not fail in use. These two roles are covered fully in other documents and ASTM standards F 1717–96 and F 1798–97, and are common to all spinal instrumentation devices. They will not be addressed further here.

Possible test protocols

Whilst there are a large number of finite element and other models of spinal fixation that might be employed in a modified form to evaluate the performance of soft stabilisation devices theoretically [8, 17, 18, 39, 41], none has been validated in terms of internal loading and deformation of the affected discs. The gold standard for testing soft stabilisation devices remains for the immediate future biomechanical testing using cadaveric specimens.

Specimen loading

As discussed above, it is important to ensure that the spinal device is tested under conditions that simulate the loading conditions that are likely to occur in life. How these loads are applied to the specimen depends upon the nature of the specimen, which in turn depends upon the configuration of the fixation device.

In the case of short segments, all the necessary compressive forces and bending moments can be applied using one or two rollers (see Fig. 1). For longer segments, this form of loading will lead to unstable buckling. To provide stable compressive loading of longer segments, the 'follower load' arrangement illustrated in Fig. 1d has become popular [7, 26, 36, 37, 43]. This arrangement is very flexible in the ways that loads can be placed on the specimen, since the compressive load, bending moments and location of the wire guides on the vertebral bodies can be changed independently. A good investigation of the biomechanical effects of the placement of loading wires guides is given by Cripton et al. [7].

A more contentious issue is the application of axial rotations. In the lumbar spine, axial rotation is limited to about 2° by intact facet joints; however, recent measure-

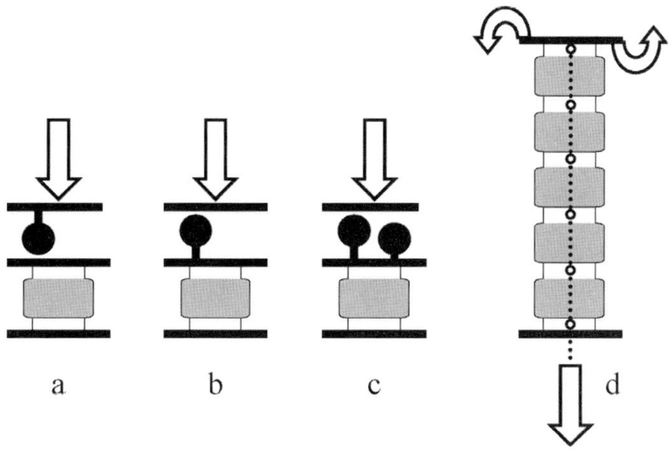

Fig. 1a–d Schematic diagrams of possible loading configurations. All the diagrams will apply compressive loading and bending towards the left. In **a** a small shear component to the right (relative to the disc) will additionally be applied, in **b** the shear component will be towards the left. The arrangement in **c** is good for applying controlled angular rotations (rather than controlled bending moments). Longer segments will not be stable under the arrangements illustrated in **a–c**; the 'follower load' arrangement illustrated in **d** will provide stable compressive loading whilst bending couples can be applied to the upper segment

ments of internal disc mechanics suggest that even rotations as small as 0.5° can significantly affect the internal mechanics of the disc [48]. Careful thought should therefore be given as to how the experimenter wishes to test the spinal device.

In terms of general guidelines for the magnitudes of applied loads and moments, the experimenter should base these on the evaluation objectives. For example, Wilke et al. [49] give a sensible set of bending moments to simulate everyday loading, e.g., 7.5 Nm bending moment for the lumbar spine. Corresponding axial compressive loads for the lumbar spine might be of the order of 1–2 kN [29] for moderate activities. If it is required to simulate more extreme activities, such as the sudden application of large, but unknown, loads, higher forces and moments should be used [19].

Measurement of internal loading

A key to understanding the effects of a fixation device on disc mechanics is the measurement of the internal distribution of load within the disc, and how this is affected by the device to be evaluated. This information can be used to give information about the relative load sharing of the disc and fixator [9, 42], but if measured correctly it can give much more information about the behaviour of the disc tissues themselves.

Disc loading has been measured by a wide range of devices, from injection pressure [34], static-fluid coupled catheters [40] and membrane-covered fluid-filled catheters [30] to needle-mounted solid-state transducers [22]. Such needle-mounted transducers are now commercially available and are recommended for their convenience of use and stability.

Frequently the measurement of disc loads has been restricted to the centre of the nucleus pulposus [27, 28, 29]. Since the centre of the disc is normally under uniform hydrostatic loading [2, 21], such measurements are very good at giving a quantification of overall disc loading, whilst being insensitive to small changes in disc positioning. However, in severely degenerate discs with positive pain reproduction on discography, the centre of the nucleus is often completely depressurised [24]. It is therefore more useful to measure loading in other locations within the disc.

There have been two basic approaches to measurement of loading patterns within the disc: simultaneous measurement from a number of transducers [47] and recording measured stress with position in the disc using a single transducer [21]. The former method is good for measuring the effects of rapidly applied loads to the specimen, but is sensitive to movement of the transducers within the disc tissue. The latter, termed stress profilometry, requires a static load to be applied for 10–20 s, but gives a continuous measurement of stress across the diameter of a disc.

Considerable information can be gained from stress profilometry. For example, in regions where the stress is anisotropic and forms sharp peaks, shear stress will be high and likely to result in fissuring [23]. Other patterns can suggest inward bulging of the inner annulus [24], whilst the loading over the whole profile can be integrated to assess total disc and facet joint loads [38].

Measurement of internal deformation

Of equal importance to the measurement of internal loads is the measurement of internal deformations. Such measurements have been more challenging, since they require the imaging of internal disc structure in intact discs.

Deformation of the outer surface has allowed, for example, disc bulging to be quantified very precisely [3, 4]. Similarly surface strain has been measured using both optical markers and strain gauges [46]. These techniques are very good at measuring surface behaviour and would be excellent for determining whether a fixation device reduced disc bulging. However, they cannot give any information about the deformations within the disc. Similarly measurements have been made of endplate deflections [5, 11].

High-resolution magnetic resonance imaging (MRI) has been used to study the internal structure of the disc under load [6, 51]. In order to perform such an investigation, it is necessary to construct a non-magnetic loading device that can be introduced into the bore of the imaging system without interfering with the radio frequency excitation or MR signals. Image acquisition also takes a finite

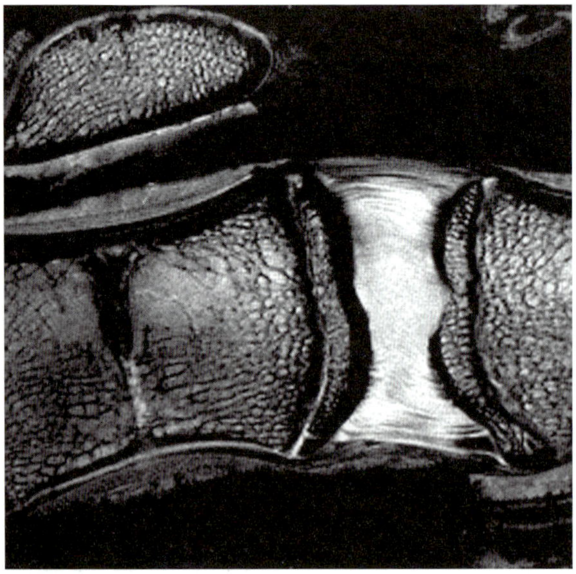

Fig. 2 High-resolution magnetic resonance (MR) image of a bovine caudal segment, showing clearly the laminate structure of the annulus. (Courtesy of Dr. M. Clemence, Department of Physics, University of Exeter)

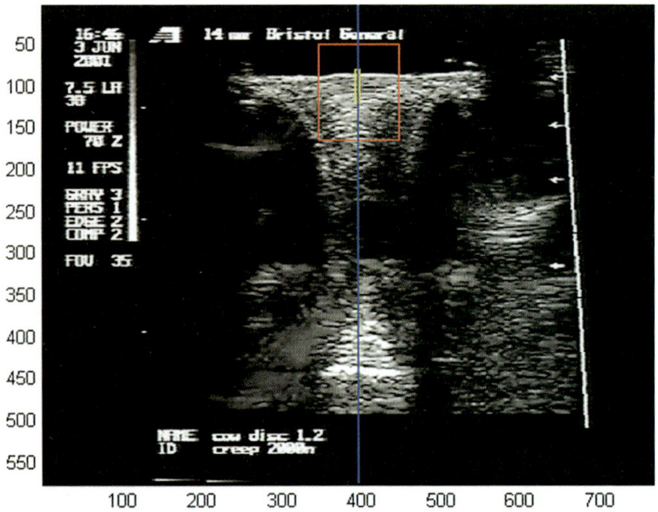

Fig. 3 In vitro image of a bovine caudal intervertebral disc in the mid-sagittal plane, showing clearly the laminate structure of the annulus. (Courtesy of Miss C. Naish, Department of Anatomy, University of Bristol and Dr. M. Halliwell, Department of Medical Physics and Bioengineering, University of Bristol)

time (normally of the order 10 min), so it is only possible to observe the effects of fairly static loads. Figure 2 gives an indication of the level of detail that can be obtained on the lamellar structure of the disc. This means that it is only possible to study equilibrium mechanics using this technique. More conventional radiographic techniques have been used to quantify internal disc deformations by imaging radiopaque targets (such as wires and balls) implanted into the disc tissue [16, 45].

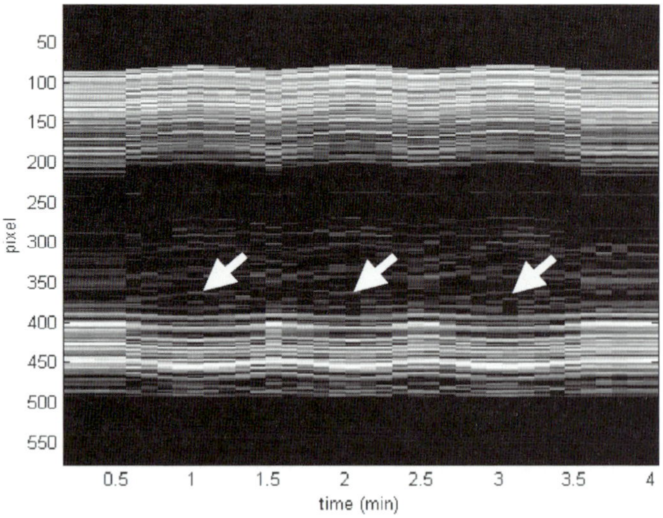

Fig. 4 Diagram showing radial deformation of the mid-sagittal diameter of the bovine caudal disc shown in Fig. 3, on application of three 1-min-duration loading cycles. It can be seen that the anterior annulus (pixels 90–210) and outer posterior annulus bulge outwards, whilst the inner posterior annulus bulges inwards. *Arrows* mark the transition point between outward and inward bulging, where a dark 'fissure' can be seen to open up. (Courtesy of Miss C. Naish, Department of Anatomy, University of Bristol and Dr. M Halliwell, Department of Medical Physics and Bioengineering, University of Bristol)

Ultrasound at clinical imaging frequencies (3–7.5 MHz) gives good detail of the laminate structure of the disc, both in vitro [31] and in vivo [25]. Such imaging in vitro can be used to detect and quantify disc pathologies such as circumferential tears and fissuring [31]. Figure 3 shows an example of the type of image that can be obtained using a 7.5 MHz clinical imaging system.

The considerable advantage of this technology over other forms of imaging is the speed of image acquisition. It is possible to record ultrasound images at 15 frames per second. Hence it is possible to observe internal deformations in response to realistic dynamic loads. Figure 4 shows how the mid-sagittal diameter of the disc shown in Fig. 3 (indicated by the blue line) deforms radially. Figure 4 can be thought of as a compilation of vertical strips of pixels taken from sequential images. (Some image analysis has been performed to ensure that the mid-sagittal diameter is always selected irrespective of axial compression of the disc.) It can be seen that the deformation of individual lamellae is clearly visible and that, in the posterior annulus, there is a point (indicated by arrows) where the annulus changes from bulging outwards to bulging inwards. It is therefore possible to use clinical frequency ultrasound imaging as a tool to optimise stabilisation device performance in terms of modification of the internal deformation to achieve a biomechanical goal for the device.

The principle alignment of the collagen fibre bundles has been inferred using diffusion tensor imaging [12].

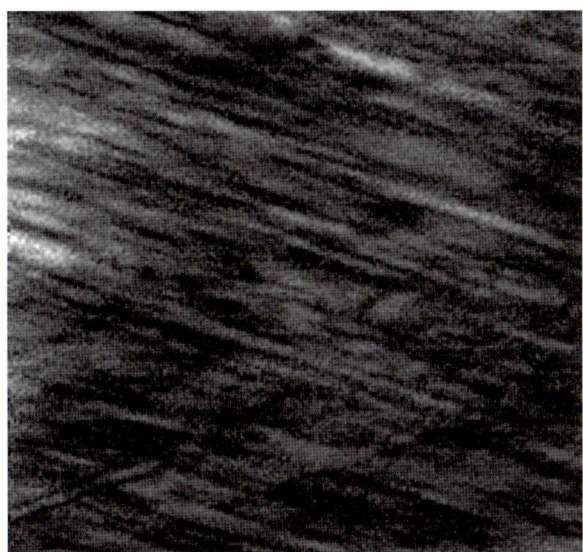

Fig. 5 Acoustic microscope image of a tangential plane within the second lamella of an intact porcine coccygeal disc. The fibre bundle paths are clearly visible. (Courtesy of Mr. S. Johnson, School of Mechanical, Materials, Manufacturing Engineering and Management, University of Nottingham, and Dr. M. Halliwell, Department of Medical Physics and Bioengineering, University of Bristol)

However, this technique requires a large number of separate relaxation time measurements to be made, and hence acquisition times are large (approx. 3.4 h). Alternatively, fibre angle has been quantified using X-ray diffraction [10, 32], and has been used to demonstrate changes in orientation resulting from mechanical loading [14, 15]. Unfortunately, the exposure times required for analysis of intact discs is very large, and there is poor spatial localisation of the tissue interrogated.

A new technique that can be used to image fine structure within intact intervertebral discs is acoustic microscopy [13]. This can be used to image and quantify collagen fibre bundle directions (see Fig. 5) in three dimensions. Hence, it is possible to quantify the effect of a stabilisation device on the local mechanics of the fibre bundles themselves. Acoustic microscopy can also be used to give very detailed images of the lamellar structure and pathology of intact discs (see Fig. 6). This figure illustrates how it is possible to identify and quantify disc structure and also large- and small-scale pathological features. It is therefore possible to assess how a stabilisation device affects, say, opening a peripheral annular tear or how it prevents fissure propagation.

Conclusions

We need to reconsider the reasons for, and goals of, biomechanical testing non-rigid stabilisation devices that are designed to modify disc mechanics rather than to replace the discs.

Before biomechanical evaluation is considered, it is important to set a mechanical objective for the device to fulfil. This objective must take into account the aspect of internal disc mechanics that needs to be modified by the device and the condition of the segment in terms of existing disc, ligament and facet joint injury and degeneration. It is then possible to design a biomechanical evaluation to confirm that this objective has been met or to optimise the performance of the device against the objective.

To perform such biomechanical evaluation, it is important to simulate the loading conditions that the spinal segment/implant will experience in life.

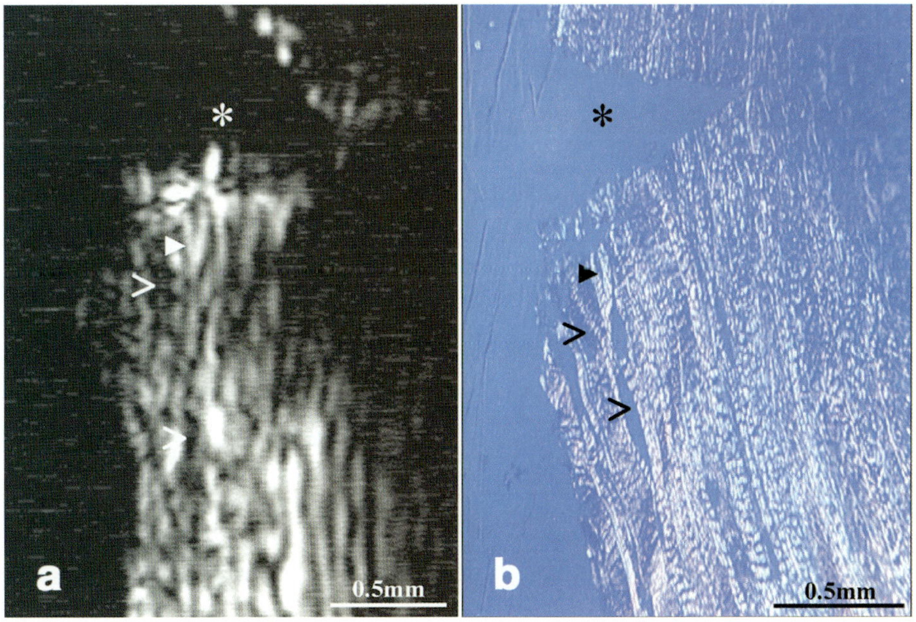

Fig. 6 Comparison of **a** an acoustic image of a region of annulus from an intact porcine intervertebral disc with **b** a corresponding polarised light micrograph of a section taken from the same region. The triangular region marked with an *asterisk* corresponds to a scalpel cut made to localise the region for comparison with histology. The *closed arrowheads* indicate a bifurcation of a lamella that is clearly visible in both images. The *open arrowheads* indicate small regions of delamination that are again visible in both images. (Courtesy of Mr. S. Johnson, School of Mechanical, Materials, Manufacturing Engineering and Management, University of Nottingham, and Dr. M. Halliwell, Department of Medical Physics and Bioengineering, University of Bristol)

The technology required to make measurements of internal loading and deformation within intact discs exists.

Acknowledgements The author wishes to thank the following for their contribution to obtaining images used in this paper: Dr. M. Clemence, University of Exeter; Dr. M. Halliwell and Miss C. Naish, University of Bristol; Mr. S. Johnson, University of Nottingham.

References

1. Abumi K, Panjabi MM, Duranceau J (1989) Biomechanical evaluation of spinal fixation devices. III. Stability provided by six spinal fixation devices and interbody bone graft. Spine 14: 1249–1255
2. Adams MA, McNally DS, Dolan P (1996) 'Stress' distributions inside intervertebral discs. The effects of age and degeneration. J Bone Joint Surg Br 78:965–972
3. Brinckmann P, Grootenboer H (1991) Change of disc height, radial disc bulge, and intradiscal pressure from discectomy. An in vitro investigation on human lumbar discs. Spine 16:641–646
4. Brinckmann P, Horst M (1985) The influence of vertebral body fracture, intradiscal injection, and partial discectomy on the radial bulge and height of human lumbar discs. Spine 10:138–145
5. Brinckmann P, Frobin W, Hierholzer E, Horst M (1983) Deformation of the vertebral end-plate under axial loading of the spine. Spine 8:851–856
6. Chiu EJ, Newitt DC, Segal MR, Hu SS, Lotz JC, Majumdar S (2001) Magnetic resonance imaging measurement of relaxation and water diffusion in the human lumbar intervertebral disc under compression in vitro. Spine 26:E437–444
7. Cripton PA, Bruehlmann SB, Orr TE, Oxland TR, Nolte LP (2000) In vitro axial preload application during spine flexibility testing: towards reduced apparatus-related artefacts. J Biomech 33: 1559–1568
8. Duffield RC, Carson WL, Chen LY, Voth B (1993) Longitudinal element size effect on load sharing, internal loads, and fatigue life of tri-level spinal implant constructs. Spine 18:1695–1703
9. Edwards AG, McNally DS, Mulholland RC, Goodship AE (1997) The effects of posterior fixation on internal intervertebral disc mechanics. J Bone Joint Surg Br 79:154–160
10. Hickey DS, Hukins DWL (1980) X-ray diffraction studies of the arrangement of collagenous fibres in human fetal intervertebral disc. J Anat 131:81–90
11. Holmes AD, Hukins DW, Freemont AJ (1993) End-plate displacement during compression of lumbar vertebra-disc-vertebra segments and the mechanism of failure. Spine 18:128–135
12. Hsu EW, Setton LA (1999) Diffusion tensor microscopy of the intervertebral disc anulus fibrosus. Magn Reson Med 41:992–999
13. Johnson S, Halliwell M, Jones M, McNally D (2001) Visualisation of collagen fibre bundles in the intact intervertebral disc. J Biomech 34:S12–S13
14. Klein JA, Hukins DWL (1982) Collagen fibre orientation in the annulus fibrosus of intervertebral disc during bending and torsion measured by X-ray diffraction. Biochim Biophys Acta 719:98–101
15. Klein JA, Hukins DWL (1982) X-ray diffraction demonstrates reorientation of collagen fibres in the annulus fibrosus during compression of the intervertebral disc. Biochim Biophys Acta 717: 61–64
16. Krag MH, Seroussi RE, Wilder DG, Pope MH (1987) Internal displacement distribution from in-vitro loading of human thoracic and lumbar spinal motion segments: experimental results and theoretical predictions. Spine 12:1001–1007
17. Lim TH, Goel VK, Weinstein JN, Kong W (1994) Stress analysis of a canine spinal motion segment using the finite element technique. J Biomech 27:1259–1269
18. Maiman DJ, Kumaresan S, Yoganandan N, Pintar FA (1999) Biomechanical effect of anterior cervical spine fusion on adjacent segments. Biomed Mater Eng 9:27–38
19. Mannion AF, Adams MA, Dolan P (2000) Sudden and unexpected loading generates high forces on the lumbar spine. Spine 25:842–852
20. Marras WS, Davis KG, Ferguson SA, Lucas BR, Gupta P (2001) Spine loading characteristics of patients with low back pain compared with asymptomatic individuals. Spine 26:2566–2574
21. McNally DS, Adams MA (1992) Internal intervertebral disc mechanics as revealed by stress profilometry. Spine 17:66–73
22. McNally DS, Adams MA, Goodship AE (1992) Development and validation of a new transducer for intradiscal pressure measurement. J Biomed Eng 14:495–498
23. McNally DS, Adams MA, Goodship AE (1993) Can intervertebral disc prolapse be predicted by disc mechanics. Spine 18:1525–1530
24. McNally DS, Shackleford IM, Goodship AE, Mulholland RC (1996) In-vivo stress measurement can predict pain on discography. Spine 21:2580–2587
25. McNally DS, Naish C, Halliwell M (2000) Intervertebral disc structure: observation by a novel use of ultrasound imaging. Ultrasound Med Biol 26:751–758
26. Miura T, Panjabi MM, Cripton PA (2002) A method to simulate in vivo cervical spine kinematics using in vitro compressive preload. Spine 27:43–48
27. Nachemson AL (1963) The influence of spinal movements on the lumbar intradiscal pressure and on the tensile stresses in the annulus fibrosus. Acta Orthop Scand 33:183–207
28. Nachemson AL (1966) Mechanical stresses on lumbar disks. Current Practice in Orthopaedic Surgery 3:208–224
29. Nachemson AL (1981) Disc pressure measurements. Spine 6:93–97
30. Nachemson AL, Morris JM (1963) Lumbar discometry: lumbar intradiscal pressure measurements in-vivo. LancetMay 25:1140–1142
31. Naish C, Mitchell R, Innes J, Halliwell M, McNally D (2001) Ultrasound imaging of the intervertebral disc. Proceedings of the 47th Meeting of the Orthopaedic Research Society, San Francisco, p 881
32. Naylor A, Happey F, Macrae T (1954) The collagenous changes in the intervertebral disk with age and their effect on its elasticity. BMJ September:570–573
33. Panjabi MM (1988) Biomechanical evaluation of spinal fixation devices. I. A conceptual framework. Spine 13: 1129–1134
34. Panjabi M, Brown M, Lindahl S, Irstam L, Hermens M (1988) Intrinsic disc pressure as a measure of integrity of the lumbar spine. Spine 13:913–917
35. Panjabi MM, Abumi K, Duranceau J, Crisco JJ (1988) Biomechanical evaluation of spinal fixation devices. II. Stability provided by eight internal fixation devices. Spine 13:1135–1140
36. Panjabi MM, Miura T, Cripton PA, Wang JL, Nain AS, DuBois C (2001) Development of a system for in vitro neck muscle force replication in whole cervical spine experiments. Spine 26: 2214–2219

37. Patwardhan AG, Havey RM, Ghanayem AJ, Diener H, Meade KP, Dunlap B, Hodges SD (2000) Load-carrying capacity of the human cervical spine in compression is increased under a follower load. Spine 25:1548–1554
38. Pollintine P, Dolan P, Adams M (2001) The load bearing function of apophyseal joints increases with age and disc degeneration. Proceedings of the 47th Annual Meeting of the Orthopaedic Research Society, San Francisco, p 872
39. Puttlitz CM, Goel VK, Traynelis VC, Clark CR (2001) A finite element investigation of upper cervical instrumentation. Spine 26:2449–2455
40. Quinnell RC, Stockdale HR, Willis DS (1983) Observations of pressures within normal discs in the lumbar spine. Spine 8:166–169
41. Rohlmann A, Calisse J, Bergmann G, Weber U (1999) Internal spinal fixator stiffness has only a minor influence on stresses in the adjacent discs. Spine 24:1192–1195; discussion 1195–1196
42. Rohlmann A, Claes LE, Bergmannt G, Graichen F, Neef P, Wilke HJ (2001) Comparison of intradiscal pressures and spinal fixator loads for different body positions and exercises. Ergonomics 44:781–794
43. Rohlmann A, Neller S, Claes L, Bergmann G, Wilke HJ (2001) Influence of a follower load on intradiscal pressure and intersegmental rotation of the lumbar spine. Spine 26:E557–561
44. Sato K, Kikuchi S, Yonezawa T (1999) In vivo intradiscal pressure measurement in healthy individuals and in patients with ongoing back problems. Spine 24:2468–2474
45. Seroussi RE, Krag MH, Muller DL, Pope MH (1989) Internal deformations of intact and denucleated human lumbar discs subjected to compression, flexion, and extension loads. J Orthop Res 7:122–131
46. Shah JS, Hampson WGJ, Jayson MIV (1978) The distribution of surface strain in the cadaveric lumbar spine. J Bone Joint Surg Br 60:246–251
47. Steffen T, Baramki HG, Rubin R, Antoniou J, Aebi M (1998) Lumbar intradiscal pressure measured in the anterior and posterolateral annular regions during asymmetrical loading. Clin Biomech 13:495–505
48. van Deursen DL, Snijders CJ, Kingma I, van Dieen JH (2001) In vitro torsion-induced stress distribution changes in porcine intervertebral discs. Spine 26: 2582–2586
49. Wilke HJ, Wenger K, Claes L (1998) Testing criteria for spinal implants: recommendations for the standardization of in vitro stability testing of spinal implants. Eur Spine J 7:148–154
50. Wilke HJ, Rohlmann A, Neller S, Schultheiss M, Bergmann G, Graichen F, Claes LE (2001) Is it possible to simulate physiologic loading conditions by applying pure moments? A comparison of in vivo and in vitro load components in an internal fixator. Spine 26:636–642
51. Wisleder D, Werner SL, Kraemer WJ, Fleck SJ, Zatsiorsky VM (2001) A method to study lumbar spine response to axial compression during magnetic resonance imaging: technical note. Spine 26:E416–420

Matthew D. Garner
Steven J. Wolfe
Stephen D. Kuslich

Development and preclinical testing of a new tension-band device for the spine: the Loop system

Abstract Wire sutures, cerclage constructs, and tension bands have been used for many years in orthopedic surgery. Spinous process and sublaminar wires and other strands or cables are used in the spine to re-establish stability of the posterior spinal ligament complex. Rigid monofilament wires often fail due to weakening created during twisting or wrapping. Stronger metal cables do not conform well to bony surfaces. Polyethylene cables have higher fatigue strength than metal cables. The Loop cable is a pliable, radiolucent, polyethylene braid. Creep of the Loop/locking clip construct is similar to metal cable constructs using crimps. Both systems have less creep than knotted polyethylene cable constructs.

Keywords Tension band · Spinous process · Sublaminar wires · Polyethylene cable · Creep · Fatigue strength

The testing for this study was carried out at the Phillips Plastics Technical Center, N4660 1165th Street, Prescott, WI 54021, USA. The study was funded by Spineology Inc.

M.D. Garner · S.J. Wolfe
S.D. Kuslich (✉)
Spineology, 1815 Northwestern Ave., Stillwater, MN 55082, USA
e-mail: skuslich@spineology.com,
Tel.: +1-651-3511011,
Fax: +1-651-3510712

S.D. Kuslich
St. Croix Orthopedics,
Stillwater, Minnesota, USA

Introduction

Wire sutures, cerclage constructs, and tension bands have been used for many years to re-appose bone fragments, to tether ligaments or tendons to bone, and to improve stability in weakened constructs following trauma or surgery. Closure of a sternotomy following cardiovascular surgery, trochanteric reattachment in reconstructive hip surgery, and stabilization of long bone fragments are a few examples of procedures utilizing tension-band systems [5, 14, 26, 48, 50, 57, 59, 65].

The natural posterior spinal tension member is comprised of several ligaments that are attached to the bones of the spine lying dorsal to the spinal canal: the inter- and supra-spinous ligaments, the ligmentum flavum, the facet capsular ligaments, and the posterior longitudinal ligament [3, 4, 36, 37, 41, 42]. When intact, the posterior spinal ligamentous structures function to limit flexion, rotation, and anterior and posterior translation of the spine [27, 42]. In spine surgery, wire and other strands and cables have been widely used to re-establish stability of the posterior spinal ligament complex [7, 11, 12, 24, 30, 34, 39, 60, 62].

Although much of the compression load of the spine is borne by the vertebral bodies and intervertebral discs of the anterior column [3, 40], attaching posterior tension bands around the laminae, spinous processes, or transverse processes can improve stability [12, 22, 24, 31, 39, 46, 49]. Easy surgical access to the spinous processes allows the surgeon to pass wires around these bony appendages or through holes prepared in individual spinous processes. However, variable strength of the bone and the relatively small surface area of the wire can cause the wire to cut through the spinous process, leading to loosening of the construct and loss of stability [6, 43, 65]. Inventors

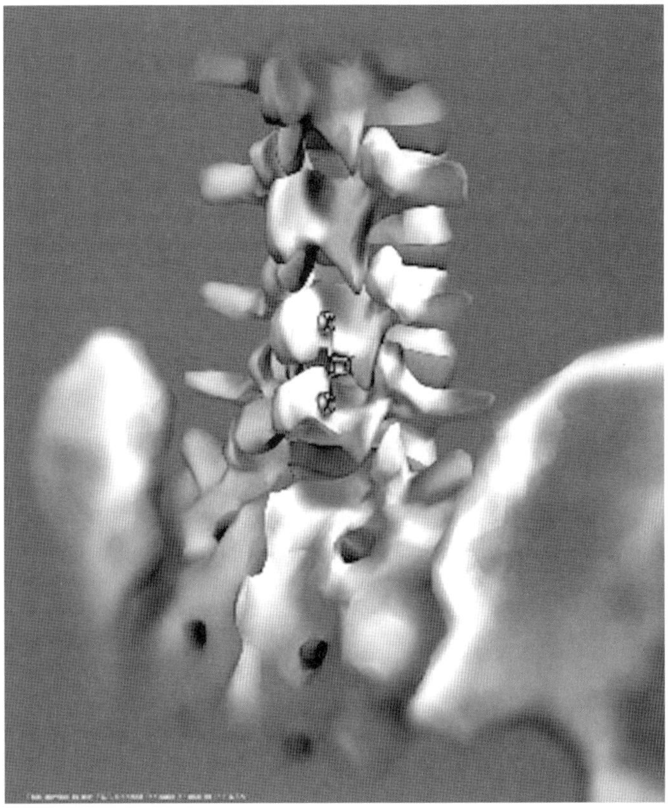

Fig. 1 The Loop system uses a braided polyethylene cable that is passed through two ferrules placed at the base of the spinous process. After tension is applied by use of the tensioning tool (Fig. 3), the locking clip (Fig. 2) secures the construct

have developed techniques and devices to address this problem. Examples include the "Wisconsin technique," wherein the Drummond Button is placed on the sides of the spinous process, and K-wires are passed through the spinous process [21, 28, 47].

When the spinous process is weak, fractured, or missing, the lamina can be utilized for wiring one spinal segment to another. The lamina is a stronger point of attachment than the spinous process [12, 20, 23, 25, 53, 64]. However, passing a wire or cable into the sublaminar space can lead to injury of the dura or spinal cord [18, 51, 54, 60, 61]. In spite of this possibility, sublaminar wiring techniques have been widely used for segmental fixation of spinal instrumentation to the posterior spine, in most cases, without nervous system injury [2, 33, 35, 45, 58, 65].

Rigid monofilament wires (Ethicon wire, Codman Sof'wire) often fail due to weakening created during twisting or wrapping [10, 15, 19, 20, 23, 51]. To address these deficiencies, multi-strand cables (Acromed Songer cable, Sofamor Danek Axis cable), which have better static yield, and tensile and fatigue strength, have been developed [12, 13, 29, 32, 38, 54, 55, 56, 63]. More recently, polyethylene cables (e.g., Smith & Nephew Richards SecureStrand), which are soft, flexible, and radiolucent, have become available. Tests indicate that they have tensile strength equivalent to multi-strand cables [8, 9, 16, 19, 38, 56, 63]. The soft polyethylene cables are easier to handle than wires or metal cables, and they conform to the bone surfaces, leading to a distribution of loads over a greater contact area [15, 18].

The Loop system

The Loop system (Spineology Inc., Stillwater, Minn.) consists of a braided polyethylene cable, a locking clip, and an optional ferrule that can be placed in the spinous process (Fig. 1). The Loop cable is a polyethylene braid with material properties similar to SecureStrand [68]. The Loop system is supplied in two versions: small cable and small locking clip for the cervical and upper thoracic spine, and large cable and large locking clip for the lower thoracic and lumbar spine.

Table 1 Physical properties of single constructs. Properties were determined with the construct held between two "S" hooks on the testing machine

	AcroMed Songer titanium cable [a]	Smith & Nephew SecureStrand [b]	Spineology Loop [a]
Mean tensile failure load (N)	2068	1565	Large – 1953 Small – 1301
Construct stiffness (N/mm)	477	322	Large – 438 Small – 410
Construct creep maximum (mm) at % of construct strength	1.8 mm @ 75%	3.7 mm @ 75% 2.8 mm @ 50% 2 mm @ 30%	2.4 mm @ 75% 1.9 mm @ 50% 1.4 mm @ 30%
Fatigue strength (N) @ 3 million cycles	<44	578	Large – 578 Small – 333

[a] Data from testing at Phillips Plastics Technical Center
[b] Data from Dickman et al. [19]

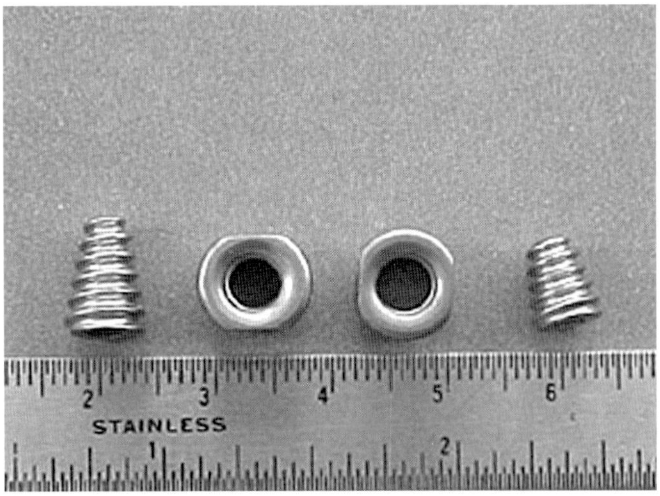

Fig. 2 The Loop locking clip utilizes friction between the female outer shell and the male inner cone, both of which are smoothly threaded. Once the male portion is secured in place, with the cable wedged between the male and female parts, the construct is exceptionally secure, with very little creep

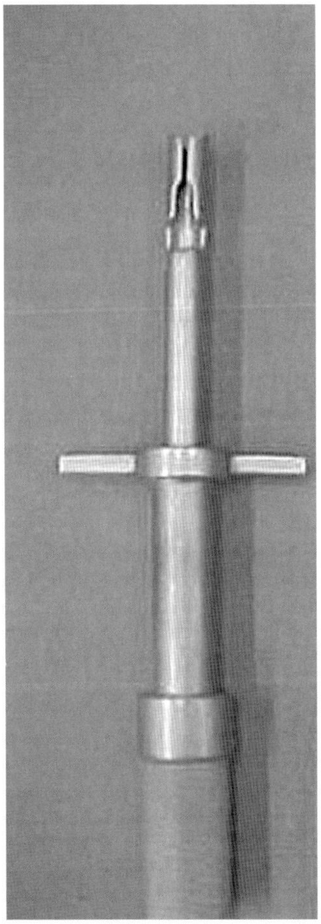

Fig. 3 The tensioning tool allows the surgeon to apply the desired degree of tension before securing the construct with the male portion of the locking clip

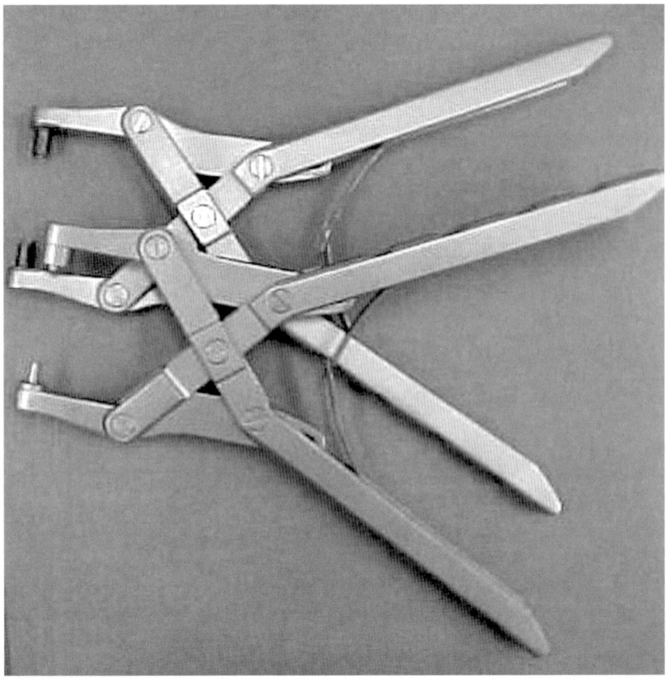

Fig. 4 The ferrule punch allows the surgeon to create a precise hole for placement of the ferrule using the ferrule inserter

Posterior spinal ligaments range in strength from approximately 67–208 lb (300–927 N) in the cervical and upper thoracic spine to about 145–321 lb (647–1432 N) in the lower thoracic spine and the lumbar spine [44]. The testing setup for the Loop construct was designed to conform to the test setup used by Dickman et al. [19], in which multiple tension-band constructs were tested. Dickman found the tensile strength of the Songer titanium cable system to be 465 lb (2068 N), which was superior to that of the SecureStrand, at 352 lb (1565 N) [19]. The Loop construct (cable and locking clip) was found to have a tensile strength of about 293 lb (1301 N) for the small cable and small clip construct and about 439 lb (1953 N) for the large cable and large clip construct [68] (Table 1). Both Loop systems exceed the expected failure loads of the spinous processes and laminae in their respective areas of use in the spine [12, 25].

The Loop locking clip consists of two mating pieces of titanium alloy that secure the polyethylene cable without the need for knots (Fig. 2). Testing of the construct for creep, again compared to testing done by Dickman [19] on several different constructs, shows that the creep of the Loop construct is comparable to the Songer cable with metal crimp lock, and superior to the weave and knotted lock of the SecureStrand [67]. The Loop tensioner (Fig. 3), used to create tension in the construct prior to locking, allows the surgeon to precisely control the degree of tension on the band material [55]. The male portion of the Loop clip is locked into the female portion of the clip using a self-limiting torque wrench.

The Loop ferrule is designed to distribute stress over a broad surface area. The smooth internal surface of the ferrule provides for passage of the cable without damaging the fibers. A standard towel clip, dental drill, or curved awl is used for making a hole in the spinous process for some wiring procedures or for passing a K-wire through the bone [1, 17, 47, 48, 52, 54, 60]. The Loop ferrule hole cutter prepares a clean, precise hole for a press fit of the ferrule in the bone. The ferrule is positioned into place using the ferrule inserter tool Fig. 4.

Mechanical properties of spinal cable and wire fixation systems

The new Loop polyethylene cable system was tested and compared to published performance values for currently available metallic spinal cable fixation systems.

Materials and methods

Published data on nine different spinal cable and wire fixation systems were reviewed: titanium and stainless steel Codman, Danek and AcroMed cable, polyethylene Smith & Nephew SecureStrand, and Ethicon 20 and 22-gauge stainless steel monofilament wire. Static tensile and fatigue strength, stiffness, and creep properties were evaluated. In all systems, a loop of the cable or wire was formed and connected, using the manufacturers suggested method. The Loop device was tested on the EnduraTec SmartTest system.

Results

The new Loop polyethylene cable system proved to be stronger in tensile strength, 1953 N, than all the other systems by 10–89% (P=0.01), except for the AcroMed Songer titanium system using end loop attachment, with a strength of 2068 N. For all systems, the fatigue limit ranged from 44.8 N to 578 N. The Loop fatigue strength is 578 N [66].

The creep behavior breaks down into two parts:

1. Change due to initial settling of the system (conformance to bone and tightening of fastener, and
2. True system creep (cutting at the bone/band interface, slipping of the fastening method, stretch in the tension band)

Creep during the initial stretch of the new Loop tension band was 19.36 µm/m/N, compared to an average of 22.12 µm/m/N for metal cables, and 113.33 µm/m/N for 20-gauge and 106.35 µm/m/N for 22-gauge monofilament wires. Initial creep of the SecureStrand polyethylene band was 35.92 µm/m/N. After initial stretch on application of the load, none of the multifilament metal cables exhibited appreciable creep during the 24-h test period. The two polyethylene cables did stretch after initial loading. The SecureStrand stretched an additional 24.22 µm/m/N versus 7.4µm/m/N for the Loop tension band.

Discussion

In comparisons, the new tension band has equivalent strength to all band types, and has higher fatigue strength than the metal bands. Metal cables and wire systems easily cut through bone and are opaque on radiographs. The polyethylene systems are radiolucent and afford better radiographic observation of the fixation site. They also provide better conformation to the bone to distribute the load more evenly.

The creep behavior of the new tension-band system is more like that of the metal cable systems. Both polyethylene cable systems creep initially while the band conforms to the tissues. The SecureStrand has additional creep because the connecting knot continues to tighten over time. Additional creep of the new system is lower than the SecureStrand, because the creep is only due to the stretching of the polymer fibers. The unique, "no-slip clip" is designed to limit damage to the band while providing a secure lock for the construct. Unlike a knot, this lock will not slide.

Conclusion

Tension bands have been used in general orthopedics and spine surgery for many years. The Loop System has strength similar to titanium cable systems and has a no-slip locking clip designed to maintain construct tension. It combines the advantages of the metallic systems (lower creep) with the advantages of the polymer cables (high fatigue strength) without sacrificing strength, stiffness or ease of use.

References

1. Al Baz MO, Mathur N (1995) Modified technique of tension band wiring in flexion injuries of the middle and lower cervical spine. Spine 20:1241–1244
2. Allen BL, Ferguson RL (1986) Neurological injuries with the Galveston technique of L-rod instrumentation for scoliosis. Spine 11:14–17
3. Andersson GBJ, Ortengren R, Nachemson A, et al (1974) Lumbar disc pressure and myoelectric back muscle activity during sitting. I. Studies on an experimental chair. Scand J Rehabil Med 6:104
4. Andersson GBJ, Chaffin DB, Pope MH (1991) Occupational biomechanics of the lumbar spine, in occupational low back pain: assessment, treatment, and prevention. Mosby Year Book, St. Louis
5. Arnold PG, Pairolero PC (1984) Chest wall reconstruction. Experience with 100 consecutive patients. Ann Surg 199:725–732
6. Bernard TN, Johnston CE, Roberts JM, et al (1983) Late complications due to wire breakage in segmental spinal instrumentation: report of two cases. J Bone Joint Surg Am 65:1339–1345

7. Bernard TN, Whitecloud TS, Haddad RJ (1983) Segmental spinal instrumentation in the management of fractures of the thoracolumbar spine: a preliminary report. Orthop Trans 7:227
8. Bernhardt A (1993) Tensile testing of UHMWPE Spectra-1000 braid. In: Smith & Nephew Spine Technical Report SP-93–11
9. Bernhardt A, Taylor M (1993) Cyclic creep testing of Spectra-1000 braid and titanium cable constructs. In: Smith & Nephew Spine Technical Report SP-93–12
10. Boeree NR, Dove J (1993) The selection of wires for sublaminar fixation. Spine 18:497–503
11. Brodsky AE, Khalil MA, Sassard WR, et al (1992) Repair of symptomatic pseudoarthrosis of anterior cervical fusion. Posterior versus anterior repair. Spine 17:1137–1143
12. Coe JD, Warden KE, Sutterlin CE, et al (1989) Biomechanical evaluation of cervical spinal stabilization methods in human cadaveric model. Spine 14: 1122–1131
13. Cooper PR (1993) Posterior stabilization of the cervical spine. Clin Neurosurg 40:286–320
14. Cordoso A, Tajonar F, Luque ER (1976) Osteotomy of the spine, new concepts, preliminary report (in Spanish). Anal Orthop Traumatol 12:105–113
15. Crawford RJ, Sell PJ, Ali MS, et al (1989) Segmental spinal instrumentation: a study of the mechanical properties of materials used for sublaminar fixation. Spine 14:632–635
16. Daigle K, Cassidy J, Holbrook J (1992) Fatigue testing of braided Spectra UHMWPE surgical cable. In: Smith & Nephew Orthopedic Research Report OR-92–49
17. Davey JR, Rorabeck CH, Bailey SI, et al (1985) A technique of posterior cervical fusion for instability of cervical spine. Spine 10:722–728
18. Dickman CA, Sonntag VKH (1993) Wire fixation of the cervical spine biomechanical principles and surgical techniques. BNI (Barrow Neurological Institute) Quarterly 9:2–16
19. Dickman CA, Papadopoulos SM, Crawford NR, et al (1997) Comparative mechanical properties of spinal cable and wire fixation systems. Spine 22:596–604
20. Dove J (1989) Segmental wiring for spinal deformity: a morbidity report. Spine 14:229–231
21. Drummond DS (1999) Segmental spinal instrumentation with spinous process wires. In: An HS, Cotler JM (eds) Spinal instrumentation, 2nd edn. Lippincott Williams & Wilkins, Philadelphia
22. Ferguson RL, Allen BL, Seay GB (1982) The evolution of segmental spinal instrumentation in the treatment of unstable thoracolumbar spine fractures. Orthop Trans 6:346
23. Guadagni JR, Drummond DS (1986) Strength of surgical wire fixation: a laboratory study. Clin Orthop 209:176–181
24. Hambly M, Lee CK, Gutteling E, et al (1989) Tension band wiring-bone grafting for spondylolysis and spondylolisthesis. Spine 14:455–459
25. Heller KD, Prescher A, Schneider T, et al (1998) Stability of different wiring techniques in segmental spinal instrumentation. An experimental study. Arch Orthop Trauma Surg 117:96–99
26. Herzwurm PJ, Walsh J, Pettine KA, et al (1992) Prophylactic cerclage: a method of preventing femur fracture in uncemented total hip arthroplasty. Orthopedics 15:143–146
27. Kazarian LE (1972) Dynamic response characteristics of the human vertebral column. Acta Orthop Scand Suppl 146: 1–186
28. Lange F (1986) The classic. Support for the spine by means of buried steel bars attached to the vertebrae, by Fritz Lange, 1910. Clin Orthop 203:3–6
29. Lange E, Bernhardt A (1994) Construct tensile testing of UHMWPE braid with comparison of titanium cable. In: Smith & Nephew Orthopedic Research Report OP-94–71
30. Lee CK, Rosa R, Fernand R (1986) Surgical treatment of tumors of the spine. Spine 11:201–208
31. Lin PM (1985) Posterior lumbar interbody fusion technique: complications and pitfalls. Clin Orthop 193:90–102
32. Lovely TJ, Carl A (1995) Posterior cervical spine fusion with tension-band wiring. J Neurosurg 83:631–635
33. Luque ER (1982) Segmental spinal instrumentation for correction of scoliosis. Clin Orthop 163:192–198
34. Luque E (1986) Segmental spinal instrumentation of the lumbar spine. Clin Orthop 203:126–134
35. Luque ER, Cassis, Nelson, et al (1982) Segmental spinal instrumentation in the treatment of fractures of the thoracolumbar spine. Spine 7:312–317
36. Marras WS (1987) Predictions of forces acting upon the lumbar spine under isometric and isokinetic conditions: a model experiment comparison. Int J Ind Ergonomics 3:19–27
37. Marras WS, Reilly CH (1988) Network of internal trunk loading activities under controlled trunk conditions. Spine 13:661–667
38. Martin RJ (1996) SecureStrand Cable System. Neurosurgery 38:842–843
39. McAfee PC, Bohlman HH, Wilson WL (1985) The triple wire fixation technique for stabilization of acute fracture-dislocations: a biomechanical analysis. Orthop Trans 9:142
40. McGill SM (1990) Loads on the lumbar spine and associated tissues. In: Goel VK, Weinstein JN (eds) Biomechanics of the spine: clinical and surgical perspective. CRC Press, Boca Raton, pp 66–94
41. McGill SM, Norman RW (1986) Partitioning of the L4-L5 dynamic moment into disc, ligamentous and muscular components during lifting. Spine 11: 666
42. Morris JM, Lucas DB, Bresler B (1961) Role of the trunk in stability of the spine. J Bone Joint Surg 43:327
43. Munson G, Satterlee C, Hammond S, et al (1984) Experimental evaluation of Harrington rod fixation supplemented with sublaminar wires in stabilizing thoracolumbar fracture-dislocations. Clin Orthop 189:97–102
44. Mykleburst JB, Pintar F, Yoganandan N, et al (1988) Tensile strength of spinal ligaments. Spine 13:526–531
45. Olson SA, Gaines RW (1987) Removal of sublaminar wires after spinal fusion. J Bone Joint Surg Am 69:1419–1423
46. Papp T, Porter RW, Aspden RM, et al (1997) An *in-vitro* study of the biomechanical effects of flexible stabilization on the lumbar spine. Spine 22:151–155
47. Resina J, Ferreiira-Alvez A (1977) A technique for correction and internal fixation for scoliosis. J Bone Joint Surg Br 5:159–169
48. Rhinelander FW, Stewart CL (1983) Experimental fixation of femoral osteotomies by cerclage with nylon straps. Clin Orthop 179:298–307
49. Schlegel KF, Pon MA (1985) Biomechanics of posterior lumbar interbody fusion (PLIF) in spondylolisthesis. Clin Orthop 193:115–119
50. Schopfer A, Willett K, Powell J, et al (1993) Cerclage wiring in internal fixation of acetabular fractures. J Orthop Trauma 7:236–241
51. Scuderi GJ, Greenberg SS, Cohen DS, et al (1993) Biomechanical evaluation of magnetic resonance imaging-compatible wire in cervical spine fixation. Spine 18:1991–1994
52. Segal D, Whitelaw GP, Gumbs V, et al (1981) Tension band fixation of acute cervical spine fractures. Clin Orthop 159:211–222
53. Sheperd DE, Leahy JC, Mathias KJ, et al (2000) Spinous process strength. Spine 25:319–323
54. Songer M (1996) Posterior cervical arthrodesis using the Songer cable system. In: Richard G. Fessler RG, Regis W, Haid RW (eds) Current techniques in spinal stabilization. McGraw-Hill, New York

55. Songer MN (1996) The role of cables in lumbosacral fusion. In: Margulies JY, Floman Y, Farcy JPC, Neuwirth MG (eds) Lumbosacral and spinopelvic fixation. Lippincott-Raven, Philadelphia
56. Songer MN, Spencer DL, Meyer PR, et al (1991) The use of sublaminar cables to replace luque wires. Spine 16:S418–S421
57. Stevens SS, Irish AJ, Vachtesevanos JG, et al (1995) A biomechanical study of three wiring techniques for cerclage-plating. J Orthop Trauma 9:381–387
58. Sullivan JA (1984) Sublaminar wiring of Harrington distraction rods for unstable thoracolumbar spine fractures. Clin Orthop 189:178–185
59. Tscherne H, Haas N, Krettek C (1986) Intermedullary nailing combined with cerclage wiring in the treatment of fractures of the femoral shaft. Clin Orthop 212:62–67
60. Vaccaro A, Singh K (1999) Principles of spinal instrumentation for cervical spinal trauma. In: An HS, Cotler JM (eds) Spinal instrumentation, 2nd edn. Lippincott Williams & Wilkins, Philadelphia
61. Watts C, Smith H, Knoller N (1993) Risks and cost-effectiveness of sublaminar wiring in posterior fusion of cervical spine trauma. Surg Neurol 40: 457–460
62. Weiland DJ, McAfee PC (1991) Posterior cervical fusion with triple-wire strut graft techniques; one hundred consecutive patients. J Spinal Disord 4:15–21
63. Weis JC, Cunningham BW, Kanayama M, et al (1996) In vitro biomechanical comparison of multistrand cables with conventional cervical stabilization. Spine 21:2108–2114
64. Wenger D, Miller S, Wilkerson J (1982) Evaluation of fixation sites for segmental instrumentation of the human vertebrae. Orthop Trans 6:23–24
65. Wilson PD, Straub LR (1952) Lumbosacral fusion with metallic-plate fixation. AAOS Instructional Course Lectures, vol IX. JW Edwards, Ann Arbor, pp 53–57
66. Wolfe S (2000) Comparative ferrule/tension band system testing. In: Spineology Inc. Internal Documents (41–012)
67. Wolfe S (2001) The Loop system verification testing. In: Spineology Inc. Internal Documents (41–026)
68. Zindrick MR, Knight GW, Bunch WH, et al (1989) Factors influencing the penetration of wires into the neural canal during segmental wiring. Joint Bone Joint Surg Am 71:742–750

S. Caserta
G. A. La Maida
B. Misaggi
D. Peroni
R. Pietrabissa
M. T. Raimondi
A. Redaelli

Elastic stabilization alone or combined with rigid fusion in spinal surgery: a biomechanical study and clinical experience based on 82 cases

S. Caserta (✉) · G.A. La Maida
B. Misaggi · D. Peroni
Spine Division,
Gaetano Pini Orthopaedic Institute,
Piazza Cardinale Andrea Ferrari no. 1,
20122 Milan, Italy
e-mail: caserta@g-pini.unimi.it

R. Pietrabissa · M.T. Raimondi
A. Redaelli
Politecnico di Milano,
Bioengineering Department, Laboratory
of Biological Structure Mechanics,
Piazza L. da Vinci, 32, 20133 Milan, Italy

Abstract The authors report their experience with the treatment of lumbar instability by a kind of spine stabilization. The elastic stabilization, which follows a new philosophy, is obtained by an interspinous device, and should be used alone in degenerative disc disease, recurrent disc herniation and in very low grade instability, or in association with rigid fusion for the prevention of pathology of the border area. In collaboration with bioengineers, we carried out an experimental study on a lumbar spine model in order to calculate stresses and deformations of lumbar disc during simulation of motion, in physiological conditions and when elastic stabilization is combined with rigid fusion. Results suggest that elastic stabilization reduces stresses on the adjacent disc up to 28° of flexion. Based on this preliminary result, we began to use elastic stabilization alone or combined with fusion in 1994. To date, we have performed 82 surgical procedures, 57 using stabilization alone and 25 combined with fusion, in patients affected by degenerative disc disease, disc herniation, recurrence of disc herniation or other pathologies. Clinical results are satisfactory, especially in the group of patients affected by recurrent disc herniation, in whom the elastic device was used alone.

Keywords Elastic stabilization · Discopathy · Disc herniation recurrence · Border area

Introduction

One of the biggest problems in spinal surgery is the treatment of vertebral instability.

The diagnostic instruments used to identify instability are standard and dynamic X-rays, and magnetic resonance (MR) images, on which early disc degeneration can be identified by so-called Modic signs [9]. Discography is the only investigational device that can identify the pain source (memory pain) through a provocative test. Computed tomography (CT) is important for the detection of bone diseases and analysis of the status of facet joints.

Many different surgical procedures are employed to treat vertebral instability: postero-lateral fusion (PLF), intersomatic fusion (ALIF or PLIF) and posterior instrumented fusion alone (screw fixation) or combined with intersomatic fusion (circumferential fusion). All these procedures may achieve the goal of fusion, with good radiological results; however, at the same time they can create a pathology of the level adjacent to the fused area.

Butler et al. [1] performed a study to determine the relationship between facet joint osteoarthritis and disc degeneration in subjects in whom both MR images and CT scans had been obtained. The MR images were used to determine disc degeneration, the CT scans to determine the presence of facet joint osteoarthritis. The authors hypothesized that disc degeneration would sometimes occur without the presence of facet joint osteoarthritis, but that facet joint osteoarthritis would only occur in the presence of disc degeneration. They concluded, on the basis of their results, that disc degeneration occurs before facet joint osteoarthritis, which may be secondary to mechanical changes in loading of the facet joints. If this concept is true for a non-instrumented spine, imagine applying this to a functional spinal unit near a fused area, in which stresses are more concentrated.

Elastic stabilization could be a good alternative to fusion in cases in which arthrodesis is an excessive procedure. It should also be used in addition to lumbar stabilization in cases in which the disc adjacent to the fused area is initially degenerated. We call this a combined stabilization.

Indications for elastic stabilization alone are very low grade instability, initial disc degeneration in young people, recurrent disc herniation with or without scar tissue formation and lumbar stenosis.

Using the interspinous device, we increase the stability of the segment, we discharge the posterior facets, and we obtain an increase in the neuroforamina size. Senegas, with his work, confirmed these concepts [10].

Before starting with the in vivo application of the device, we performed a biomechanical study, in collaboration with bioengineers of the Politecnico di Milano. The aim of the study was to understand better the efficacy of the Bronsard's ligament when applied on a model simulating the lumbar spine.

Materials and methods: biomechanical model

We conceived a schematic representation of lumbar spine (Fig. 1) composed of contiguous segments representing the spine in a sagittal plane.

To simplify the scheme, we decided to consider the spine as formed by elastic discs, with a circular hollow section interposed to rigid bodies with a circular full section. We did not consider the nucleus pulposus properties. All data regarding mechanical and geometrical characteristics were deduced from other mechanical models reported in literature [3, 8].

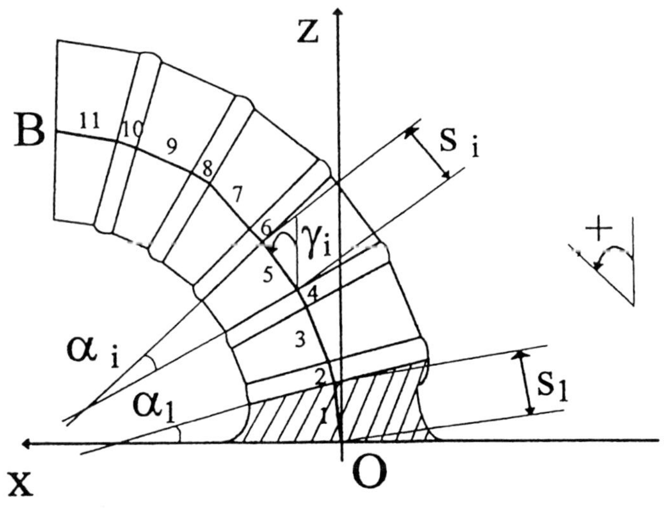

Fig. 1 Schematic representation of the lumbar spine: αi is the angle between two adjacent discs; γi is the angle of inclination of each vertebral body; Si is the height of the vertebral body

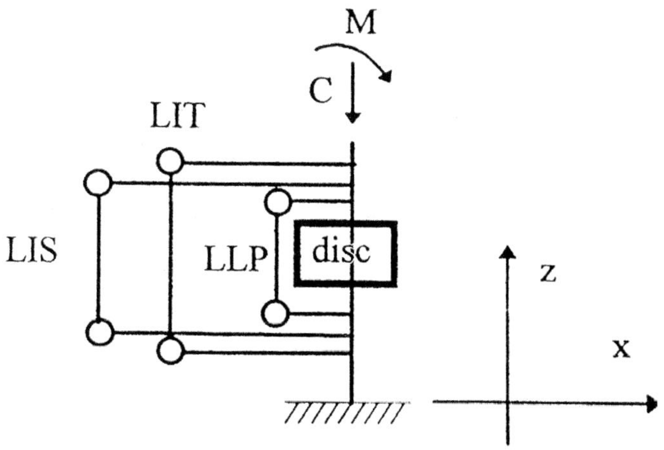

Fig. 2 Scheme of a vertebral body unit during anterior flexion. C and M represent the weight and muscular forces. LLP represents the posterior longitudinal ligament, LIT the ligamentum flavum and the intertransverse ligament, LIS the interspinous and supraspinous ligaments

We studied the lumbar spine in a standing position; our purpose was to evaluate stress and deformation of intervertebral disc during flexion.

We decided to consider only flexion, at first, to simplify the evaluation, which could be very complex for other movements owing to the different components included. During forward flexion some torsion components are present, but they are so slight that we can consider the flexion movement as a pure one, completely contained in the median plane of the subject.

The lumbar spine is subject to a system of loads in which body weight, muscle and ligament actions are all involved, maintaining the trunk's balance in all degrees of flexion.

In Fig. 2 we present a schematic representation of a vertebral motion segment during flexion, showing the various forces involved.

By means of a classic technique normally used in engineering for hyperstatic structures, we analysed the internal actions and the main stresses and deformations of intervertebral discs that develop at different degrees of flexion up to 40°.

The simulations carried out concerned physiological movement, movement at one or two levels with rigid stabilization and finally the movement at one level with rigid stabilization combined with the elastic stabilization outlined above, using Bronsard's ligament.

Results: biomechanical model

Figure 3 presents the results of the simulation, showing the maximal stress values in the L3-L4 disc (y-axis) for angles of lumbar flexion up to 40° (x-axis).

The graph shows maximal solicitation in the disc adjacent to a fused area increases by more than the values calculated in physiological conditions, and much more if there is a two-level fixation. If we put an elastic stabilization on the disc above, this value reduces, but only if lumbar flexion is less than 28°. For a higher grade of flexion, the value increases.

Elastic stabilization seems to reduce the concentration of stresses applied on the bordering disc during flexion by up to about 30°.

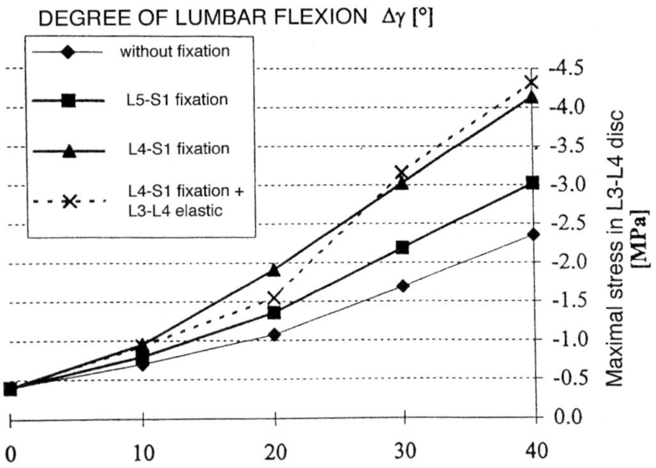

Fig. 3 The y-axis shows that the maximum strain is at the L3-L4 intervertebral disc; the *x*-axis shows the angle of lumbar flexion

The increase in stresses for higher grades of flexion is probably due to the mechanical properties of the Bronsard's ligament. This could mean that the artificial ligament we used may be too stiff.

We now use the DIAM interspinous device, which is less stiff than the Bronsard one, and we intend to test it on the same biomechanical model.

Materials and methods: patient series

From January 1994 to December 2001 we performed 82 surgical procedures; 57 were elastic stabilization alone and 25 were associated with instrumentation and fusion (combined stabilization). The mean age was 43 years and the admission diagnosis was degenerative disc disease in 50% of the cases, disc herniation in 25.6%, recurrent disc herniation in 11% and some other diagnosis in 13.4% of the cases (Table 1).

Two patients were affected by L5 spondylolisthesis. We performed a reduction and a combined stabilization in both cases. Fusion was performed from L4 to S1, associated with an elastic stabilization in L3-L4 because of initial degeneration of the disc.

Four patients suffered from a lumbar stenosis. We performed a one- or two-level laminectomy associated with elastic stabilization.

Fifty-seven patients (57/82) underwent elastic stabilization alone (Table 2). In 61.4% of these cases we performed a one-level L4-L5 elastic stabilization. Six patients underwent a two-level procedure, four of them had an L3-L4 and L4-L5 stabilization. In one case we performed an L5-S1 stabilization using the Dynasys system with an L4-L5 interspinous device (DIAM).

Table 1 Admission diagnosis

Admission diagnosis	*N*
Degenerative disc disease	41
Disc herniation	21
Recurrent disc herniation	9
Lumbar instability	5
Spondylolisthesis	2
Lumbar stenosis	4
Total	82

Table 2 Elastic stabilization alone

Level	*N*
L2-L3	6
L3-L4	10
L4-L5	35
L1-L2 and L2-L3	1
L3-L4 and L4-L5	4
L4-L5 and L5-S1	1
Total	57

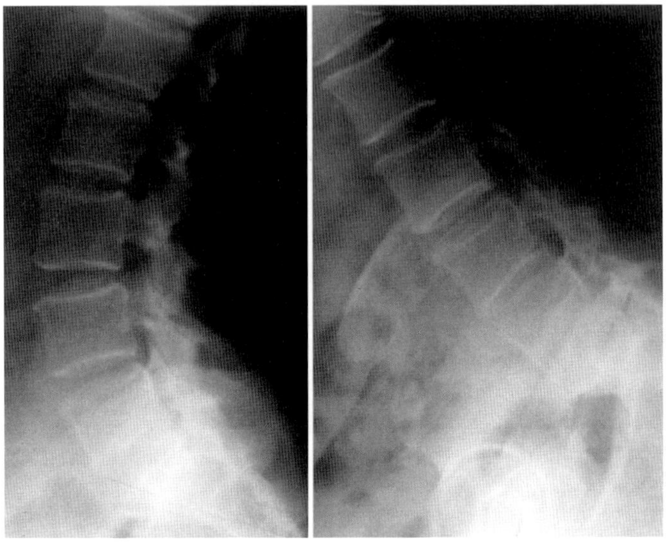

Fig. 4 Dynamic radiographs of a 35-year-old woman affected by L4-L5 degenerative disc disease. Low-grade L4-L5 instability is evident

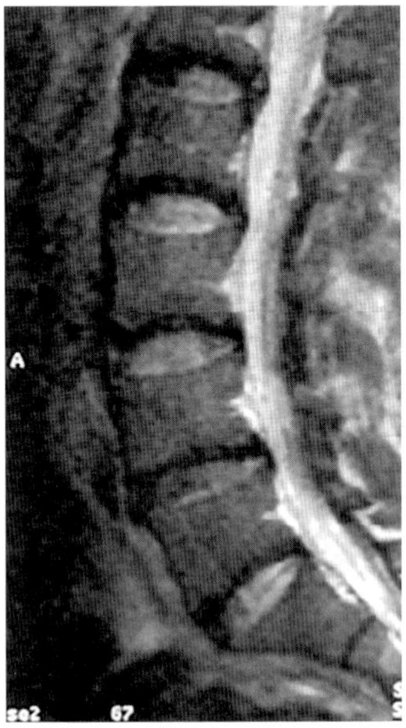

Fig. 5 Magnetic resonance (MR) image shows an L4-L5 bulging disc

In Fig. 4 we present the case of a 35-year-old woman affected by L4-L5 degenerative disc disease with initial signs of instability on dynamic radiographs. MR images (Fig. 5) demonstrate the presence of a bulging disc. She suffered from persistent back pain, and

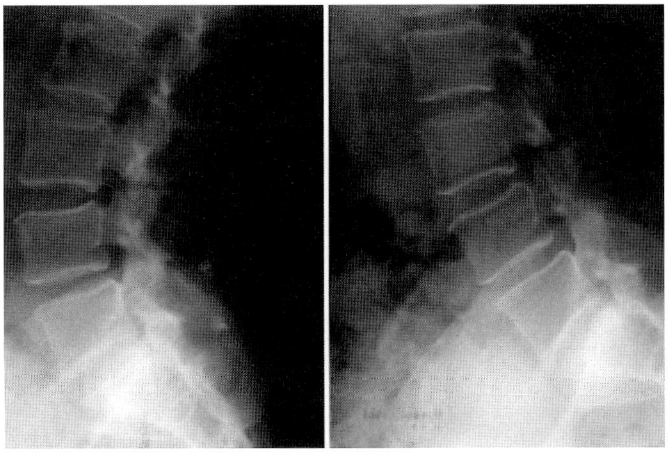

Fig. 6 One-year follow-up dynamic radiographs after implantation of the L4-L5 interspinous device

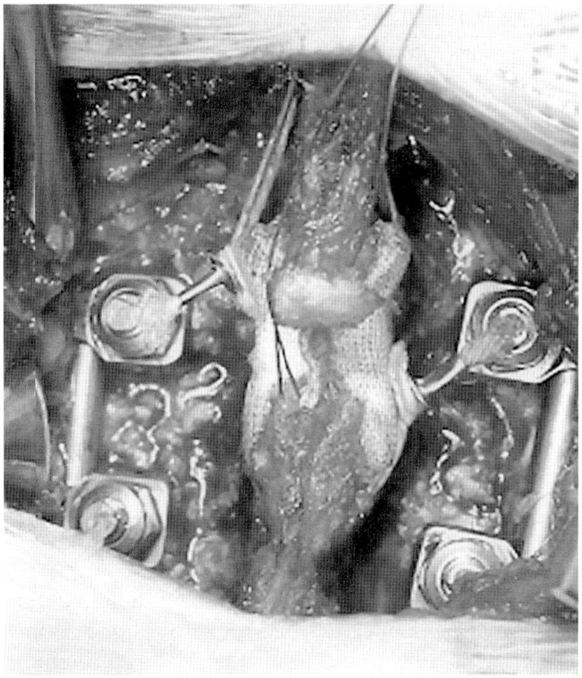

Fig. 7 Intraoperative view of an L5-S1 fusion combined with an L4-L5 elastic stabilization

Table 3 Elastic stabilization combined with fusion (combined stabilization)

Fused area	Elastic stabilization	*N*
L5-S1	L4-L5	6
L4-S1	L3-L4	11
L4-L5	L3-L4	4
L4-L5	L2-L3 and L3-L4	1
L3-L4	L2-L3	1
L3-L4	L2-L3 and L4-L5	1
L5-S1	L3-L4 and L4-L5	1
Total		25

we decided to perform an L4-L5 elastic stabilization. The dynamic radiographs taken at 1-year follow-up (Fig. 6) demonstrate the good position of the device and increased stability of the segment. The patient is pain free.

In twenty-five patients (25/82) we performed a combined stabilization (Table 3).

L4-S1 rigid stabilization with fusion associated with an L3-L4 elastic stabilization was performed in 44% of these cases. Three patients underwent spinal fusion associated with two-level elastic stabilization; in one of them we performed a one-level fusion with interspinous devices on the level above and below.

Figure 7 shows the intraoperative view of an L5-S1 fusion combined with an L4-L5 elastic stabilization. The suture of the supraspinous ligament follows the interspinous device placement.

Figure 8 and Fig. 9 show a 60-year-old man affected by multilevel disc disease and lumbar instability. At 4 years of follow-up (Fig. 10) good bone fusion from L4 to S1 and a restored height of the L3-L4 space are evident.

Results: patient series

We reviewed 61 patients (61/82) with a mean follow up of 20 months (minimum 12 months; maximum 6 years). Clinical results are highly satisfactory, especially in the group of patients affected by recurrent disc herniation, in whom the elastic device was used alone.

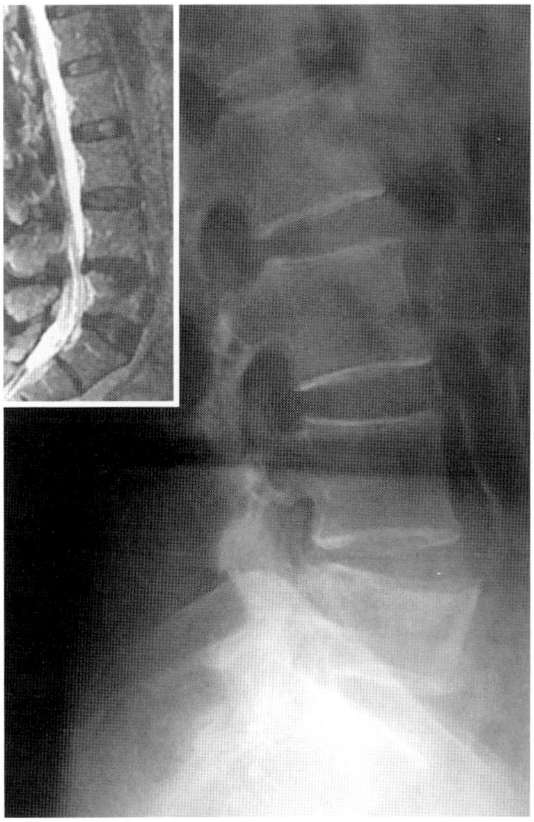

Fig. 8 Lateral radiograph and MR image of a 60-year-old man, showing multilevel disc disease

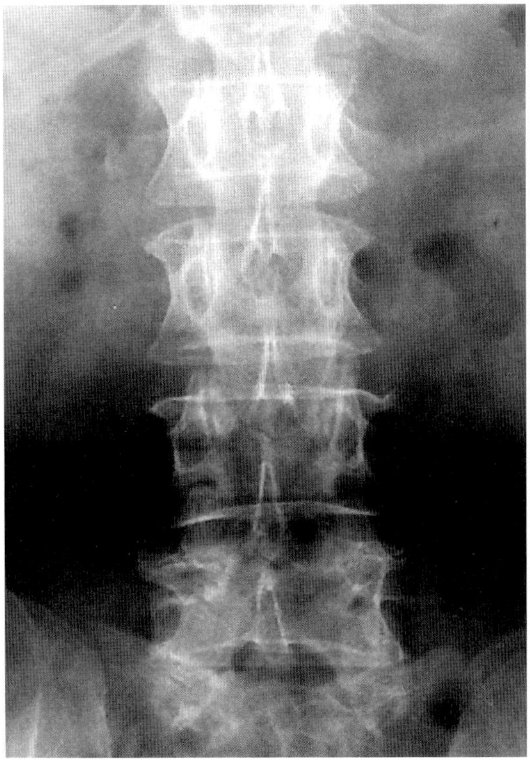

Fig. 9 Anteroposterior radiograph shows the presence of L4-S1 degenerative processes

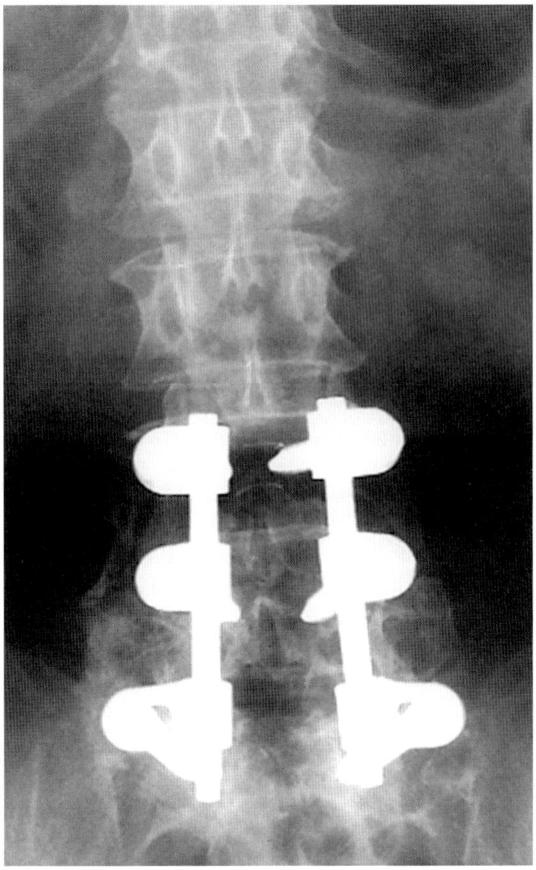

Fig. 10 At the 4-year follow-up after L4-S1 fusion associated with L3-L4 elastic stabilization, good bone fusion from L4 to S1 and a restored height of the L3-L4 space are evident

No complications related to the material were detected.

Although elastic stabilization with an interspinous device seems able to prevent the recurrence of disc herniation [11], in our series one patient developed a recurrence 2 years after the intervention of elastic stabilization. Our mean follow-up period is too short to reach any conclusion on this.

The best results were for a single-level elastic stabilization positioned at L4-L5. No differences in results were observed if two devices were placed one above the other. The L5-S1 level should be avoided because of the poor quality of the S1 spinous process.

Discussion

Freudiger et al. [6] published an in vitro study on dynamic neutralization of the lumbar spine. They concluded that the dynamic neutralization system they used reduces bending angles and horizontal translations, but increases vertical translations. They also concluded that the bulging of the posterior anulus was reduced.

Some authors [5, 7] have used elastic stabilization for the treatment of initial lumbar instability, with satisfactory results, while Dubois et al. [4] classified dynamic destabilization into phases in order to facilitate recognition of the early signs and symptoms of lumbar instability. Based on their classification they operated on 57 consecutive patients with the Dynasys system. They concluded that their dynamic stabilization system is applicable to a wide range of nonstructural lumbar instability.

From our experience, we believe that elastic stabilization with an interspinous device (DIAM) is a safe procedure with good clinical results, especially in patients affected by recurrent disc herniation.

It can also be used with good results in patients affected by degenerative disc disease, lumbar stenosis and very low grade instability.

When used in association with lumbar stabilization arthrodesis, we think that elastic stabilization reduces the mechanical stresses applied on the disc above. In this way the bordering area can be protected from accelerated degenerative process [2].

This is an hypothesis, which requires a scientific demonstration. We are therefore carrying out a radiological study (X-rays and MRI) on patients operated, in order to obtain evidence on whether a minor rate of precocious degenerative processes is detected in this group compared to a control group.

References

1. Butler D, Trafimow JH, Andersson GB, McNeill TW, Huckman MS (1990) Discs degenerate before facets. Spine 15:111–113
2. Caserta S, Misaggi B, Peroni D, La Maida GA (2001) Elastic stabilization combined with rigid fusion: a prevention of pathology of the border area. Proceedings of the 24th National Congress of the Italian Spine Society. Eur Spine J 10:352–362
3. Chazal J, Tanguy A, Bourges M, Gaurel G, Escande G, et al (1985) Biomechanical properties of spinal ligaments and a histological study of the supraspinal ligament in traction. J Biomech 18:167–176
4. Dubois G, de Germay B, Schaerer NS, Fennema P (1999) Dynamic neutralization: a new concept for restabilization of the spine. In: Szpalski M, Gunzburg R, Pope MH (eds) Lumbar segmental instability. Lippincott Williams & Wilkins, Philadelphia, pp 233–240
5. Fassio B, Cohen R, Beguin C, Jucopilla N (1991) Traitement des instabilités lombaires dégénératives L4-L5 par ligamentoplastie inter-épineuse. Rachis 3: 464–474
6. Freudiger S, Dubois G, Lorrain M (1999) Dynamic neutralization of the lumbar spine confirmed on a new lumbar spine simulator in vitro. Arch Orthop Trauma Surg 119:127–132
7. Graf H (1992) Instabilité vertébrale. Traitement à l'aide d'un systéme souple. Rachis 4:123–137
8. Kapandjj IA (1994) Fisiologia articolare, vol 3, 5th edn. Monduzzi, pp 78–121
9. Modic M, Pavlicek W, Weinstein M, et al (1984) Magnetic resonance imaging of intervertebral disc disease. Radiology 152:103–111
10. Senegas J (1991) Surgery of the intervertebral ligaments: alternative to arthrodesis in the treatment of degenerative instabilities. Acta Orthop Belg 57 [Suppl 1]:221–226
11. Voydeville GP, Feldmann L (1992) Ligamentoplastie intervertébrale avec cale souple dans les instabilités lombaires. Etude préliminaire. Orthop Traumatol 2:259–264

Robert C. Mulholland
Dilip K. Sengupta

Rationale, principles and experimental evaluation of the concept of soft stabilization

Abstract The apparent clinical success of spinal stabilization methods that restrict rather than abolish movement in relieving mechanical back pain indicates that the concept of the aetiology of back pain should be reviewed. Further understanding of how degeneration affects disc biomechanics, and an understanding of how current soft stabilization systems alters them, may allow us to define more precisely what are the essential requirements of an ideal soft stabilization system. It appears that abnormal patterns of loading rather than abnormal movement are the reason that disc degeneration causes back pain in some patients. Abnormal load transmission is the principal cause of pain in osteoarthritic joints, and both osteotomy and, indeed, joint replacement succeed because they alter the load transmission across the joint. This concept is supported by the fact that abnormal patterns of stress distribution measured across the disc correlate with painful discs on discography. Clinically, it is often noted that back pain is primarily related to position or posture, rather than movement of the lumbar spine. Clinical success after solid fusion is unpredictable because it does not necessarily prevent painful loading across the disc, and also it may interfere with maintenance of sagittal balance in varying postures. The Graf ligament restricted flexion, and was modestly successful. It unfortunately increased the load over the posterior annulus. The Dynesys system reduces movement both in flexion and extension, and appears to be more successful. However, often it also unloads the disc to a degree that is unpredictable. The authors believe that this unloading of the disc is an important feature of a flexible stabilization system. A new a design of a flexible stabilization system has recently been described in an in vitro study, which unloads the disc by introduction of a load-sharing fulcrum near the axis of movement together with an elastic posterior ligament. This design produces maximal unloading of the disc, whilst allowing a restricted range of movement, which serves the important purpose of allowing the patient to maintain sagittal balance in varying postures.

Keywords Soft stabilization · Disc degeneration · Low-back pain

R.C. Mulholland (✉) · D.K. Sengupta
Centre for Spinal Studies and Surgery,
Queen's Medical Centre,
University Hospital Nottingham,
Nottingham, UK
e-mail: rcmulholland@hotmail.com,
Tel.: +44-115-9609389,
Fax: +44-151-9245993

R.C. Mulholland
34 Regent Street, Nottingham NG1 5BT,
UK

Back pain: movement or load related?

It is difficult to find any basis for the concept of instability as a cause of low back pain. It was a phrase that came into use in the middle of the last century, and was used by clinicians to imply that there was some non-specific mechanical failure of the spine, as opposed to an arthritis or infection. When bioengineers became involved in trying to sort out the biomechanics of the spine [5], they embraced the term. They interpreted instability in a purely literal bioengineering sense, validated to some extent in other joints like the knee and shoulder. Thus, despite the pioneering work of Nachemson and Schultz [27], who demonstrated that pain was related to disc pressures and posture, but not movement, the era of back pain being due to a disorder called "instability" was born, and fusion was seen as the appropriate solution.

Role of the disc

It is generally recognized that morphological changes in the disc play a major role in low-back pain, although it is also recognized that there is no correlation between the degree of degeneration and the severity of back pain. The disc has two biomechanical roles, it must transmit load and it must allow a controlled range of movement, so that such movement does not compromise the adjacent neural elements. It is generally accepted that the effect of disc degeneration is to reduce movement [6, 7], not to increase it, as the term "instability" would imply.

It may be argued that, unfortunately, this reduction of movement is associated with abnormal patterns of movement, and this is the meaning of "instability". However, despite considerable efforts over many years, using flexion/extension films, no clear relationship has been established between pain and such abnormal movements. In other words, patients with degenerative disc disease may exhibit abnormal patterns of movement, yet have no pain. The one new movement that may be present in some patients with degenerative disc disease is translational movement [6, 7], as is seen in patients with degenerative spondylolisthesis. It is this movement that is often regarded as an important abnormality in patients with so called instability. In the lumbar spine such translational movement can only occur if the facet joints become incompetent, but this is not a feature in many patients with back pain. It is a common clinical experience that at re-exploration after failed posterior fusion, even if there is demonstrable flexion-extension movement and a clear pseudoarthrosis, translation movement is very seldom present.

The second role of the disc is that it must transmit load. It is well designed for this purpose. The normal disc is isotropic [12], that is to say that it behaves liked a fluid-filled bag, and transmits load uniformly across the surface of the disc and to the endplate [16, 17]. This has a number of important biomechanical consequences.

Key among these is that in any position of the spine, be it flexion, extension or lateral-bending, the load is transmitted uniformly over the endplates. There is no high spot-loading related to different positions of the spine. It may be recalled that this is the case in a normal diathrodial joint. Here, the design of the joint ensures an even pattern of load transmission. Disturbance of anatomy of the joint, such as a menisectomy in the knee, or destruction of the cartilage by disease (infection/arthritis) in other joints, leads to a disturbance in the normal weight transmission, producing pain. It was recognized many years ago that an appropriately planned osteotomy, which altered the load transmission, might result in pain relief. We are all familiar with radiographs showing the high spot-loading in a subluxing hip, and are also aware that an appropriate osteotomy, which reduces spot-loading by containing the hip, relieved pain. Similarly, in a varus or valgus deformity of knee joint, abnormal distribution of load may lead to unicompartmental osteoarthritis, and an appropriate osteotomy, especially if done early with minimal cartilage loss, would produce a satisfactory long-term result. We emphasize that the biomechanical effect was to alter the loading pattern, and the resultant clinical effect was pain relief. If we accept that in load-bearing joints overall an altered loading pattern produces pain, then we can more easily accept this concept also applies to the disc.

Another important consequence of the uniformity of distribution of load transmission across the surface of the disc is that it transmits load to the annulus, producing a tension in the annulus, and converting it into a load-bearing structure. It is established that disc degeneration alters the isotropic nature of the disc [13, 17] and, as a consequence, load transmission over the endplate becomes irregular, leading to high spot-loading, particularly associated with certain positions.

The concept of load-related pain and its clinical significance

It is curious that instability or movement abnormalities are blamed for back pain. Whenever a history is taken of chronic back pain, it is clear that the problems experienced are postural, rather than related to the process of movement. It is pain whilst bent down, it is pain whilst leaning forward, and it is pain whilst sitting. As the loads on the back are mostly produced by muscle action rather than body weight, activities that involve strong muscle action, such as lifting, are associated with pain. Standing perfectly still with a heavy load is a painful experience for some patients with a painful back, quite unrelated to any movement. We are all aware that lying down flat and reducing the load relieves pain. Nachemson [22], in his classic work, showed very clearly the close relationship of posture and load in the disc, and later Schultz and Nachemson and their co-workers [27] demonstrated the important effects of muscle action on these loads.

Exercise and physiotherapy

When we consider the use of physiotherapy in the treatment of chronic back pain, there is again a curious illogicality in our concept of how it might work. If instability were indeed the cause of chronic back pain, then the use of corsets, much used in the past, would not now be derided. If one is going to treat an unstable joint by encouraging movement, then one has to be confident that the movement one encourages is the normal pattern, and not the abnormal one. As we are not clear what abnormal patterns we are planning to prevent, it is not truly possible to plan a treatment that will specifically allow normal movement, and stop the abnormal ones. Let us suppose that it is the translation movement that we are concerned about. It is difficult to conceive that strengthening muscles, most of which are at right angles to the line of translational movement, will have any effect. But of course physiotherapy, rehabilitation and manipulation do succeed in alleviating back pain [31], presumably not by stopping abnormal movement, but by altering the loading pattern of the degenerated disc. How they might do so becomes clearer if we look more closely at the anatomy of the degenerate disc, and the effect of the altered anatomy on the biomechanical functioning.

Macro- and micro-anatomy of disc degeneration

In a clinicopathologic study on degenerated disc tissue collected from surgery and from cadaveric spines, Moore and Vernon-Roberts et al. [21] described:

> Nuclear desiccation and fragmentation leads to the eventual formation of clefts in the annulus, followed by the extrusion of mainly nuclear material through these preexisting annular clefts. Isolated fragments of annulus and endplate are much less common than nucleus in extruded material and probably also originate as part of the degenerative process.

Normal nucleus consists of a homogeneous gel of collagen and proteoglycan. In a degenerated disc, it changes to a non-homogeneous mixture of fragmented and condensed collagen, areas of fluid, and indeed areas of gas on occasion. If the load is transmitted through such a fragment within the degenerated disc, it will lead to a high focal load being transmitted to the endplate cartilage and the subchondral bony trabeculae. This results in corresponding endplate changes, apoptosis of cells and destruction and thinning of the cartilaginous endplate [2, 30].

As the nucleus become desiccated and depressurized, an increasingly larger load is transmitted through the annulus. Now the area of the disc through which most of the load is transmitted depends on the posture: in flexion the anterior annulus, in extension the posterior annulus. Loading the annulus, unprotected by the supporting pressure of the nucleus, will lead to splitting and inward folding of the annulus. This altered pattern of load transmission leads to changes in the cancellous bone architecture in the vertebral body. In a study on cadaver degenerated disc, Simpson et al. [30] observed significant architectural changes in the anterior regions of the vertebral body, with increases in the number and thickness of bony trabeculae. Minimal alterations were found at posterior regions. Bone loss was observed in central regions (most distant from the cortex) as disc disorganization increased, a reduction in both number and thickness of trabeculae. They concluded that this might be a response to a redistribution of load to the vertebral body periphery as a result of disc disorganization. What is clear is that the loading pattern is immensely variable, and that physical movement and position will alter this.

Clinical experience in support of abnormal loading as a cause of pain

An acute attack of sciatica due to disc herniation is often preceded by recurrent episodes of 'lumbago', lasting for a few days or longer. Often these patients are relatively asymptomatic between the episodes. When such cases are treated with discectomy to relieve sciatica, discrete fragments of disc materials are removed at operation, and this relieves sciatica, as well as the episodes of lumbago.

This well-observed clinical scenario may be explained by the experimental work reported by Brinckmann and Porter [4]. They produced models of incomplete radial tears in cadaver discs. In addition, fragmented tissue pieces that resembled those retrieved at surgery for prolapse were created in the centre of the disc. They could reproduce disc protrusion by loading such a model within physiological range when the fragment was present, but not without a fragment. They concluded that disc protrusion had to be preceded by generation of radial fissures and tissue fragmentation within the disc, and that prolapse was a late event during the course of a long-term degenerative process. In the clinical scenario alluded to, it seems probable that the fragment is present prior to the protrusion for some time. As its removal commonly cures the recurrent attacks of lumbago, is it not likely that such attacks are related to the fragment? Is it not likely that its presence, mobile in the disc space, causes on occasion an abnormal loading pattern?

Another clinical observation is the undoubted effect that manipulation can have in acute episodes of lumbago. It seems most likely that this must be related to a movement of tissues within the disc, suggesting that the internal morphology can be acutely altered. The best analogy for the discomfort is the "stone in the shoe" concept. As the stone moves to a position of lesser weight bearing area under the foot, one can walk comfortably again.

The "stone in the shoe" hypothesis – a degenerated disc is painful only at abnormal load transmission

The random nature of recurrent lumbago is difficult to tie in with a concept of instability. How would one explain relatively symptom-free periods between the episodes of acute disabling back pain on the basis of instability? Does it suddenly become stable? However, if we accept the "stone in the shoe" analogy, then the randomness and indeed the variable response to manipulation becomes explicable. By altering the distribution of fluid/fragments within the disc, one may alter the way it transmits load, and pain goes.

The concept that the actual arrangement of tissues in the disc affects load transmission also explains the fact that there is no clear correlation between degree of disc degeneration and pain.

With advanced degeneration the disc tissues become progressively more collagenized, and homogeneous, so that once again loading becomes even over this homogeneous mass, leading to spontaneous relief of pain.

Experimental work in support of the hypothesis – pressure profile across the disc and pain in discography

Although some doubt has been cast on the value of discography in identifying a painful disc, it is a common practice to perform a discogram prior to spinal fusion. This provided us with the opportunity to examine the loading patterns of degenerate discs, prior to spinal surgery [18]. Fifteen patients who were candidates for spinal fusion, and were having discograms to determine the segmental level to be fused, had a pressure profilometry study, as described by McNally and Adams [17], at the same time. In this technique, a stress transducer, mounted on a needle, is drawn through the disc so that a graph of stress against position within the disc can be plotted. Stress is a complex mechanical parameter that can vary with the direction of measurement (horizontal or vertical), the directional dependence resulting from the mechanical properties of the disc. In a normal disc, which is isotropic, the stress is the same in both directions, but in a degenerated disc, which is anisotropic, stresses vary both in their direction and across different parts of the disc. The plot of stress against position is termed a "stress profile" of the disc. All the 31discs studied were abnormal on MRI, but some were painful on discography, and others were not. It was found that the discs painful on discography had particular patterns of stress profile. The nucleus was depressurized and was not taking load. The posterior annulus was taking increased load. A number of painful discs had a very high level of focal loading in the disc. A painful disc could be predicted by an abnormal annulus in 90% of levels ($P<0.001$). Pain was predicted by a depressurized nucleus in 63% of levels ($P<0.017$). There was extensive variability of stress distribution (and therefore the mechanical function of the different areas of the disc) even in discs showing the same degree of radiographic degeneration. This demonstrated that the radiographic or MRI appearance of a disc is not a direct indicator of its mechanical competence, and fits in with the clinical observation that degree of disc degeneration is not related to pain.

This study showed that pattern of loading, rather than absolute levels of loading, was related to pain in a degenerated disc. Clearly, if this was the case, then surgery that alters loading patterns alone, without significant reduction of movement, may be an appropriate alternative to fusion.

Results of fusion

If indeed instability was the main cause of back pain, one would have expected that spinal fusion would be more successful than it has been. Improvement in the instrumentation technique resulted in increase in successful fusion rate, but this has not been reflected by a corresponding increase in the rate of successful clinical outcome [3]. Despite the introduction of pedicle screws in the late 1980s, and cages in the late 1990s, and the frequent use of circumferential fusion in association with cages, the clinical efficacy of fusion has remained the same. Indeed with more recent sophisticated methods of assessing clinical success, the so-called "excellent" results of fusion are in the region of 30% [8]!

Sagittal balance and fusion

It will be appreciated that a fusion may well produce a normal loading pattern. This may explain the successful clinical outcome in some cases. It may also be possible that a successful fusion may interfere with normal sagittal balance, especially if it involves more than one level, and may force a person to assume a position that produces abnormal load on an adjacent segment. Lazennec et al. [14] observed that a common complaint of fusion patients is that they get sitting pain. When one looks at the sitting lateral radiographs of the lumbo-sacral spine and observes the posture that is adopted, it is often seen that, if a patient has a stiff segment from L4 to S1 fusion, sitting imposes considerable postural stresses on levels above the fusion and also on the limited rotatory capacity of the sacroiliac joint, which forces both joints to their extreme limits.

Clearly a posterior fusion does not stop loading on the disc. It will reduce it and may alter its pattern. It may at the same time prevent the spine taking up a position where normal loading pattern occurs. However, in any particular patient, we are commonly not aware of the precise loading pattern and in what position it occurs, so the effect of fusing a spine in one position will be somewhat random as regards clinical success. We may fuse it in a position where the remaining loading on the disc may indeed be a painful loading position! This may explain an unsuccessful clinical outcome after a successful fusion.

One would anticipate that an anterior fusion would be more likely to produce a normal loading pattern, and indeed the results of anterior fusion are better than those of posterior fusion, which still allows endplate loading [26, 34]. However, experience with cages produces some indication as to why anterior fusion is not necessarily successful.

McAfee, in his extensive review of the results of cage fusion [15], indicated that the clinical results were little better than those of other methods of fusion, and Whitecloud et al. [33] demonstrated that, even after a circumferential fusion using cages, the rate of excellent results was only 30%. Agazzi et al. [1] reported that, again using cages, the rate of excellent or good results was only 39%, and there was no relation between clinical outcome and the success of the fusion.

Of course, with an anterior fusion with a cage, body load has to be taken by the cage and transmitted to the vertebrae below. Many of the cages had a small "footprint", and essentially loaded through the soft cancellous bone at the centre of the vertebrae, over a limited area only. Polikeit and Nolte [24] showed that the enormous loads thus produced may amount to some 500% higher than the endplate would normally experience. McAfee [15] had pointed out that clinical success was associated with the development of bone around the cage, inevitably increasing the area for load transmission and reducing the contrast between an area loaded, and one not loaded. Clearly, the clinical results of cage fusion will be improved if the cage and adjacent bone does indeed transmit load over a wide area onto the vertebrae below.

If we accept that stopping movement is not a factor in clinical success, but creating a normal loading pattern is, then we are empowered to look at other methods of changing loading patterns, without the disadvantages of producing a stiff segment.

Where is the pain arising from?

We initially thought that an abnormal loading pattern over the endplate, which is highly innervated (much more so than the disc), was the explanation of the pain. However, recent work with vertebroplasty for osteoporotic fractures demonstrates that bone itself is a source of pain, and this pain can be alleviated if the internal mechanics of the bone are strengthened by cement, without any correction of deformity. Bone is very sensitive to pressure within it, as one can see in acute osteomyelitis. The high pressures produced by small cages are presumably the reason for their clinical failure. Much research has been devoted to identify pain sources in the posterior annulus. However, if indeed the posterior annulus was a major player as a pain source, it is difficult to see why disc degeneration would not always be associated with pain, as the annulus is invariably deformed, and has various tears and fissures, despite the segment being painless.

Flexible stabilization

Flexible stabilization is a commonly used term to describe various systems that have been developed which allow spinal movement, but restrict its range. They were based on the concept that they permitted only restricted movement within the range of normal movement. We believe that they work either because they restrict movement to a zone or range where normal or near normal loading may occur, or they prevent the spine adopting a position where abnormal loading may occur.

Graf ligament

The Graf ligament system was one of the first relatively widely practiced methods of soft stabilization (Fig. 1). It consists of a non-elastic band as a ligament to connect the pedicle screws across the segment to be stabilized, to lock the segment in full lordosis. The concept was that, once the facet joints were locked, it would stop rotation. The inventor Henri Graf [10] was of the view that "instability" was related to the development of an abnormal rotatory movement, and if this were stopped, the system would still allow limited flexion, but within the range of normal flexion, which would therefore probably not be painful. There was no clinical or experimental basis for his views as to the cause of instability, but despite this, a clinical review and a biomechanical study carried out by our team at the Centre for Spinal Studies and Surgery in Nottingham

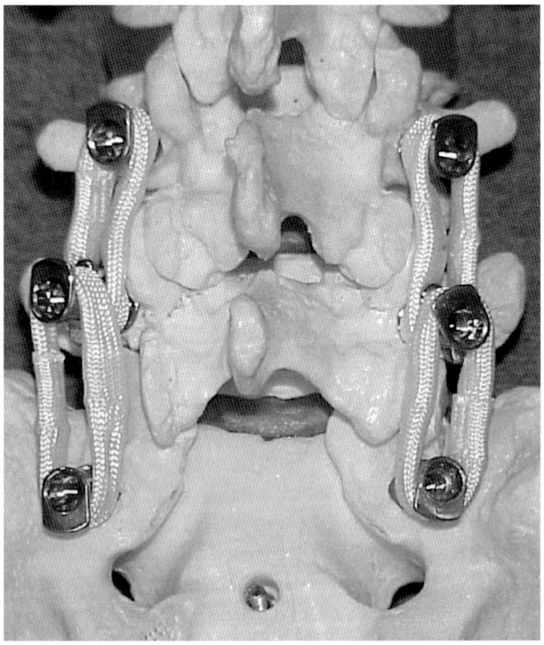

Fig. 1 Graf ligament system, applied to two adjacent motion segments in a spine model

showed that the Graf ligamentoplasty procedure had significant clinical success, with results similar to fusion [11]. It has the theoretical disadvantage that it overloads the posterior annulus, which, according to our earlier disc pressure profilometry study [18], was associated with a painful disc. It is somewhat uncertain as to whether success was related to the restriction of motion, or to the transfer of load to the posterior aspect removing loading from the anterior part of the disc. Our study [11] demonstrates that application of Graf ligament certainly transfers the load to the posterior annulus, and this may well be the explanation of its late failure! Graf ligamentoplasty procedure also produces a significant increase in lateral canal stenosis, especially if there is any preexisting degenerative change in the facet joints or in-folding of the ligamentum flavum, owing to the marked lordosis of the segment instrumented, and indeed early clinical failure was often associated with this surgical complication.

Dynesys

In the recently introduced Dynesyssystem (Sulzer Spine-Tech) (Fig. 2), the stabilization is achieved by connecting the pedicle screws with a non-elastic ligament, very similar to the Graf system, except that there is a plastic cylinder around the ligament. The plastic cylinder between the screw heads limits the degree of lordosis that can be created. The ligament is threaded through the cylinder and pulled tightly, with 300 N force, approximating the two screw heads to the extent that the interposed cylinder allows. As the posterior ligament is not elastic, flexion compresses the disc, and the axis of flexion is the posterior ligament, well posterior to the normal axis of flexion. Active extension will open up the anterior annulus without compression of the posterior annulus. Theoretically, lordosis can be achieved by the action of the spinal extensor muscles, and in extension the cylinder will take increasing load.

The early results of the Dynesys are promising. There are reports of some dramatic successes and some failures. The developers of the system claim it works by preventing so-called "parasitic" or "abnormal" movement. However, in addition to restricting the range of movement, it may also unload the disc if the patient achieves a position of lordosis, so that the plastic cylinder becomes weight bearing. However, lordosis and load sharing by the plastic cylinder depends very critically on the placement of the implant, and on the ability of the patient to achieve lordosis with his extensor muscles. Rajaratnam and co-workers recently reviewed [25] a group of 60 patients treated with Dynesys, with postoperative standing films with a plumb line. These patients did not achieve lordosis at the stabilized segments, although in some patients appropriate sagittal balance was achieved by extension above the instrumented segments. Of greater potential consequence, it was noted that, where the cylinder was placed with too much distraction, it leads to kyphosis of the segment. It is a common experience that kyphosis, if seen after disc excision, is associated with a higher incidence of back pain.

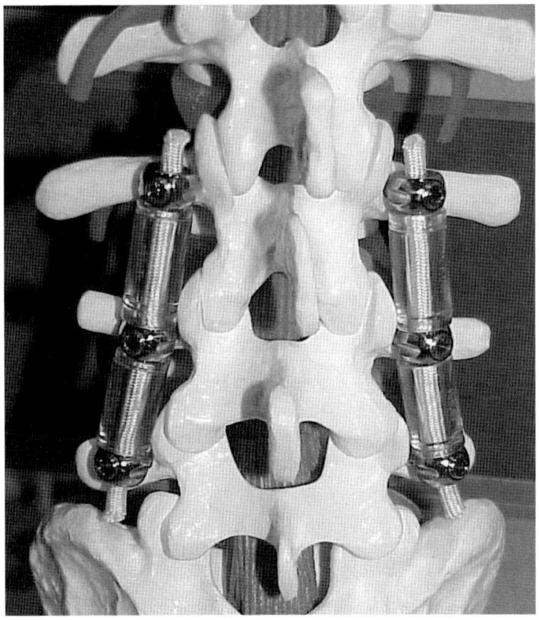

Fig. 2 Dynesis system, applied to two motion segments in a spine model

Leeds-Keio ligamentoplasty for spondylolisthesis

Mochida et al. [19, 20] reported an innovative method of posterior stabilization in which the Leeds-Keio artificial ligament was used as a nonrigid implant to stop movement in degenerative spondylolisthesis. They used fabric ligament, originally developed for reconstruction of anterior cruciate ligament, to tie it round drill holes through the pars of the adjacent vertebrae. In a biomechanical study on a porcine model [32], they found the system could effectively stop movement of the affected spinal segment even after cyclical loading of up to 1500 cycles. In a subsequent report [20], they compared the results of syndesmoplasty with ligament with that of instrumented fusion in a group of patients, and found no difference in outcome. They concluded that the non-rigid stabilization can produce an equally good result as compared to fusion, in patients with degenerative spondylolisthesis.

Fulcrum-assisted soft stabilization (FASS)

The fulcrum-assisted soft stabilization (FASS) system [28] (Fig. 3) was developed to address what was perceived as disadvantages of the Graf system. In this system, a fulcrum is placed between the pedicle screws, in front of the

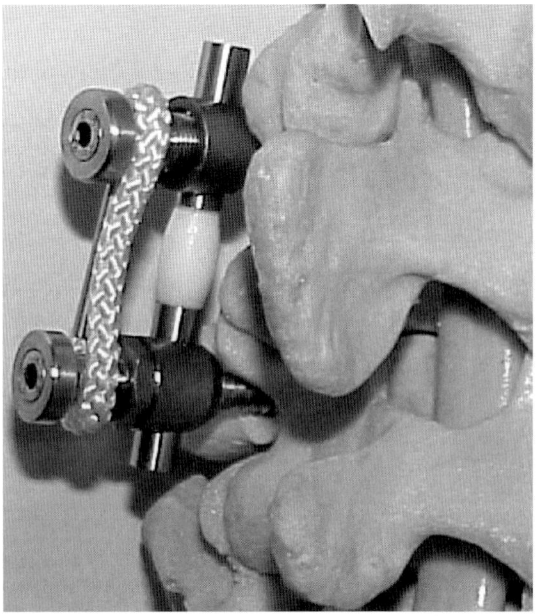

Fig. 3 Fulcrum-assisted soft stabilization system (FASS), applied here to the left side of one motion segment in a spine model. The ligament is elastic. The two fulcrums are fully flexible and each is placed anterior to the ligament and between the pedicle screws on either side, to permit flexion-extension, lateral bending and rotation of the motion segment, but resist axial compression. The compression force applied by the elastic ligament is converted by the fulcrum into a distraction force in front, thereby unloading the disc. The fulcrum shares the load with the disc. The system is still under development

ligament. The fulcrum distracts the posterior annulus. When the elastic ligament is placed posterior to the fulcrum, to compress the pedicle screw heads, the fulcrum transforms this posterior compression force to an anterior distraction force, which distracts the anterior annulus. The ligament creates the force that produces a lordosis, and it is not dependent on active muscle action, unlike in the Dynesys system. It is imperative that the FASS device should be inserted with sufficient tension in the ligament to create the required lordosis.

There are two problems commonly experienced with the Graf system:

1. The lordosis that the Graf ligament system invariably produces results in narrowing of the lateral recess, leading to root entrapment, especially if there was any preexisting facet arthropathy.
2. The Graf system increases the loading of the posterior annulus, which is a feature of the painful degenerate disc.

The presence of the fulcrum prevents both these problems.

FASS system can unload the disc, unaided by the posture or muscle action. It addresses a major defect of the Dynesys system, insofar as it does not allow the segment to be put into kyphosis. The lordosis is created by the implant, and is not dependent on the patient's ability to achieve lordosis with his or her own muscles.

The implant experimentally does unload the disc. It was found in the cadaver experiment that the degree of unloading is directly related to the stiffness produced by the system [29]. In other words, more flexibility is lost as greater unloading of the disc is achieved by adjustment of the tension in the ligament and the fulcrum. Clearly, if a very stiff system is implanted, then screw loosening and implant failure is more likely to occur in the long term. To maintain the normal physiological environment in the disc, it may desirable to unload the disc partially, and allow the segment a mobility as close to normal as possible. The fulcrum is thus only a load-sharing device. The system is still under development and a clinically applicable prototype is yet to be available.

Summary

In summary, there is enough evidence in the literature and support in common clinical experience to justify the hypothesis that chronic low-back pain is load related and not movement related, as the term "instability" would suggest. The concept of spinal ligamentoplasty or flexible stabilization is that it allows movement of the segment, and unloads the disc to a degree. The partial clinical success of the Graf and the Dynesys systems clearly show that back pain can be alleviated despite allowing movement. These systems may succeed in those patients where pain is related to abnormal loading in flexion. It is hypothesized that a desirable flexible stabilization system should combine overall disc unloading with restricting movement to a range where abnormal loading does not occur. The advantage of preserving movement is not related to the clinical need to bend one's back, but the need of the spine to be able to achieve sagittal balance in the varying postures required for daily living.

Philosophically, the true cure of a degenerative disc disease is a reversal of the degenerative process. This requires that the disc is rehydrated, and regains its height, mobility and load-bearing function. The only therapeutic approach towards this goal at present is gene therapy [9, 23], which aims at rejuvenating the chondrocytes in the nucleus of the disc. Unfortunately, the hostile and somewhat anoxic environment in a degenerate and fully loaded disc may not allow the rejuvenated cells inserted to survive and function. Soft stabilization may provide a sufficiently favourable environment in the disc for a gene therapy to achieve its goal.

References

1. Agazzi S, Reverdin A, May D (1999) Posterior lumbar interbody fusion with cages: an independent review of 71 cases. J Neurosurg 91 [2 Suppl]:186–192
2. Ariga K, Miyamoto S, Nakase T, Okuda S, Meng W, Yonenobu K, Yoshikawa H (2001) The relationship between apoptosis of endplate chondrocytes and aging and degeneration of the intervertebral disc. Spine. 26:2414–2420
3. Boos N, Webb JK (1997) Pedicle screw fixation in spinal disorders: a European view. Eur Spine J 6:2–18
4. Brinckmann P, Porter RW (1994) A laboratory model of lumbar disc protrusion. Fissure and fragment. Spine. 19:228–235
5. Dvorak J, Panjabi MM, Chang DG, Theiler R, Grob D (1991) Functional radiographic diagnosis of the lumbar spine. Flexion-extension and lateral bending. Spine. 16:562–571
6. Fujiwara A, Tamai K, An HS, Kurihashi T, Lim TH, Yoshida H, Saotome K (2000) The relationship between disc degeneration, facet joint osteoarthritis, and stability of the degenerative lumbar spine. J Spinal Disord 13:444–450
7. Fujiwara A, Lim TH, An HS, Tanaka N, Jeon CH, Andersson GB, Haughton VM (2000) The effect of disc degeneration and facet joint osteoarthritis on the segmental flexibility of the lumbar spine. Spine 25:3036–3044
8. Gibson JN, Grant IC, Waddell G (1999) The Cochrane review of surgery for lumbar disc prolapse and degenerative lumbar spondylosis. Spine 24: 1820–1832
9. Goupille P, Jayson MI, Valat JP, Freemont AJ (1998) Matrix metalloproteinases: the clue to intervertebral disc degeneration? Spine 23:1612–1626
10. Graf H (1992) Lumbar instability. Surgical treatment without Fusion. Rachis 412:123–137
11. Grevitt MP, Gardner AD, Spilsbury J, Shackleford IM, Baskerville R, Pursell LM, Hassaan A, Mulholland RC (1995) The Graf stabilisation system: early results in 50 patients. Eur Spine J 4:169–175; [discussion p 135]
12. Hukins DW (1992) A simple model for the function of proteoglycans and collagen in the response to compression of the intervertebral disc. Proc R Soc Lond B Biol Sci 249:281–285
13. Krag MH, Seroussi RE, Wilder DG, Pope MH (1987) Internal displacement distribution from in vitro loading of human thoracic and lumbar spinal motion segments: experimental results and theoretical predictions. Spine 12:1001–1007
14. Lazennec JY, Ramare S, Arafati N, Laudet CG, Gorin M, Roger B, Hansen S, Saillant G, Maurs L, Trabelsi R (2000) Sagittal alignment in lumbosacral fusion: relations between radiological parameters and pain. Eur Spine J 9:47–55
15. McAfee PC (1999) Interbody fusion cages in reconstructive operations on the spine. J Bone Joint Surg Am 81: 859–880
16. McMillan DW, McNally DS, Garbutt G, Adams MA (1996) Stress distributions inside intervertebral discs: the validity of experimental "stress profilometry". Proc Inst Mech Eng [H]. 210: 81–87
17. McNally DS, Adams MA (1992) Internal intervertebral disc mechanics as revealed by stress profilometry. Spine 17:66–73
18. McNally DS, Shackleford IM, Goodship AE, Mulholland RC (1996) In vivo stress measurement can predict pain on discography. Spine 21:2580–2587
19. Mochida J, Toh E, Suzuki K, Chiba M, Arima T (1997) An innovative method using the Leeds-Keio artificial ligament in the unstable spine. Orthopedics 20:17–23
20. Mochida J, Suzuki K, Chiba M (1999) How to stabilize a single level lesion of degenerative lumbar spondylolisthesis. Clin Orthop 368:126–134
21. Moore RJ, Vernon-Roberts B, Fraser RD, Osti OL, Schembri M (1996) The origin and fate of herniated lumbar intervertebral disc tissue. Spine 21: 2149–2155
22. Nachemson A (1975) Towards a better understanding of low-back pain: a review of the mechanics of the lumbar disc. Rheumatol Rehabil 14:129–143
23. Nishida K, Kang JD, Suh JK, Robbins PD, Evans CH, Gilbertson LG (1998) Adenovirus-mediated gene transfer to nucleus pulposus cells. Implications for the treatment of intervertebral disc degeneration. Spine 23:2437–2442; [discussion 2443]
24. Polikeit A, Nolte L-P (2000) Factors affecting the behaviour of interbody cages in the lumbar spine – finite element analysis. Proceedings of the ISSLS Annual Meeting, Adelaide, 2000, p 215
25. Rajaratnam SS, Mueller M, Shepperd JAN, Mulholland RC (2002) Dynesis stabilization of the lumbo-sacral spine. Poster presentation presented at Britspine 2002, The Second Combined Meeting of the BSS BASS BCSS SBPR, Birmingham, 27 February – 1 March
26. Schofferman J, Slosar P, Reynolds J, Goldthwaite N, Koestler M (2001) A prospective randomized comparison of 270 degrees fusions to 360 degrees fusions (circumferential fusions). Spine 26:E207–212
27. Schultz A, Andersson G, Ortengren R, Haderspeck K, Nachemson A (1982) Loads on the lumbar spine. Validation of a biomechanical analysis by measurements of intradiscal pressures and myoelectric signals. J Bone Joint Surg Am 64:713–720
28. Sengupta DK, Guyer RD, Hochschuler S, Mulholland RC (1999) Fulcrum assisted soft stabilisation in the treatment of low back pain – a new concept. Proceedings of the ISSLS Annual Meeting, Hawaii, 1999, p 20
29. Sengupta DK, Webb JK, Mulholland RC (2001) Can soft stabilization in the lumbar spine unload the disc and retain mobility? A biomechanical study with fulcrum assisted soft stabilization on cadaver spine. Proceedings of the ISSLS Annual Meeting, Edinburgh, 2001, p 129
30. Simpson EK, Parkinson IH, Manthey B, Fazzalari NL (2001) Intervertebral disc disorganization is related to trabecular bone architecture in the lumbar spine. J Bone Miner Res 16:681–687
31. Smith D, McMurray N, Disler P (2002) Early intervention for acute back injury: can we finally develop an evidence-based approach? Clin Rehabil 16:1–11
32. Suzuki K, Mochida J, Chiba M, Kikugawa H (1999) Posterior stabilization of degenerative lumbar spondylolisthesis with a Leeds-Keio artificial ligament. A biomechanical analysis in a porcine vertebral model. Spine. 24:26–31
33. Whitecloud TS 3rd, Castro FP Jr, Brinker MR, Hartzog CW Jr, Ricciardi JE, Hill C (1998) Degenerative conditions of the lumbar spine treated with intervertebral titanium cages and posterior instrumentation for circumferential fusion. J Spinal Disord 11:479–486
34. Zdeblick TA (1993) A prospective, randomized study of lumbar fusion. Preliminary results. Spine 18:983–991

Timothy M. Ganey
Hans Joerg Meisel

A potential role for cell-based therapeutics in the treatment of intervertebral disc herniation

T.M. Ganey (✉)
6104 River Terrace,
Tampa, Florida 33604, USA
e-mail: Timganey@Tampabay.rr.com,
Tel.: +1-813-2328794,
Fax: +1-561-3650441

H.J. Meisel
Bergmannstrost-Klinik, Halle, Germany

Abstract Lower back pain and disc degeneration negatively affect quality of life and impose an enormous financial burden. An extensive body of scientific work has evolved that characterizes the disc, demonstrating spinal anatomy and morphology that contribute to risk and likely promote failure. Ultimately, matrix failure is responsible for mechanical failure, which in turn results in spinal compromise anatomically and subsequent pain. One intervening approach to breaking this sequence has been to repopulate the anatomy with autologous disc chondrocytes – cells capable of restoring the matrix and retaining the mechanical balance by which the disc functions. This strategy has been implemented both in patients and in animal models, and early results, although preliminary, support the premise as a positive approach.

Keywords Spine · Intervertebral disc · Intervertebral disc degeneration · Cell-based therapeutics · Tissue engineering

Introduction

The structure of the spine has been conserved in basic design across several classes of living organisms. Although inter-species variation accounts for a differing number of individual vertebrae, the metameric nature of spine has evolved to permit continued axial growth. Humans' uniqueness in upright posture accommodates an opportunity for unparalleled forelimb dexterity, but comes at the price of spine instability.

Spine degeneration and low back pain affects the adult population to a sufficient extent that personal risk should be considered only an ancillary basis of the etiology. This is not to discount previous studies validating genetic predisposition [1, 12, 20, 23] or disc nutrition [22] as factors in the degenerative process, but to suggest that the high prevalence reflects a myriad of yet-unidentified risks that effect similar symptoms. Over the course of a lifetime, the human disc undergoes marked changes in shape, volume, and composition – all factors that affect performance and mechanical function. Even in asymptomatic patients, 93% of individuals older than 60 years demonstrate evidence of degenerative change [4]. In another retrospective analysis of cadaver material, a comparable prevalence indicates degenerative anatomical change as a progressive, age-dependent phenomenon that is present in 97% of individuals who are 50 years old [15]. Ultimately, it is a loss of correct anatomical structure that potentiates disc herniation and leads to pain and the subsequent need for surgical intervention.

Numerous scientific studies have provided observations that lend to understanding the biochemistry and biomechanics of the disc itself, offering insights into structure-function relationships that attribute inclusive cause-effect relationships [5]. General agreement has it that intervertebral discs lose water over time, and in doing so reduce the functional capacity to resist axial loading [3]. What remains challenging is to intercept the water loss as a function of matrix binding, addressing composition and decomposition in terms of binding capacity, and ultimately to examine loading as an incendiary to shifting metabolic capacity. Knowing that intervertebral disc degeneration leads to slow but insidious desiccation and

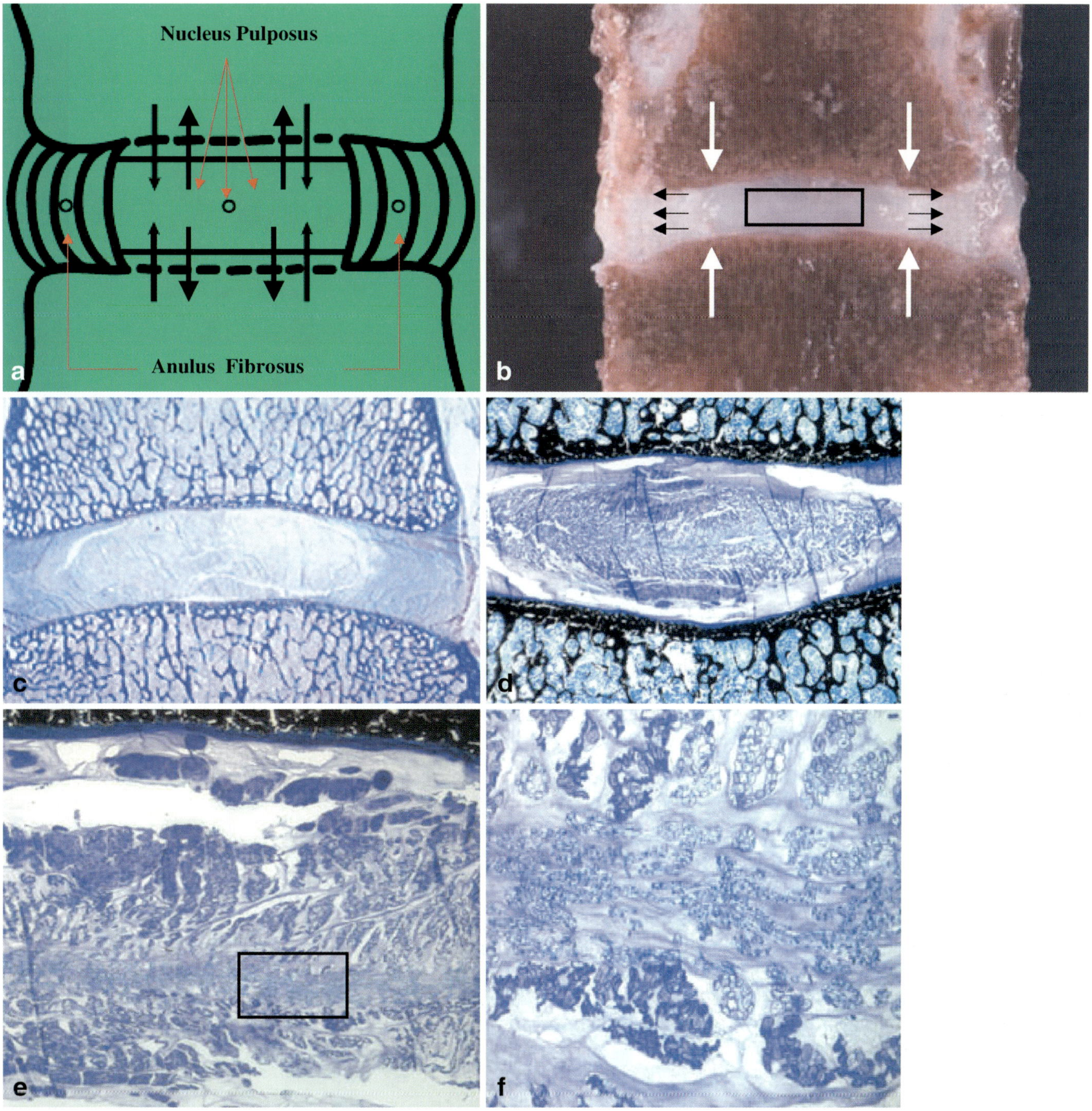

Fig. 1 **A** The intervertebral disc consists of two basic components: a central proteoglycan-rich nucleus pulposus and an outer series of concentric lamellae known collectively as the anulus fibrosis. The anular fibers insert directly into adjacent vertebral endplates, thereby constraining the central region of the intervertebral disc. **B** A cut section of the spine is represented. The *white arrows* indicate axial compression loads that the human spine would be subjected to. The *black lines* represent the lateral deforming direction of the nucleus and its central constraint within the anulus fibers. **C** Histology of the normal motion segment demonstrates the subchondral margins of adjacent vertebrae and the axial confinement imposed by a non-deformable vertebral body. **D** At higher magnification, variations in cell morphology within the nucleus can be seen (4×, MacNeal's Toluidine Blue). **E** Further magnification reveals different cell lines, and different morphologies within the nucleus (10×, MacNeal's Toluidine Blue). **F** The *area outlined in* ***E*** represents a central repository of nucleus cells which proliferate and reorient themselves in the direction of the axial load. These cells are capable of high matrix production, as indicated by the intense staining, and are also proliferative as clonal expansions within the nucleus material

eventual loss of morphology associated with the disc itself, the inherent challenge in seeking a remedy will be to recognize aspects of the causal condition and redress changes that will relieve symptoms and effect conditions that will maintain functional morphology. Although cells form only 1% of the adult disc tissue by volume, their role in balancing constitutive expression of matrix synthesis and metabolic turnover is vital. Most assessments of intervertebral disc failure have focused on degenerative change – changes in morphology that affect the biomechanical performance of the motion segment. In this consideration, mechanical failure is little more than a corollary of matrix structure, which in turn depends on balanced cell metabolism for efficient maintenance of the disc matrix. Given the value of cells to the metabolic health of the disc, one therapeutic strategy would be to either replace, regenerate, or in some other manner augment the intervertebral disc cell complement, with a goal of correcting matrix insufficiencies and restoring normal segment biomechanics. Understanding the basis for structure in the context of degeneration is critical to appreciating the potential value of cells as a means of therapy.

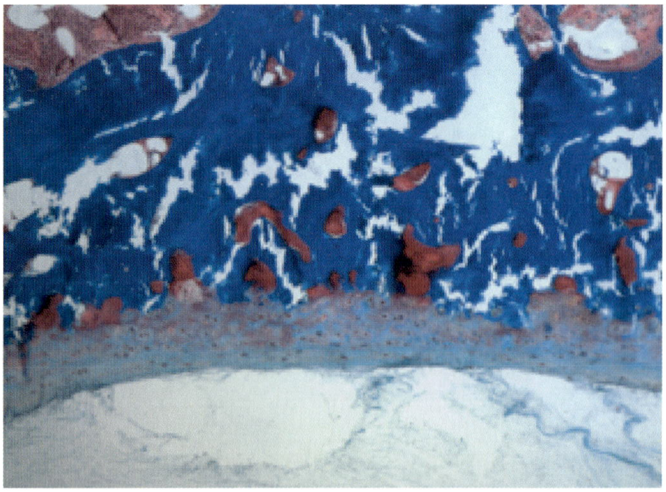

Fig. 2 The central subchondral interface and the hyaline cartilage covered endplate directly interface with the central nucleus pulposus (100×, Goldner tri-chrome)

Intervertebral disc gross structure

It is impossible to discuss an intervertebral disc without defining the integral unit of a motion segment. The term "motion segment" was coined to denote two vertebrae and the disc connecting them. Within the motion segment, each intervertebral disc is composed of two parts: a central, deformable nucleus pulposus, and an outer ring of connective tissue described as the anulus fibrosis (Fig. 1). Together the two components function to dissipate axial loading by using the tensile properties of collagen, the principal component of the anulus fibrosis. In balance the force exchange is efficient, coupling progressive recruitment of collagenous fibers radially in response to central deforming action of the nucleus. Within the context of the two components lies a more subtle balance, with anatomical differences between the two components – more a spectrum than an interface. Separate from these two main components lies the vertebral endplate of each vertebra, which itself has distinctions along its entire margin.

Anulus fibrosis

The anatomy of the disc is often described from its central structures to its peripheral components. While such descriptions respect the ontogeny of the development process, they fail to fully explain the basis of action or how imbalance results in tissue failure. The anulus fibrosis is characterized in the literature as a series of concentric laminae connecting two intervertebral discs [5]. The anulus inserts into the periphery of the superior and inferior vertebrae, isolating a central disc of the endplate that resembles articular cartilage in many regards. In almost every respect the anulus fibrosis is a ligament – connective tissue in composition connecting two bones in function. Ligaments insert into bone as series of distinct laminations, themselves varying in both collagen and mineral content as a continuum in transition [6].

The central disc of cartilage underlying the nucleus pulposus resembles in every respect articular cartilage at the end of long bones (Fig. 2). This central cartilage demonstrates an interface with the subchondral base different from that of the areas where the anulus fibers insert. As more an articular than a fibrous cartilage, a key difference of the central plate is that it has a lower density of types I and III collagen, instead featuring type II, a nonfibrillar cartilage [8, 17]. Being more an articular component (biomechanical buffer) than an interface for tendon insertion, the central region is less calcified and has a thinner subchondral plate. These variations are important in the context of the intervertebral disc, and the nucleus in particular, because of its metabolic demands and its structural morphology.

Nucleus pulposus

The nucleus pulposus is the central component of the intervertebral disc, demonstrating a high matrix to cell ratio as the most striking feature. This central area exists without blood supply, innervation, or lymph drainage in the adult spine, although during development it has both. Chondrocytes make a matrix that is highly charged due to its proteoglycan content, thereby creating a tissue capable of structuring water. This biochemical formulation offers the central matrix a unique capacity, in essence creating a hydraulic space of fixed volume and alterable dimension. When this sphere is loaded axially, it carries with it the capacity to deform the anulus on account of the axial force, progressively recruiting additional fiber in an attempt to retain water. When the loading history of the spine matches the force, the mechanical function is elastic, restoring and retaining previous morphometric and biochemical balances.

Unfortunately, it is not always possible either for the human body as a whole, or for the intervertebral disc, to maintain the ideal hydration-force balance. When forces exceed the balance of tissue design, then either water is extruded, or tissue fails. Several reports have confirmed the differences in disc height that accompany enhanced or prolonged loading [10, 11, 13]. During sustained imbalance over an extended period of time, force imbalance results in a slow ebbing of water content, focal increases of charge within the extracellular matrix, and reduced metabolic production. These long-term sustained imbalances result in a loss of disc height, and a change in the basic paradigm of structure-function efficiency. Short-term variations in metabolic process are correctable, in many cases full disc height recovers overnight [14].

Sustained loss of water, however, changes the height of the disc, and results in not only a loss of matrix, but of the nucleus cells responsible for making the matrix. As the peripheral anulus fibers are capable of holding less water than the central proteoglycan matrix of the nucleus, water flows centrally from the periphery in addition to flowing across the subchondral endplate directly into the nucleus. Articular cartilage is extremely functional as an aqueous sieve, thereby precipitating a lake of calcium that accompanies relative levels of hydration.

In a somewhat destructive cycle, exaggerated loading first distends and then pushes water peripherally. If not replenished, the imbalance of water alters the compression-extension balance, and peripheral anulus fibers that developed with a load history to accommodate tension are placed into a physical condition of axial compression. Previous studies show that tension promotes homeostasis in tendons and ligaments, and that a reduction in tension or a condition of slack promotes collagenase expression [16]. The outcome of the imbalance then has repercussions separate from the mere loss of water, effecting morphology changes that in turn change metabolic properties.

Vertebral endplate thickening has been suggested to be part and party to nutritional imbalance, reducing water flow into the intervertebral disc and thereby contributing to a "nutritional desert" [21]. Considering the basic chemistry of diffusion and osmosis, water tends to flow from areas of higher concentration to areas of lower concentration, diluting ions to equilibrium. In that consideration, water should flow into the nucleus and the anulus and the subchondral vertebral plate should thin to effect more rapid transport of water. The reduction in water flowing into the disc and the accompanying thickening of bone instead supports the hypothesis that the reduction in water content in the anulus and the nucleus functionally shifts the interstitial precipitation point of calcium, leaving a lake of mineral in the wake of receding water concentration. Tide marks and changing tidemarks are always found more adjacent to the subchondral bone than near the surface of hyaline cartilage.

As the subchondral base thickens, the ability for water to be differentially shed through the endplate changes, and water moving from the nucleus to the anulus as a means of force dissipation occurs in a more constrained environment. Respecting the fact that the ligamentous anulus is a strong fibrous material, it will yield to focused peripheral force before the mineralized endplate will fail in shear. Basing anulus response on known outcomes in ligaments in other areas of the body, the anulus fibrosis would be predictably weaker, less stiff, more compliant and less viscous, resulting in elongation and potentiating ligament failure [7].

This model accounts for herniation of the nucleus peripherally, rather than a pushing of the nucleus through the endplate. Extrusion of the nucleus through the endplate does occur and is defined by the morphology and pathology of the Schmorl node, a condition prevalent but masked by the lack of nerve receptors in the central cartilaginous disc. Separate from the topic in this discussion, these perforations of the endplate have been noted in 46% of patients seen at autopsy [25]. Few were symptomatic, and although all nodes were detectable by radiographic study, such screening would be an unacceptable procedure for unsymptomatic individuals.

In the early stages of mechanical force, particularly in intervertebral discs with limited degeneration, the weakest component is the subchondral plate. Under sustained imbalance, anulus degeneration accompanied by subchondral thickening shifts the most susceptible anatomy to the anular fibers. The perceptible difference to the patient is immediate, with the nerve roots anything but a benign interface for the bulging anulus. Nuclear herniation through the anulus is generally posterolateral, and the juncture of nerve and nucleus results in pain. This important distinction of functional anatomy is critical to formulating attempts to reconstitute the anatomy, remove pain, and restore function to the spinal motion segment.

Nucleus replacement (cell-based therapeutics)

Failure of the disc results from overloading, and the type of failure is closely correlated with the nature of the force. Chronic forces will result in slow but sure desiccation, in many cases paralleled by "pains of aging" rather than sudden and disabling lower back problems. In incidences of acute overload [cartilage is velocity dependent (viscoelastic)], the force (nucleus extrusion) will be neutralized either through the plate or through the peripheral anulus fibers. Knowing that the hydraulic has a limited capacity for compression, tissues with lesser water content will yield before the more hydraulic tissue deforms.

Understanding the basis for disc failure, the goal must be two-fold: first to regain disc height to reduce the axial nerve compression and restore the tissue dynamics of the anulus, and second, to reconstitute the central nucleus with a matrix that can hold water and effect a different balance of nutritional flow. One technology that has emerged in this context is the hydrogel implant, or prosthetic disc nucleus (PDN). The PDN was designed to restore disc height, and to fluctuate in diurnal flow, conceptually the same as the human disc. It is composed of a hydrogel within a biologically inert jacket, and is surgically implanted in pairs. With rigid dimensions, it does not fully simulate the plasticity of the original disc in terms of its deformability, and its size requires a fairly invasive procedure. Instead of restoring height with an amorphic prosthetic, a second goal and consideration has been to engender the nucleus with a complement of its original cells, and to allow these cells to reconstitute a matrix that will change the metabolic balance as well as restore disc kinematics.

Autologous disc chondrocyte transplantation (ADCT)

Disc chondrocyte cultivation has been approved as a therapeutic drug in Germany since 1997. German law permits physicians to address clinical projects from the purview of their own experience, and regulates therapy-controlled studies rather than requiring prospective clinical trials. Such a regulatory architecture permits promising technologies to be implemented at a faster pace, and offers a current basis for the most advanced interpretation to date. Applications that show clinical promise continue under carefully controlled clinical parameters so that they will meet standards of acceptable practice for worldwide clinical treatment. The procedure for ADCT is straightforward when surgical discectomy is indicated for the treatment of disc herniation and spinal cord or nerve root compression. Instead of fixing the tissue in formalin, sectioning, identifying, and storing the information, the material recovered in surgery is sent for tissue culturing, and returned at a later date for percutaneous transplantation. As one might suspect, it is impossible to differentiate the tissue recovered in surgery into either all nucleus or all anulus (Fig. 3). It is clear from published studies that co-culture actually enhances the matrix production and accelerates the proliferation rate of nucleus pulposus cells [19]. The standard interval between discectomy and transplantation has yet to be optimized, but it is important to affirm anulus healing prior to transplanting cells. Our experience has determined that a time interval of 8–12 weeks has been acceptable to the outcome.

Cells are carefully cultured under conditions of good manufacturing practices, ensuring that autologous cells are returned to the patient and that process validation is accountable from harvest to return. This is a critical aspect of the cell process, ensuring correct receipt and optimal conditions for cell growth and phenotypic maintenance.

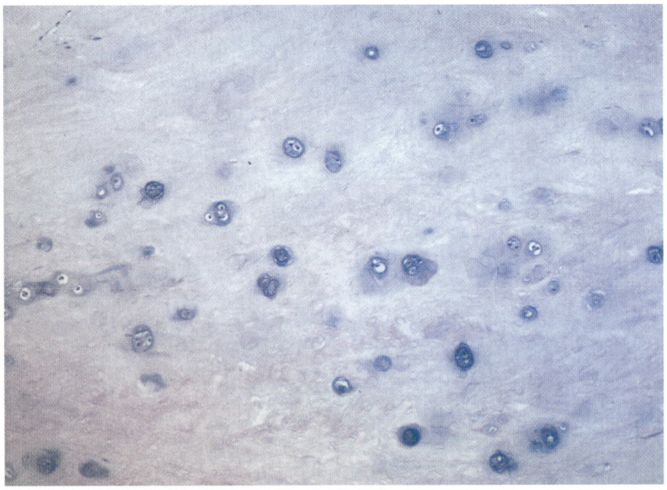

Fig. 3 Tissue removed during discectomy has cells that resemble both nucleus and anulus within its matrix (250×, H&E)

The first studies to look at the feasibility of the procedure have been performed in Switzerland and Germany. Patients participating in the studies were carefully selected to reflect acute traumatic herniation, in effect to still have active and viable nuclear morphology, albeit it displaced posteriorly as a herniated disc. Although the groups are small, patients from the Swiss group have responded in a positive fashion, remaining asymptomatic several years following transplantation. Magnetic resonance (MR) images of two of the patients demonstrates a restructuring of the spine and a lack of Modic changes at the subchondral plate (Fig. 4). Signal intensity associated with substantial matrix enhancement is not apparent, but considering the extent of damage that accompanies surgical dissection, the repair and conformation of the signal is acceptable. A lack of pain and functional recovery are the chief measures of clinical efficacy, and were demonstrated by all patients participating.

A second study was instituted and performed at the Bergmannstrost Clinic in Halle, Germany, by one of the authors (H.J.M.). Similar to the first study, the goal of this project was to develop confidence that the technology was sound in principle, and could achieve symptomatic relief and functional recovery. Patients in this study were evaluated clinically and also by MRI, demonstrating anatomical recovery in some cases with heightened nuclear signal. Moreover, prior to the cells being transplanted, the internal pressure of the disc was evaluated (Fig. 5). An inline pressure gauge was developed specifically for this study, to provide an assurance that the cells would be placed into a fixed space, and not leak through another

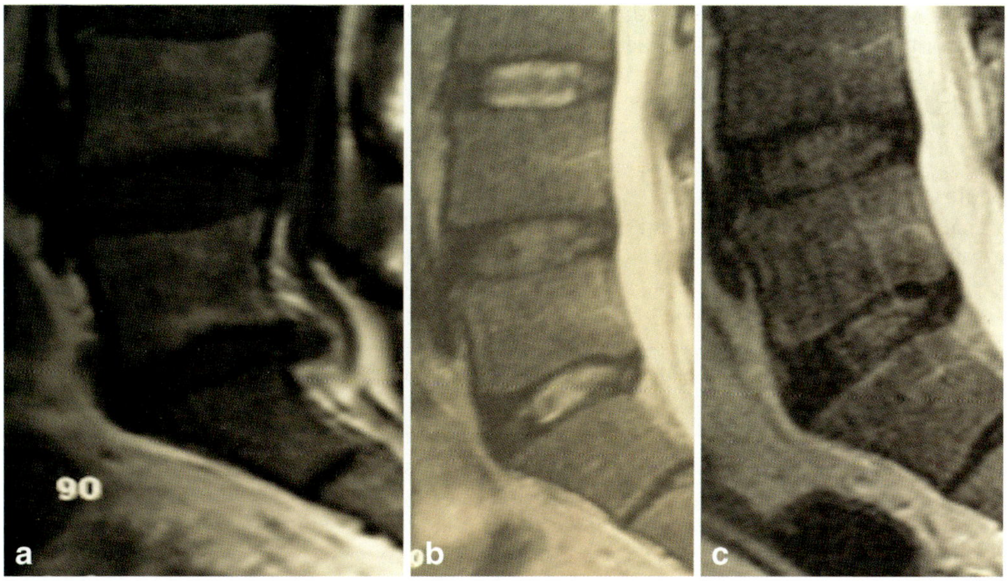

Fig. 4A-C **A** 38-year-old woman undergoing discectomy. **A** At presentation, **B** 15 months after transplantation, and **C** 30 months after transplantation

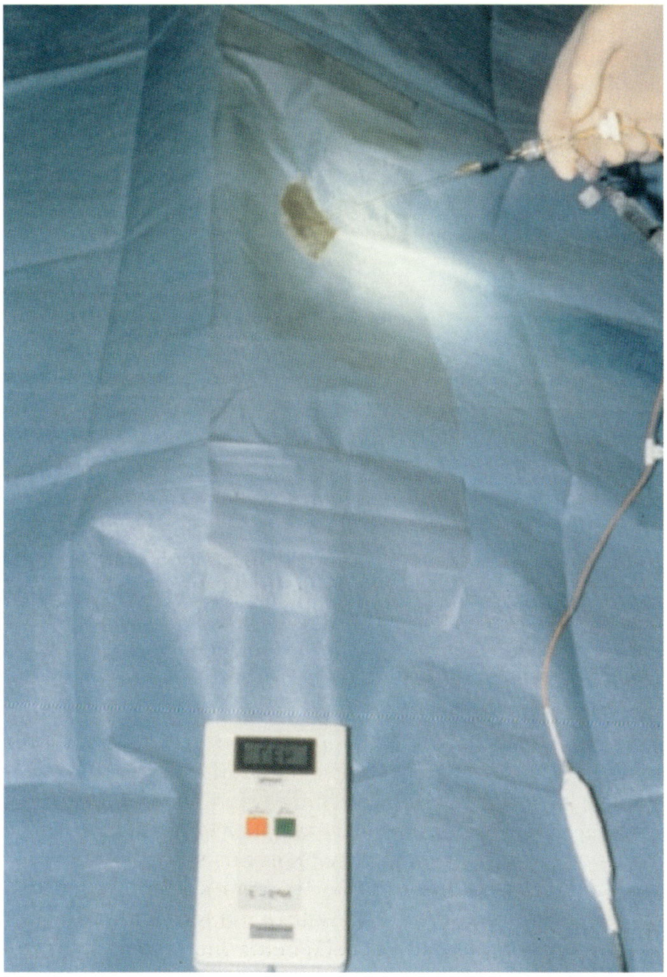

Fig. 5 Pressure was measured prior to inserting the cells to ensure that cells would not leak. Normal saline was injected to a pressure of 600 mm Hg for 3 min, and if no decay of pressure occurred, the saline was withdrawn and the cells were transplanted

fissure in another area of the anulus under mechanical load. Pressure was held for 3 min, and only after an assurance that no pressure decay had occurred were the cells transplanted.

What remains encouraging from both of these studies is the sustained symptomatic relief that the patients have attained from this procedure. Encouraged by the results in these clinical treatments, additional studies were designed to look more closely at the biological mechanism underlying the apparent surgical success. Studies were performed in canine models to examine biological healing by radiography, histology, and MRI along a 1-year time course, and using labeled cells to demonstrate the cells responsible for the activity.

Canine study

A study was designed to directly show the effect of the cells, contrasting a degeneration model with an area in the same dog that had been treated by chondrocyte transplantation. All transplantations were done during a single 2-day session. In all animals vertebrae L1–L4 served as the experimental site, with disc levels L1-L2 and L3-L4 serving as biopsy sites and L2-L3 acting as the control level. Cells were transplanted into L3-L4, but not into L1-L2, to demonstrate the effects of cell transplantation over spontaneous healing.

Several variables in this study provided a strong basis for accepting the results as positive. It was impossible to standardize the debridement of the tissue during the sampling for the biopsy. Individual dogs demonstrated different growth curves for their chondrocytes in culture and differences in the number of cells that were transplanted, both in indexed number and in fluid volume that could be injected. Additionally, some dogs received their trans-

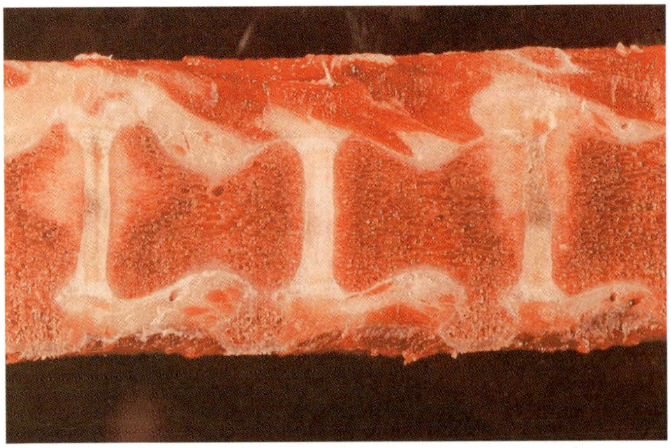

Fig. 6 Appearance of tissue grossly 3 months after transplantation. From *left to right* L4–L1. Note the marked difference in level L3-L4, which received cells, compared to the changes in tissue at the level that did not receive the cells

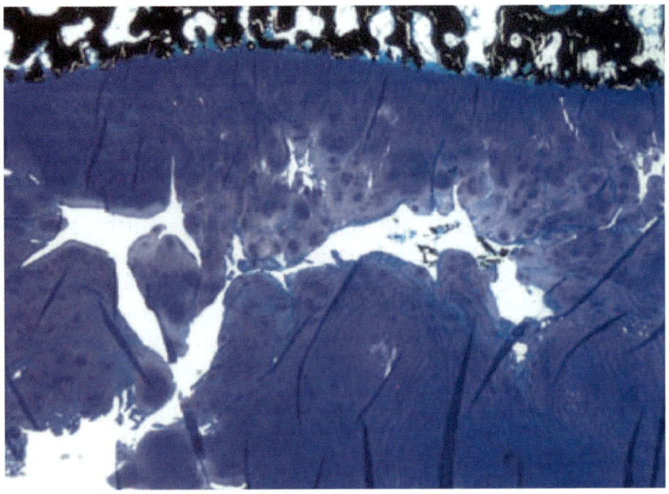

Fig. 7 Cells that had been transplanted at 12 months demonstrated abundant matrix formation, although the morphology was not directly comparable to normal nucleus pulposus (40×, MacNeil's Toluidine Blue)

plantation at 5 weeks, while others received cell therapy at 12 weeks. The goal was to better understand the interval in setting a time to surgery and the value of anular healing in the success of the cell therapy. Several conclusions could be drawn from this study, but the positive change in tissue morphology with time was the most encouraging aspect.

At the 3-month timepoint, much of the matrix was still in flux from the biopsy procedure. This was true whether cells were transplanted at 5 weeks or held until 12 weeks, as was the case for all the autologous cell transplantations (Fig. 6). The biopsy procedure was particularly aggressive, and resulted in a model that related more to damage than to degeneration. However, in this model the presence of cells positively affected the development of a clear subchondral margin.

The surgical biopsy was a causal factor in osteophyte formation, and was present in all animals on the lateral aspect of the vertebral articulation and therefore considered a response to periosteal inflammation. Differences in the amount of bone formation varied with the level that had received the cells. Intervertebral discs receiving cells displayed less osteophyte formation.

During the remodelling process of the vertebral endplate, marrow fibrosis was a common occurrence. This was not unexpected, as both bone remodelling and inflammatory responses to surgical injury are known to increase tissue and matrix permeability. Intervertebral disc levels that had received cells showed a tendency for less scarring, evident as a deep-yellow color grossly in intervertebral discs that had not received cells. Histology supporting chondrocyte transplantation offered evidence that nucleus pulposus-like cells were within the region of the injection, were surrounded by matrix, and exhibited phenotypic characteristics consistent with normal cell morphology (Fig. 7).

Disc height varied considerably, from obvious collapse in some animals that had not received cells, to a slight diminution despite the addition of transplanted chondrocytes. In some cases, thicker intervertebral discs actually displayed poorer morphology, but at some point function and form must mediate mechanical and morphometric balance in active locomotion. Disc height could be shown to have a positive trend associated with cell transplantation, but the larger the number of variables, including cell number injected, the more difficult it became to see the positive trend. The longer the dogs were examined (clinical durability), the greater the healing and the stronger the differences between the level transplanted and that left to degenerate.

All of the dogs gained a separation of the subchondral plate and clear delineation of the separate morphologies. In no cases was a morphotypic "nucleus pulposus" generated, but in every case cells comparable to and appropriate for consideration as chondrons could be found. These cells displayed characteristic territorial matrix surrounding each group of cells. No evidence of necrotic change was present. The lack of active vascularization, formation of bone in the intervertebral space, and the general "normal" gain of the matrix suggests that active remodeling is guided by some innate patterning principle capable of effecting an anatomical basis separate from either cell- or matrix-directed regenerative change.

Progressive changes in regenerative potential could be seen through changes over time in the various aspects of the healing process, e.g. marrow vascularity, sclerotic changes in bone, disc height, inflammatory cellularity. At the 3-month time point, much of the matrix was still undergoing changes in response to the original biopsy procedure and the on-going mechanical demands (and changing demands at that). This was true whether cells were transplanted at 5 weeks or held until 12 weeks. With the exception of a single dog, no gross instability was evident. It seems that subchondral resolution was the primary positive change that was positively associated with time. Accompanying the formation and clear margins of the subchondral bone, marrow fibrosis seen at early analysis time points no longer factored in the potential for vascularizing and fusing the disc. Unfortunately, osteophyte formation was also associated with increasing time following transplantation. Even though osteophytes were stimulated by aggressive debriding of tissue, they did not interfere with matrix deposition or in the basic pathology of the disc. Over time, it would be expected that lateral bridging would impart a bias to mechanical loading, which in turn will precipitate biochemical changes, that will likely affect both matrix composition and matrix performance.

What appears to be the ultimate driver is the initial damage sustained in taking the biopsy. Second most important is the time over which the animal and spinal level in particular has to heal. Finally, no evidence could be found that would indicate that time to transplant could be positively correlated with outcome.

Models of cell transplantation

Other considerations of nucleus replacement have taken into account the interdependence and potential importance of anulus cells in stimulating nucleus cells in culture [19]. Using a rabbit model, and measuring cell proliferation as a function of DNA synthesis, Okuma and co-workers reported that co-culturing stimulated cell proliferation, inhibited degeneration, and enhanced the synthesis of type-II collagen in the matrix. Additionally, they were able to show that increases in type-II collagen were coupled with BrdU incorporation of the transplanted cells. They cautiously interpret these findings as showing that the positive results of cell proliferation in the presence of disc degeneration do not always indicate regeneration. Their results differ slightly from those of Wang et al., who concluded that nucleus pulposus cells are insensitive to culture conditions [24].

Cell culture in alginate, three-dimensional matrix is engaging for several reasons, not the least of which is the limitations the cross-linked matrix imposes on cell proliferation. Achieving a tissue in phenotype consistent with the in situ nature of the cells is attractive for obvious reasons, most critically the ability of cells in alginate to reflect collagen and proteoglycan synthesis that mirrors gene expression in disc tissue [2]. While placement continues to be an issue needing resolution, it does appear that transplanted cells can retain a phenotypic appearance and attain cellular capacity in vivo.

Other studies have demonstrated the sand rat as an effective model of spontaneous disc degeneration and have shown histochemical and morphologic changes to support cell transplantation [9] and maintenance of disc height and significant differences in matrix expression. The propensity for spontaneous degeneration and the general poor health of this animal relative to its kidney function and water transport axis offers two sentiments for consideration. The first, of course, is the challenge in demonstrating active regeneration in an animal model that has been shown to have active endocrine bias (diabetes) and poor kidney and water shunting. Being able to demonstrate active recovery against a gradient of failure offers strong assurances of potential success in other systems.

The second point, and a critical one, is the fact that small rodents actively grow throughout their lives, maintain an active apophyseal architecture at the end of each spine, and, as such, have inner dampening through the vertebral body growth plate. This anatomy changes the dynamic of axial loading compared to the humans', and imparts some bias in considering the results. Still, this and other studies in rats and lagomorphs [18] demonstrate the capacity of cell transplantation to stave off further degeneration, where that in itself may be a mediator of a protective advantage in the timeframe of effective remedy.

All of the cell studies demonstrate a capacity to buffer degeneration, those cells placed with attendant matrix demonstrating a greater capacity. Cells appear to be viable, retain a capacity for proliferation, and demonstrate an ability to make appropriate matrix, to undergo gene expression consistent with the phenotypic demands of the anatomy, and, in our hands at least, to facilitate clinical durability.

A capacity for improvement will be the hallmark of the acceptability of this technology as a clinical therapeutic. At the current time, autologous transplant in controlled conditions presents the least challenging option to the clinic. It complies with the standard of least manipulation of a cell line, imposes little chance of immune rejection, and, as a terminally differentiated lineage, also puts an emphasis on cells and intention. Still to be proven is whether the tissue morphology over time will retain the new form and to what extent cells could be given as a prophylactic to reduce vertebral compromise before it becomes symptomatic. The human spine is most unusual, and the scientific desire for remedy strong. Under these conditions, the potential for regenerative repair of the motion segment will become a contending option for stabilization procedures, which today offer fusion as an option to unstable and painful motion.

References

1. Annunen S, Paassilta P, Lohiniva J, Perala M, Pihlajamaa T, Karppinen J, et al (1999) An allele of COL9A2 associated with intervertebral disc disease. Science 285:409–412
2. Baer AE, Wang JY, Kraus VB, et al (2001) Collagen gene expression and mechanical properties of intervertebral disc cell-alginate cultures. J Orthop Res 19:2–10
3. Bibby SRS, Jones DA, Lee RB, Yu J, Urban JPG (2001) The pathophysiology of the intervertebral disc. Joint Bone Spine 68:537–542
4. Boden SD, Davis DO, Dina TS, Mark AS, Wiesel S (1990) Abnormal magnetic resonance scans of the lumbar spine in asymptomatic subjects: a prospective investigation. J Bone Joint Surg Am 72:1178–1184
5. Doers TM, Kang JD (1999) The biomechanics and biochemistry of disc degeneration. Curr Opin Orthop 10: 117–121
6. Frank C (1997) The biology of ligament reconstruction. In: Niwa S, Yoshino S, Kurosaka M (eds) Reconstruction of the knee joint. Springer, Tokyo, pp 7–27
7. Gelberman R, Goldberg V, An K-N, Banes A (1998) Tendon. In: Woo Sl-Y, Buckwalter JA (eds) Injury and repair of musculoskeletal soft tissue. American Academy of Orthopaedic Surgeons, Park Ridge, pp 5–40
8. Ghosh P, Bushell GR, Taylor TFK, Akeson WH (1977) Collagens, elastins and noncollagenous protein of the intervertebral disc. Clin Orthop 129:124–132
9. Gruber HE, Johnson T, Norton HJ, Hanley EN Jr (2002) The sand rat model for disc degeneration: radiologic characterization of age-related changes: cross-sectional and prospective analyses. Spine 27:230–234
10. Hutton WC, Elmer WA, Boden SD, Hyon S, Toribatake Y, Tomita K, Hair GA (1999) The effect of hydrostatic pressure on intervertebral disc metabolism. Spine 24:1507–1515
11. Hutton WC, Ganey TM, Elmer WA, Kozlowska E, Ugbo JL, Doh ES, Whitesides TE Jr (2000) Does long-term compressive loading on the intervertebral disc cause degeneration? Spine 25:2993–3004
12. Kawaguchi Y, Osada R, Kanamori M, Ishihara H, Ohmori K, Matsui H, et al (1999) Association between an aggrecan gene polymorphism and lumbar disc degeneration. Spine 24:2456–2460
13. Lotz JC, Colliou OK, Chin JR, Duncan NA, Liebenberg E (1998) Compression-induced degeneration of the intervertebral disc: An in vivo mouse model and finite-element study. Spine 21: 2493–2506
14. Malko JA, Hutton WC, Fajman WA (2002) An in vivo MRI study of the changes in volume (and fluid content) of the lumbar intervertebral disc after overnight bed rest and during an 8-hour walking protocol. J Spinal Disord Tech 15:157–163
15. Miller JA, Schmatz C, Schultz AB (1988) Lumbar disc degeneration: correlation with age, sex, and spine level in 600 autopsy specimens. Spine 13: 173–178
16. Nabeshima Y, Grood ES, Sakurai A, Herman JH (1996) Uniaxial tension inhibits tendon collagen degradation by collagenase in vitro. J Orthop Res 14: 123–130
17. Nerlich AG, Schleicher ED, Boos N (1997) Immunhistologic markers for age-related changes of human lumbar intervertebral discs. Spine 22:2781–2795
18. Nomura T, Mochida J, Okuma M, Nishimura K, Sakabe K (2001) Nucleus pulposus allograft retards intervertebral disc degeneration. Clin Orthop 389:94–101
19. Okuma M, Mochida J, Nishimura K, Sakabe K, Seiki K (2000) Reinsertion of stimulated pulposus cells retards intervertebral disc degeneration: an in vitro and in vivo experimental study. J Orthop Res 18:988–997
20. Paassilta P, Lohiniva J, Goring HH, Perala M, Raina SS, Karppinen J, et al (2000) Identification of a common risk factor for lumbar disk disease. JAMA 285:1843–1849
21. Roberts S, McCall IW, Menage J, Haddaway MJ, Eisenstein SM (1997) Does the thickness of the vertebral subchondral bone reflect the composition of the intervertebral disc? Eur Spine J 6:385–389
22. Urban JP, Holm S, Maroudas A, Nachemson A (1977) Nutrition of the intervertebral disk. An in vivo study of solute transport. Clin Orthop 129:101–114
23. Videman T, Leppavuori J, Kaprio J, Battie MC, Gibbons L, Peltonen L, Koskenvuo M (1998) Intragenic polymorphisms of the vitamin D receptor gene associated with intervertebral disc degeneration. Spine 23:2477–2485
24. Wang JY, Baer AE, Kraus VB, Setton LA (2001) Intervertebral disc cells exhibit differences in gene expression in alginate and monolayer culture. Spine 26:1747–1752
25. Yasuma T, Saito S, Kihara K (1988) Schmorl's nodes. Correlation of X-ray and histological findings in postmortem specimens. Acta Pathol Jpn 38:723–733

M. Alini
P. J. Roughley
J. Antoniou
T. Stoll
M. Aebi

A biological approach to treating disc degeneration: not for today, but maybe for tomorrow

M. Alini (✉) · J. Antoniou · M. Aebi
Orthopaedic Research Laboratory,
Division of Orthopaedic Surgery,
McGill University, MUHC-RVH site,
687 Pine Avenue, Room L4.70,
Montreal H3A 1A1, Montreal, Canada
e-mail: mauro@orl.mcgill.ca,
Tel.: +1-514-8421231/35380,
Fax: +1-514-8431699

P.J. Roughley
Genetics Unit,
Shriners Hospital for Children,
McGill University, Montreal, Canada

T. Stoll
Mathys Medical, Bettlach, Switzerland

M. Alini
AO Research Institute, Davos, Switzerland

Abstract The intervertebral disc unites the vertebrae in the spine, providing the flexibility required for bending and twisting and resisting the compression inflicted by gravity when in an upright posture. The discs have a complex structure, with the outer annulus fibrosus having lamellae of organized collagen fibrils and the inner nucleus pulposus having a more random collagen organization and an abundance of aggregating proteoglycans. This composite nature endows the disc with both the tension-resisting properties of a ligament and the compression-resisting properties of articular cartilage. Unfortunately, disc structure and function does not remain optimal throughout life, but undergoes progressive degeneration, commencing in the young adult, and is particularly evident in the nucleus pulposus. With time, disc degeneration may result in clinical symptoms, such as low back pain, and require medical intervention. Such treatment may involve removal of the offending disc by surgery rather than its repair, which would be the preferred course of action. In the near future, current bioengineering techniques may offer the possibility of repairing the damaged disc, if an engineered tissue with the appropriate functional properties can be generated to augment the ailing disc. In this report, we summarized our recent results, in which disc cells were implanted into a scaffold of collagen and hyaluronan, or entrapped into a chitosan gel, and growth factors were used to modulate matrix synthesis in an attempt to produce a tissue with a similar molecular composition to native nucleus pulposus tissue.

Keywords Intervertebral disc · Degeneration · Repair · Scaffolds · Growth factors

Introduction

Intervertebral discs are characterized by their abundant extracellular matrix and low cell density, coupled with an absence of blood vessels, lymphatics, and nerves in all but the most peripheral annulus layers. In many respects, this absence leaves the disc prone to degeneration, because the cells have a large extracellular matrix to maintain without nociceptive feedback to limit and detect damage, and no source of repair through the vasculature.

Intervertebral discs are not uniform in composition, but consist of two clearly distinct regions. The outer annulus fibrosus is a fibrocartilage, and contains concentric lamellae rich in collagen, whereas the inner nucleus pulposus is a less structured gelatinous substance rich in proteoglycans. Degeneration and age-related changes in both the biochemical composition and structure of each component of the intervertebral disc have been widely reported [5, 14, 37, 40, 49]. As discs degenerate, the nucleus pulposus becomes more consolidated and fibrous, and is less clearly demarcated from the annulus fibrosus. Focal defects appear in the cartilage endplate, and there is a decrease in the number of layers of the annulus with an increase in thickness and spacing of the collagen fibrils [38]. Degeneration causes decreased hydration, especially in the nucleus [5]. Water content in the nucleus pulposus drops from about 90% of the tissue wet-weight in the infant to less than 70% in the elderly [5, 21]. In the annulus fibrosus, the water content remains relatively constant with age, accounting for approximately 60–70% of the tissue wet-weight [5, 21].

Collagen represents about 15–20% of the nucleus, and 65–70% of the annulus dry-weight [5, 17, 18]. At least seven distinct collagen types have been identified in the intervertebral disc, types I, II, III, V, VI, IX and XI. The annulus fibrosus of the intervertebral disc has been reported to contain all these collagen types, whereas the nucleus pulposus contains only types I, II, VI and IX collagen [1, 6, 7, 8, 17, 18, 62]. In addition, type X collagen has been shown to be present in discs with histomorphological alterations consistent with disc degeneration [3, 11]. Types I and II collagen constitute about 80% of the collagens in the intervertebral disc [5, 17]. Although the other collagen types identified in the disc account for a smaller proportion of the total collagen, they may make a very significant contribution to the overall function of the tissue. Recent work has shown that type II collagen degradation in the human lumbar intervertebral disc is increased with age and degeneration, and in parallel, the cell synthetic capacity is strongly suppressed with aging and degeneration [5, 20].

The trends in molecular abundance observed for collagen are reversed for proteoglycans, which represent approximately 50% of the dry-weight in the nucleus, but only 10–20% in the annulus [5, 17, 18]. The ability of the discs to resist compressive forces is largely due to their high content of the proteoglycan aggrecan and its ability to interact with hyaluronan [23, 25, 44]. Versican, another proteoglycan with the ability to interact with hyaluronan, has also been shown to be present within the intervertebral disc [58]. In addition to aggregating proteoglycans, the discs also contain decorin, biglycan, fibromodulin and lumican [29, 53, 57], which belong to the family of leucine-rich repeat proteoglycans. Ageing and degeneration of the discs are accompanied by a marked decrease in proteoglycan content in the nucleus and major alterations in proteoglycan structure [5, 12, 37].

The process of disc degeneration involves the destruction of structural proteins, including collagens and proteoglycans, within the extracellular matrix. It is generally agreed that proteinases play a major role in this process. One group of proteinases thought to be involved in the destruction of the disc matrix includes members of the matrix metalloproteinases (MMPs) [13, 19, 41, 43, 46, 47], particularly the collagenases and gelatinases. Once activated, collagenases can degrade types I and II collagen by cleavage in their helical domains, thus making these collagens susceptible to further enzymatic degradation by gelatinases. A second group of proteinases involved in matrix degradation includes members of the ADAM family [55], particularly those members with thrombospondin repeat motifs (ADAMTS) [59]. Two members of this subfamily are of particular importance because of their ability to specifically degrade aggrecan – aggrecanase-1 (ADAMTS4) and aggrecanase-2 (ADAMTS5). It has been shown that aggrecan cleavage products due to degradation by both the matrix metalloproteinases and aggrecanases are present in the intervertebral disc, suggesting that these enzymes are active in this tissue [56]. Unlike most other connective tissue cell types, little is known about the ability of disc cells to produce the different metalloproteinases. The only proteinase extracted directly from intervertebral disc appears to be a serine proteinase rather than a metalloproteinase, and it has properties similar to plasmin [15, 39]. However, human disc in organ culture has been shown to synthesize stromelysin (MMP3), which can become activated within the matrix [34]. MMP1, 2, 3, 7, 8 and 9 have also been shown to be present in degenerated human discs, suggesting a role for these metalloproteinases in disc degeneration [16, 52].

Mechanisms that may contribute to the age-related and/or degenerative changes of the disc include reduction in nutrient supply, diminished cell viability, loss of notochordal cells, cell senescence, cell apoptosis and genetic factors, which lead to biochemical alterations in the composition and structure of the extracellular matrix [2, 9, 10, 22, 24, 26, 48, 50, 51]. In addition, alterations in intervertebral disc structure are associated with, or aggravated by, mechanical factors [27, 28, 30, 31, 32, 36, 42, 45].

The degenerative disorders of the lumbar spine that require surgical intervention include herniated discs, spinal stenosis, degenerative spondylolisthesis, degenerative scoliosis, and degenerative disc disease. Among these, it is the treatment of idiopathic low back pain associated with lumbar degenerative disc disease that is the most controversial, and remains a challenge for the orthopaedic surgeon. Although, surgical procedures involving vertebral fusion produce a relatively good short-term clinical result in relieving pain, they alter the biomechanics of the spine and can lead to further degeneration of the discs at adjacent levels. In fact, the failure rate for lumbar fusions is estimated to be in the 20–40% range [60], and there is clinical and radiological evidence that spinal fusion leads to accelerated degeneration of the adjacent motion segment [33, 54].

Biological approach to repair disc damage

In general, surgical procedures try to remove rather than repair the problems associated with the degenerate intervertebral disc. Repair is, however, the ideal therapeutic approach, as it restores the normal structure and function of the intervertebral disc. We believe that future treatments will be able to effect biological repair of the damaged tissue by restoring it to a tissue of similar functional competence to the healthy native one. These are the dreams of all investigators involved in tissue engineering research, which extend from the "simple" injection of cells into the defect, to the futuristic aspiration of implanting an in-vitro-generated intact motion segment.

However, unless one is a true optimist, only two biological approaches to the treatment of disc degeneration are likely to become clinically available within the next 10 years. At the earlier stage of disc degeneration, injection of inhibitors of proteolytic enzymes or biological factors that stimulate cell metabolic activity (i.e. growth factors) can be foreseen, in order to slow down the degenerative process. Alternatively, when disc degeneration is confined to the nucleus, it is not unreasonable to propose that implantation or injection of a biomatrix embedded with cells will have the potential to restore functionality, and to retard further disc degeneration. In both cases, several problems need to be addressed before the two potential treatment modalities can be turned into clinical realities.

Our attempt to initiate biological repair of disc degeneration is based on the second of the above described approaches, namely the supplementation of the degenerated nucleus pulposus with cells seeded or embedded within a biomatrix. In principle, two types of biomatrices can be envisaged as scaffolds for use in disc repair. The first involves a preformed matrix into which isolated disc cells can be seeded, the composite maintained in vitro to attain an optimal composition, and the product then implanted into the degenerate disc. A second approach is to use a soluble polymer to which cells can be added and the mixture then injected into the disc where the scaffold can polymerize in situ. The advantages of the second approach are that the polymerized construct will conform precisely to the disc defect and that its clinical application is more straightforward, avoiding extensive surgical disruption of the annulus. However, the latter system is not readily compatible with prior in vitro culture of the construct, and requires that the cells produce an appropriate extracellular matrix in the nutritionally deprived disc milieu.

Our initial work focused on selecting a biomatrix that was able to support disc cell viability and phenotype, and allow the accumulation of an extracellular matrix rich in proteoglycans. Two biomatrices were selected: a collagen-hyaluronan scaffold from Orquest Inc. (Mountain View, Calif., USA), and a chitosan gel developed by Biosyntech (Laval, Quebec, Canada).

The first scaffold, composed of collagen and hyaluronan, was chosen because it mimicked the matrix by which disc cells are normally surrounded in their native environment [35]. Cells were isolated from the nucleus pulposus of coccygeal discs from mature bovine tails, and then imbibed by surface tension into the dry biomolecular scaffold consisting of cross-linked type I collagen and hyaluronic acid in a 9:1 ratio [61]. The cell-seeded matrices were maintained in culture on an orbital shaker in the presence of fetal calf serum (FCS) or a variety of growth factors (TGF-β1, bFGF and IGF-1). FCS was able to induce proteoglycan synthesis and produce a matrix that exhibited Safranin O staining. TGF-β1 produced similar levels of proteoglycan as FCS, whereas proteoglycan levels were reduced with either bFGF or IGF-1 (Fig. 1). Combinations of the growth factors did not greatly influence the effect of TGF-β1 alone. In contrast, cell division was stimulated to the greatest extent by the presence of IGF-1. It was also shown that by day 20 of culture the matrices not only contained aggrecan, but also the members of the small leucine-rich repeat proteoglycan family (decorin, biglycan, fibromodulin and lumican), as are found in normal disc, and that both type I and II collagen were being synthesized. However, while all the proteoglycans of a normal disc were present, it was evident that the construct was not able to retain the majority of the proteoglycans that the cells synthesized (Table 1). This resulted in a tissue that was biomechanically unable to counteract the compressive loads to which the disc is normally subjected. In future work in this area it will be important to establish conditions under

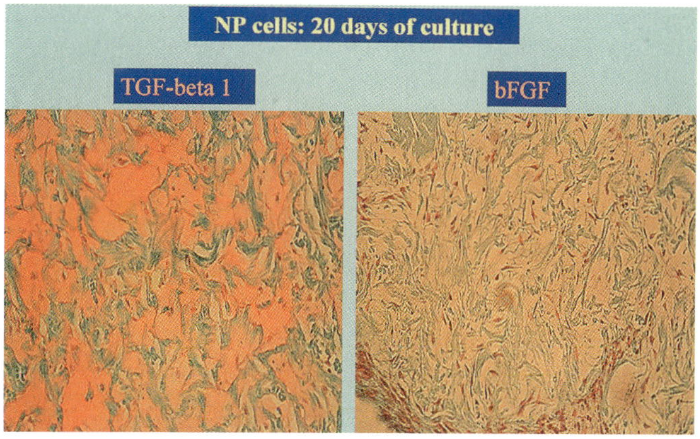

Fig. 1 Safranin O staining of nucleus pulposus cells seeded into collagen-hyaluronan scaffolds after 20 days of culture. Cells were stimulated with 10 ng/ml of TGF-β1 or 10 ng/ml of bFGF during the 20 days of culture

Table 1 Percentage of proteoglycans (PG) retained within the scaffolds and percentage of the total proteoglycans synthesized (medium + scaffolds) in vitro, compared to native mature bovine nucleus pulposus (NP) tissue. Disc cells were cultured in the presence of 10 ng/ml TGF-β1

Scaffolds	Results	
	% PG retained within the scaffold	% PG synthesized in vitro vs native NP tissue
Collagen-hyaluronan	25%	5%
Chitosan gel	75%	35%

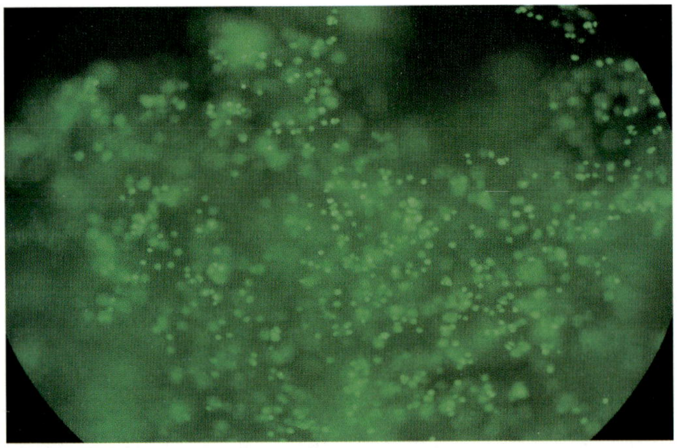

Fig. 2 Calcein AM and ethidium homodimer-1 staining of nucleus pulposus cells embedded into chitosan after 20 days of culture. Almost all the cells show a green fluorescence color, indicating excellent cell viability

which proteoglycan retention occurs efficiently, either by modifying the composition/structure of the scaffold or by treatment with more appropriate growth factors or biomechanical stimulation.

In a second approach, we used a chitosan-based polymer, which can be maintained as a soluble polymer at room temperature, and induced to gel at body temperature. Such a system might allow disc cells to be injected with the soluble polymer, which can then polymerize and entrap the cells in vivo (Fig. 2). Using identical experimental conditions to those described above for the collagen-hyaluronan scaffold, we found that the chitosan-based polymer was superior to the collagen-hyaluronan matrix, in both the synthesis and retention of proteoglycans (Table 1). This suggests that, at least in vitro, it should be feasible to generate a tissue with appropriate biochemical and mechanical properties similar to native nucleus pulposus. Thus, the disc cells can maintain their phenotype when cultured in a chitosan-based polymer, and over time are capable of producing a matrix with a proteoglycan content approaching that found in vivo [4].

Nevertheless, an important issue still requires to be addressed: the source of clinically useful cells. It is difficult to imagine that healthy nucleus cells could be obtained from the degenerated tissue that needs to be replaced. Two possible alternatives are conceivable: allogenic donor disc cells and/or autologous stem cells. While one can envisage the use of cells harvested from a donor, because of the immunologically privileged status of the nucleus pulposus, ethical considerations and the potential for spreading infectious diseases make the allogenic option less attractive. The use of stem cells as a source for generating nucleus pulposus cells would be the ideal choice, though at present there are no defined culture conditions where this differentiation process occurs. In addition, there are no well-defined cellular markers that can be used to identify disc cells and clearly distinguish them from other chondrocyte-like cells.

Furthermore, replacement of degenerate nucleus pulposus with a tissue engineered in vitro does not remove the reasons why the native tissue has degenerated. Indeed, one is attempting to repair without resolving the issue of what caused the original damage. So, what are the unidentified causes that lead to disc degeneration? Lack of an appropriate nutritional supply, and mechanical imbalance with excessive loading are possible explanatory mechanisms, together with genetic predisposition. Thus, more fundamental research investigating the possible mechanisms that lead to disc degeneration needs to be strongly supported by the scientific and industrial communities, if one is to be able to both initiate repair and prevent or retard subsequent degeneration.

Irrespective of these unresolved issues, our work does support the feasibility of generating a functional bioengineered disc matrix, and should provide optimism that biological therapy for disc degeneration may be a clinical reality in the not too distant future.

Acknowledgements We would like to thank Orquest Inc. (Mountain View, Calif., USA) for provision of the collagen/hyaluronan scaffold, and Biosyntech (Laval, Quebec, Canada) for the provision of the chitosan scaffold. Financial support was received from the Arthritis Society of Canada, the Canadian Arthritis Network and the AO/ASIF Foundation (Davos, Switzerland).

References

1. Adam M, Deyl Z (1984) Degenerated annulus fibrosus of the intervertebral disc contains collagen type II. Ann Rheum Dis 43:258–263
2. Aguiar DJ, Johnson SL, Oegema TR (1999) Notochordal cells interact with nucleus pulposus cells: regulation of proteoglycan synthesis. Exp Cell Res 246:129–137
3. Aigner T, Gresk-Otter KR, Fairbank JC, von der Mark K, Urban JP (1998) Variation with age in the pattern of type X collagen expression in normal and scoliotic human intervertebral discs. Calcif Tissue Int 63:262–268
4. Alini M, Li W, Aebi M, Roughley P, Hoemann C (2002) The use of disc cells embedded within a chitosan gel to repair degenerated intervertebral discs: a preliminary study. Canadian Connective Tissue Conference, 31 May–1 June, 2002, Sherbrooke, Quebec
5. Antoniou J, Steffen T, Nelson F, Winterbottom N, Hollander AP, Poole RA, Aebi M, Alini M (1996) The human lumbar intervertebral disc. Evidence for changes in the biosynthesis and denaturation of the extracellular matrix with growth, maturation, ageing, and degeneration. J Clin Invest 98:996–1003
6. Ayad S, Weiss JB (1986) Biochemistry of the intervertebral disc. In: Jayson MIV (ed) The lumbar spine and back pain. Pitmann, London, pp 100–137

7. Ayad S, Abedin MZ, Grundy SM, Weiss JB (1981) Isolation and characterisation of an unusual collagen from hyaline cartilage and intervertebral disc. FEBS Lett 123:195–199
8. Ayad S, Abedin MZ, Weiss JB, Grundy SM (1982) Characterisation of another short-chain disulphide-bonded collagen from cartilage, vitreous and intervertebral disc. FEBS Lett 139: 300–304
9. Ayotte D, Ito K, Tepic S, Perren SM (2000) Direction-dependent constriction flow in a poroelastic solid: the intervertebral disc valve. J Biomech Eng 122:587–593
10. Bernick S, Cailliet R (1982) Vertebral end-plate changes with aging of human vertebrae. Spine 7:97–102
11. Boos N, Nerlich AG, Wiest I, von der Mark K, Aebi M (1997) Immunolocalization of type X collagen in human lumbar intervertebral discs during ageing and degeneration. Histochem Cell Biol 108:471–480
12. Buckwalter JA (1995) Aging and degeneration of the human intervertebral disc. Spine 20:1307–1314
13. Chin JR, Murphy G, Werb Z (1985) Stromelysin, a connective tissue-degrading metalloendopeptidase secreted by stimulated rabbit synovial fibroblasts in parallel with collagenase. Biosynthesis, isolation, characterization, and substrates. J Biol Chem 260: 12367–12376
14. Cole TC, Ghosh P, Taylor TK (1986) Variations of the proteoglycans of the canine intervertebral disc with ageing. Biochim Biophys Acta 880:209–219
15. Cole TC, Melrose J, Ghosh P (1989) Isolation and characterisation of a neutral proteinase from the canine intervertebral disc. Biochim Biophys Acta 990:254–262
16. Crean JK, Roberts S, Jaffray DC, Eisenstein SM, Duance VC (1997) Matrix metalloproteinases in the human intervertebral disc: role in disc degeneration and scoliosis. Spine 15: 2877–2884
17. Eyre DR (1988) Collagens of the disc. In: Ghosh P (ed) The biology of the intervertebral disc. CRC Press, Boca Raton, pp171–188
18. Eyre DR (1989) The intervertebral disc. B. Basic sciences perspectives. In: Frymoyer JW, Gordon SL (eds) New perspectives on low back pain. American Academy of Orthopaedic Surgeons, Park Ridge, pp 147–207
19. Freije JM, Diez-Itza I, Balbin M, Sanchez LM, Blasco R, Tolivia J, Lopez-Otin C (1994) Molecular cloning and expression of collagenase-3: a novel human matrix metalloproteinase produced by breast carcinomas. J Biol Chem 269:16766–16773
20. Goudsouzian NM, Aebi M, Alini M (1999) In situ hybridization of collagen types I and II RNA expression in the bovine intervertebral disc: variation with age. Trans Orthop Res Soc 24:814
21. Gower WE, Pedrini V (1969) Age-related variations in proteinpolysaccharides from human nucleus pulposus, annulus fibrosus, and costal cartilage. J Bone Joint Surg Am 51:1154–1162
22. Gruber HE, Hanley EN (1998) Analysis of aging and degeneration of the human intervertebral disc. Comparison of surgical specimens with normal controls. Spine 23:751–757
23. Hascall VC (1977) Interaction of cartilage proteoglycans with hyaluronic acid. J Supramolec Struc 7:101–120
24. Heathfield TF, Goudsouzian NM, Aebi M, Alini M (1998) Effect of TGF-beta1 on proteoglycan synthesis in isolated intervertebral disc cells. Trans Orthop Res Soc 22:149
25. Heinegård D, Axelsson I (1977) Distribution of keratan sulfate in cartilage proteoglycans. J Biol Chem 252:1971–1979
26. Holm S, Moroudas A, Urban JPG, Sestam G, Nachemson A (1981) Nutrition of the intervertebral disc: somite transport and mechanism. Connect Tissue Res 8:101–108
27. Hutton WC, Toribatake Y, Elmer WA, Ganey TM, Tomita K, Whitesides TE (1998) The effect of compressive force applied to the intervertebral disc in vivo. A study of proteoglycans and collagen. Spine 23:2524–2537
28. Iatridis JC, Mente PL, Stokes IAF, Aronsson DD, Alini M (1999) Compression-induced changes in intervertebral disc properties in a rat tail model. Spine 24:996–1002
29. Johnstone B, Markopoulos M, Neame P, Caterson B (1993) Identification and characterization of glycanated and nonglycanated forms of biglycan and decorin in the human intervertebral disc. Biochem J 292:661–666
30. Kazarian L (1975) Creep characteristics of the human spinal column. Orthop Clin North Am 6:3–18
31. Keller T, Spengler D, Hansson T (1987) Mechanical behavior of the human lumbar spine. I. Creep analysis during static compressive loading. J Orthop Res 5:467–478
32. Kiviranta I, Jurvelin J, Tammi M, Saamanen AM, Helminen HJ (1987) Weight bearing controls glycosaminoglycan concentration and articular cartilage thickness in the knee joints of young beagle dogs. Arthritis Rheum 30:801–809
33. Lee CK (1988) Accelerated degeneration of the segment adjacent to a lumbar fusion. Spine 13:375–377
34. Liu J, Roughley PJ, Mort JS (1991) Identification of human intervertebral disc stromelysin and its involvement in matrix degradation. J Orthop Res 9: 568–575
35. Liu L-S, Thompson AY, Heidaran MA, Poser JW, Spiro RC (1999) A novel collagen/hyaluronate bone-grafting matrix. Biomaterials 20:1097–1108
36. Lotz JC, Chin SR (2000) Intervertebral disc cell death is dependent on the magnitude and duration of spinal loading. Spine 25:1477–1483
37. Lyons G, Eisenstein SM, Sweet MB (1981) Biochemical changes in intervertebral disc degeneration. Biochim Biophys Acta 673:443–453
38. Marchand F, Ahmed AM (1990) Investigation of the laminate structure of lumbar disc annulus fibrosus. Spine 15: 402–410
39. Melrose J, Ghosh P, Taylor TK (1987) Neutral proteinases of the human intervertebral disc. Biochim Biophys Acta 923:483–495
40. Miller J, Schmatz C, Schultz AB (1988) Lumbar disc degeneration: correlation with age, sex, and spine level in 600 autopsy specimens. Spine 13: 173–178
41. Murphy G, Cockett MI, Stephens PE, Smith BJ, Docherty AJ (1987) Stromelysin is an activator of procollagenase. A study with natural and recombinant enzymes. Biochem J 248: 265–268
42. Myers B, McElhaney J, Doherty B (1991) The viscoelastic responses of the human cervical spine in torsion: experimental limitations of quasi-linear theory, and a method for reducing these effects. J Biomech 9: 811–817
43. Nguyen Q, Murphy G, Roughley PJ, Mort JS (1989) Degradation of proteoglycan aggregate by a cartilage metalloproteinase. Evidence for the involvement of stromelysin in the generation of link protein heterogeneity in situ. Biochem J 259:61–67
44. Nilsson B, De Luca S, Lohmander S, Hascall VC (1982) Structures of N-linked and O-linked oligosaccharides on proteoglycan monomer isolated from the Swarm rat chondrosarcoma. J Biol Chem 257:10920–10927
45. Ohshima H, Urban JPG, Bergel DH (1995) Effect of static load on matrix synthesis rates in the intervertebral disc measured in vitro by a new perfusion technique. J Orthop Res 13:22–29
46. Okada Y, Nagase H, Harris ED Jr (1986) A metalloproteinase from human rheumatoid synovial fibroblasts that digests connective tissue matrix components. Purification and characterization. J Biol Chem 261:14245–14255

47. Okada Y, Konomi H, Yada T, Kimata K, Nagase H (1989) Degradation of type IX collagen by matrix metalloproteinase 3 (stromelysin) from human rheumatoid synovial cells. FEBS Letts 244:473–476
48. Paassilta P, Lohiniva J, Goring HH, Perala M, Raina SS, Karppinen J, Hakala M, Palm T, Kroger H, Kaitila I, Vanharanta H, Ott J, Ala-Kokko L (2001) Identification of a novel common genetic risk factor for lumbar disk disease. J Am Med Assoc 285:1843–1849
49. Pearce R (1993) Morphologic and chemical aspects of aging. In: Buckwalter JA, Goldberg VM, Woo SLY (eds) Musculoskeletal soft-tissue ageing. Impact on mobility. American Academy of Orthopaedic Surgeons, Rosemont, pp 363–379
50. Roberts S, Menage J, Eisenstein SM (1993) The cartilage end plate and intervertebral disc in scoliosis: calcification and other sequelae. J Orthop Res 11:747–757
51. Roberts S, Urban JP, Evans H, Eisenstein SM (1996) Transport properties of the human cartilage endplate in relation to its composition and calcification. Spine 21:415–420
52. Roberts S, Caterson B, Menage J, Evans EH, Jaffray DC, Eisenstein SM (2000) Matrix metalloproteinases and aggrecanase: their role in disorders of the human intervertebral disc. Spine 25:3005–3013
53. Roughley PJ, White RJ, Magny MC, Liu J, Pearce RH, Mort JS (1993) Non-proteoglycan forms of biglycan increase with age in human articular cartilage. Biochem J 295:421–426
54. Schlegel J, Smith J, Schleusener R (1996) Lumbar motion segment pathology adjacent to thoracolumbar, lumbar, and lumbosacral fusions. Spine 21: 970–981
55. Schlondorff J, Blobel CP (1999) Metalloprotease-disintegrins: modular proteins capable of promoting cell-cell interactions and triggering signals by protein-ectodomain shedding. J Cell Sci 112:3603–3617
56. Sztrolovics R, Alini M, Mort JS, Roughley PJ (1997) Aggrecan degradation in human intervertebral disc and articular cartilage. Biochem J 326:235–241
57. Sztrolovics R, Alini M, Mort JS, Roughley PJ (1999) Age-related changes in fibromodulin and lumican in human intervertebral discs. Spine 24:1765–1771
58. Sztrolovics R, Grover J, Cs-Szabo G, Shi SL, Zhang Y, Mort JS, Roughley PJ (2002) The characterization of versican and its message in human articular cartilage and intervertebral disc. J Orthop Res 20:257–266
59. Tang BL (2001) ADAMTS: a novel family of extracellular matrix proteases. Intl J Biochem Cell Biol 33:33–44
60. Turner JA, Ersek M, Herron L, Haselkorn J, Kent D, Ciol MA, Deyo R (1992) Patient outcomes after lumbar spinal fusions. JAMA 268:907–911
61. Wei L, Heidaran M, Liu S-L, Spiro R, Aebi M, Alini M (2000) Intervertebral disc cell-seeded implants: a preliminary study. Trans Orthop Res Soc 25: 754
62. Wu JJ, Eyre DR, Slayter HS (1987) Type VI collagen of the intervertebral disc. Biochemical and electron-microscopic characterization of the native protein. Biochem J 248:373–381